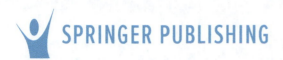

D0144302

GET THE MOST FROM YOUR BOOK

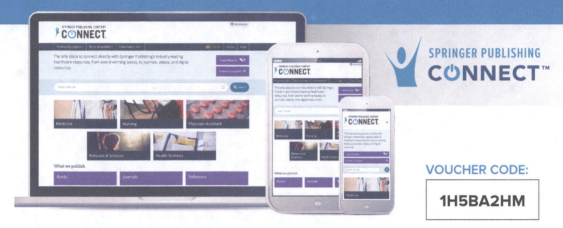

SPRINGER PUBLISHING CONNECT™

VOUCHER CODE:

1H5BA2HM

Online Access

Your print purchase of *Health Policy and Analysis, Second Edition*, includes **online access via Springer Publishing Connect™** to increase accessibility, portability, and searchability.

Insert the code at https://connect.springerpub.com/content/book/978-0-8261-8543-3 today!

*Having trouble? Contact our customer service department at **cs@springerpub.com***

Instructor Resource Access for Adopters

Let us do some of the heavy lifting to create an engaging classroom experience with a variety of instructor resources included in most textbooks SUCH AS:

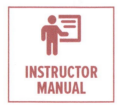

INSTRUCTOR MANUAL

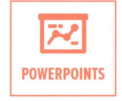

POWERPOINTS

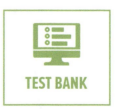

TEST BANK

Visit **https://connect.springerpub.com/** and look for the **"Show Supplementary"** button on your **book homepage** to see what is available to instructors! First time using Springer Publishing Connect?

Email **textbook@springerpub.com** to create an account and start unlocking valuable resources.

HEALTH POLICY
AND ANALYSIS

John W. Seavey, PhD, MPH, is Professor Emeritus in the Department of Health Management and Policy at the University of New Hampshire (UNH). Previously he was the Everett B. Sackett Professor (1996–2012) and Senior Fellow at The Carsey Institute (2005–2011). He received his baccalaureate degree from Bates College (1966), an MA (1968) and PhD (1973) in political science from the University of Arizona, and a Master of Public Health (MPH) from Harvard School of Public Health (1979). He came to UNH from the University of Arizona's Health Sciences Center in 1980 as an assistant professor; he was promoted to associate professor (1985) and then to professor (1992). He taught a variety of courses but focused on health policy courses at the graduate and undergraduate levels. He served as Chair of the Department for multiple terms and was the founding director of the UNH Masters in Public Health Program (MPH).

His research focus has been on rural healthcare in the United States and then on the impact of socioeconomic status on health. Publications include two other books and numerous peer-reviewed articles as well as monographs and he has served as reviewer for multiple editorial boards.

He has been the recipient of many UNH awards, among them the UNH Outstanding Associate Professor Award (1991), College of Health and Human Services Distinguished Career Research Award (2003), UNH Faculty Social Justice Award (2005), and Distinguished UNH Professor (2005). He was on the Board of Directors of the Association of University Programs in Health Administration (1989–1995) and served as the Chair (1993–1994). He was the recipient of the New Hampshire Public Health Association's Roger Fossum Lifetime Achievement Award (2011).

Semra A. Aytur, PhD, MPH, is a professor in the Department of Health Management and Policy at the University of New Hampshire (UNH). Dr. Aytur teaches courses in health policy, epidemiology, biostatistics. environmental health, health behavior, and sustainability. Prior to joining UNH, she received her baccalaureate degree from Brown University (1991), an MPH from Boston University School of Public Health (1996), and her doctoral degree (2006) and postdoctoral fellowship (2009) in cardiovascular epidemiology at the University of North Carolina, Chapel Hill. Additionally, she has served as a policy and evaluation specialist for local and state health departments. Her research focuses on policy and environmental changes to prevent obesity, diabetes, and cardiovascular disease. She is particularly interested in health disparities and in policies that influence the natural, social, and built environment to promote health equity. Dr. Aytur collaborates with researchers around the country on policy issues related to obesity prevention, physical activity, climate change, planetary health, community resilience, and environmental issues. She specializes in collaborative decision processes designed to promote civic engagement.

Dr. Aytur has received several research grants from the Robert Wood Johnson Foundation as well as from federal agencies to evaluate policy, environment, and systems change pertaining to chronic disease prevention and climate change adaptation. She enjoys collaborating with policy makers, urban planners, transportation planners, and citizens to develop strategies to promote sustainable, health-promoting community environments. Nationally, she is a member of the National Physical Activity Policy Research and Evaluation Network (PAPREN) and the American Public Health Association. She has conducted educational health policy briefings to bipartisan legislators in the state of New Hampshire and in Washington, DC. Dr. Aytur is committed to community-engaged research that supports resilience and planetary health.

Robert J. McGrath, PhD, is the current Everett B. Sacket Professor and Chair of the Department of Health Policy and Management at the University of New Hampshire. He is also currently the director of the Graduate Programs in Health Data Science. He received his baccalaureate degree (BS) from UNH in 1996, an MS (1998) from the Harvard School of Public Health, an MA (2000) from Brandeis University, and a PhD from the Heller School at Brandeis in 2006. His coursework focuses on strategic management as well as quantitative methods for health management and policy, health policy, and health policy analysis.

His academic focus surrounds health data and information issues for healthcare practice and policy. He has served in a number of academic and administrative roles and led many health IT programs, including NH Connects for Health, the NH Health Care Interoperability Project, and the Health Information Security and Privacy Project, and he helped guide the first Health Information Exchange Strategic Plan for New Hampshire. His concurrent research focuses on health disparities for treatment and outcomes in adolescents and for families. He also served as an assistant health policy advisor for former governor, now U.S. Senator, Jeanne Shaheen.

He has received a number of federal and private research grants and has worked with many state-based agencies and community partners to promote healthy child development and data-informed health modelling toward a better understanding of health.

HEALTH POLICY AND ANALYSIS

Framework and Tools for Success

Second Edition

John W. Seavey, PhD, MPH
Semra A. Aytur, PhD, MPH
Robert J. McGrath, PhD

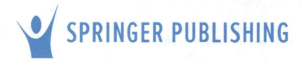

Springer Publishing Company, LLC
11 West 42nd Street, New York, NY 10036
www.springerpub.com
connect.springerpub.com

Acquisitions Editor: David D'Addona
Compositor: Transforma

ISBN: 978-0-8261-8542-6
ebook ISBN: 978-0-8261-8543-3
DOI: 10.1891/9780826185433

A robust set of instructor resources designed to supplement this text is located at http://connect.springerpub.com/content/book/978-0-8261-8543-3. Qualifying instructors may request access by emailing textbook@springerpub.com.

Instructor Chapter PowerPoints: 978-0-8261-8545-7
Instructor Manual: 978-0-8261-8544-0
Instructor Test Bank: 978-0-8261-8546-0

23 24 25 26 27 / 5 4 3 2 1

The author and the publisher of this Work have made every effort to use sources believed to be reliable to provide information that is accurate and compatible with the standards generally accepted at the time of publication. The author and publisher shall not be liable for any special, consequential, or exemplary damages resulting, in whole or in part, from the readers' use of, or reliance on, the information contained in this book. The publisher has no responsibility for the persistence or accuracy of URLs for external or third-party Internet websites referred to in this publication and does not guarantee that any content on such websites is, or will remain, accurate or appropriate.

Library of Congress Cataloging-in-Publication Data
Names: Seavey, John W., author. | Aytur, Semra A., author. | McGrath, Robert J., 1967- author.
Title: Health policy and analysis : framework and tools for success / John W. Seavey, Semra A. Aytur, Robert J. McGrath.
Other titles: Health policy analysis
Description: Second edition. | New York, NY : Springer Publishing Company, LLC, [2024] | Preceded by Health policy analysis / John W. Seavey, Semra A. Aytur, Robert J. McGrath. [2014]. | Includes bibliographical references and index. | Summary: "This textbook focuses primarily on the US federal government with additional general coverage of state and local governments. However, it is important to point out the importance of other countries, especially developing countries, as well as the Indigenous populations within the United States. Since we cannot do justice to covering these here, we have included an Appendix that provides some suggested resources to explore these important areas of public health policy further. Since public health is connected directly or indirectly to almost all public policies, the breadth of health policy is limitless. We have used multiple examples within the textbook reflecting this breadth of health policy"-- Provided by publisher.
Identifiers: LCCN 2022054322 | ISBN 9780826185426 (paperback) | ISBN 9780826185433 (ebook)
Subjects: MESH: Health Policy | Policy Making | United States
Classification: LCC RA418.3.U6 | NLM WA 525 | DDC 362.10973--dc23/eng/20230201
LC record available at https://lccn.loc.gov/2022054322

Publisher's Note: **New and used products purchased from third-party sellers are not guaranteed for quality, authenticity, or access to any included digital components.**

Printed in the United States of America by Gasch Printing.

Contents

Preface

Health policy is a dynamic field of study. Since the first edition of this textbook, much has changed in terms of the political landscape, public health, healthcare, and data analytics. No book can cover the field comprehensively because it continues to evolve and expand. The intent of this textbook is to provide an overview of concepts, tools, and resources that will open the door of public health policy analysis to students. Students can adapt the framework and foundational tools to provide a springboard for lifelong learning and inquiry.

Health policy analysis is not for the faint of heart. It is a challenging task that requires synthesizing knowledge from multiple disciplines and using many different skills. Some of that knowledge can come through textbooks and classes, and other types of knowledge come by way of experience in collaboration with others in both the political system and public health. We hope that this primer will stimulate you to explore other perspectives and other forms of knowledge. Since public health is connected directly or indirectly to almost all public policies, the breadth of health policy is limitless. We have used multiple examples within the textbook reflecting this breadth of health policy.

This textbook focuses primarily on the U.S. federal government with additional general coverage of state and local governments. However, it is important to recognize the importance of health policy in other countries as well as Indigenous populations within the United States. Since we cannot do justice to covering these here, we have included an Appendix that provides some suggested resources to explore these important areas of public health policy further.

One of our experiences from teaching classes in health policy has been that students generally lack a nuanced understanding of the U.S. political system. As a consequence, we have added several new chapters on the U.S. political system. Of course, these chapters are not a substitute for a political science textbook or classes. Instead, we attempt to provide an overview of the U.S. political structure, process, and culture with examples drawn from public health.

Health policy analysis occurs in multiple types of settings. After graduation, you may be employed by a nonprofit health organization, a member of Congress, a governmental agency at the national state or local level, a political think tank, a public or private research center, a lobbying or advocacy organization, and so on. The task of conducting a policy analysis may involve developing a policy proposal to assess one or more alternatives *a priori* or evaluating the success of a policy that has already been implemented. As such, you may be involved in analyzing health policy at various stages of the process. Readers should use this textbook to address their particular needs in context, rather than thinking of it as a "one size fits all" process. There are Breakout Boxes that provide conceptual details and practical examples in the chapters.

Chapter 1 provides an overview of major perspectives of public health that are critical to understanding how public health professionals approach health policy. For example, the chapter discusses the determinants of health, one of the major perspectives regarding the myriad factors that shape community health. The core functions of public health are delineated using the COVID-19 pandemic as an example. The chapter also discusses concepts of both population health and public health. This chapter enables the reader to understand basic concepts and terminology in the public health lexicon before engaging in policy analysis.

Chapter 2 begins with a brief explanation of the need for political systems, as well as the need to address market failures. Here we discuss many broad concepts such as the difference between law and policy, separation of powers, federalism, delegated and implied powers, and other general political concepts. To illustrate the concept of federalism there is a discussion of Medicare and Medicaid as well as an informational Breakout Box describing the passage of the Patient Protection and Affordable Care Act. This chapter leads into Chapter 3, which provides a description of the U.S. federal government's legislative, executive, and judicial branches. This chapter also highlights how state and local governments may differ in terms of some of these structures.

Chapter 4 begins by discussing the importance of the political process and other concepts that are not included in the structural elements of the system. Here we discuss procedural democracy, constitutional democracy, and democratic pluralism. We include a description of the importance of factions, political parties, the scope of decision-making, the ability to block, and incrementalism. This leads to Chapter 5, which walks you through the "political maze" of American politics. In this chapter, there are sections on legislative committees, the importance of congressional staff, and how a bill becomes a law. It also includes sections on the process of writing rules and regulations and executive orders. We discuss the importance of the judiciary as well as various processes that exist at the state and local levels (such as initiatives and referendums).

Chapter 6 deals with the critical area of political culture which generally involves the unwritten accepted norms of behavior within institutional arenas, which are constantly evolving. This is frequently overlooked in examining the political system, but it is critical to understanding the policy process and its outcomes. We provide examples of the dominant political culture in the United States. We also describe nonpartisanship and the increasingly partisan divide in the United States. How these emerging changes in our political culture will affect our constitutional democracy remains an open question.

Chapter 7 prepares you to begin exploring the process of developing a policy analysis. It starts by offering examples and templates that might be useful in organizing your analysis. It discusses the importance of utilizing peer-reviewed literature as well as grey literature and provides helpful suggestions of what to look for in these resources. In addition, we also emphasize the need to reach out to various stakeholders in the policy area you have chosen. Experts in various organizations (government agencies, nonprofits, academic institutions, community-based organizations, provider organizations, lobbying groups, etc.) that are involved in or affected by the substantive area of policy are important sources of information. Finally, this chapter provides some useful tips on writing an executive summary and provides other practical resources for making your delivery more user friendly.

Chapter 8 provides an overview of some of the history of health services research and previous health policy analysis efforts and lenses. It examines the literature in terms of effectiveness, efficiency, equity, and feasibility and some of the complications involved in those areas of analysis. It provides a detailed examination of integrative frameworks that are commonly used in public health, such as PRECEDE-PROCEED and RE-AIM. Finally, it describes some of the public and private organizations that are important sources of health policy information that you might wish to access when conducting your analysis.

Chapter 9 provides an important overview of health data science, analytical methods, and their evolution. Proprietorship, privacy, the ever-changing nature of data collection, the level of precision, interoperability, and other complexities associated with using data are discussed. The contributions of both quantitative and qualitative methods are discussed as well as the "evidence pyramid" used to assess analytical studies. Sources of public and private health data for public health policy analysis are described. The data ecosystem is discussed, along with the expansion of what is considered data. Descriptions of Big Data and artificial intelligence are also provided. There are tools provided for assistance in analysis. Finally, there is a discussion of data gaps and potential biases that may arise when conducting an analysis.

Chapter 10 provides guidance on laying out your policy topic's background and history relative to what has been tried previously in your geopolitical unit or elsewhere. We use the example of obesity to illustrate this. Paying attention to what legal authority your policy maker or organization has to affect a policy is also an important consideration. Examining model programs and the synergies between your policy topic and other policies is an important avenue of exploration. Finally, this chapter also focuses on moving your policy initiative onto the political agenda or "getting it on the radar" as it competes for attention with other policy initiatives.

Chapter 11 focuses on the explicit statement of your policy initiative and the importance of framing. It provides practical examples of a policy statement as well as framing.

Chapter 12 revisits the importance of values and perspectives in terms of understanding who is likely to support or oppose your policy. Which values are you potentially impacting by your policy? There is detailed discussion of potential stakeholders, using childhood obesity as an example. The chapter provides tools for a qualitative and quantitative analysis of stakeholders. It also provides practical examples from Washington State.

Chapter 13 discusses developing criteria one could use to determine the success of your policy. What outcomes of your policy proposal would make it successful in the short term and longer term? How would we know if a policy met its goals? This may have additional utility in attracting new stakeholders to support your initiative. It can give potential supporters talking points as to the potential benefits of a policy change. It is also useful in the implementation phase of the policy process by setting targets to determine whether the policy is on track or in need of adjustments.

Chapter 14 discusses how one might weigh the policy options and evidence that you have compiled. There is a discussion of the strengths and weakness of incrementalism and the role of a trial balloon. The importance of the precautionary principle for public health is included here. Finally, there is a discussion on how you can feel that the analysis is "complete" and that you have sufficiently addressed the policy issues.

Chapter 15 discusses the task of making your policy recommendation. The format of this will likely be determined by your policy maker or supervising organization, but we offer some examples. Since no policy is automatically adopted, there are ideas and strategies for getting the policy adopted through legislative, executive, and judicial means.

We trust that you will use this textbook for the further advancement of the public's health. As we have learned through exploring the determinants of health and the core functions of public health, health policy analysis has much to contribute to personal, population, and planetary health. There is much work to be done in health policy development, implementation, and evaluation to improve the public's health and eliminate health disparities. We wish you well in your endeavors.

John W. Seavey
Semra A. Aytur
Robert J. McGrath

Acknowledgments

The development of any textbook is a complicated task, and it takes many people. There are many authors cited in the text who have shared their analytical work and wisdom. As we have mentioned throughout the book, these citations do not exhaust the list of potential resources. What we have tried to do is to guide readers in various directions in hope that they will go deeper with academic courses, literature, and personal exploration.

We have benefited from our undergraduate and graduate students who ask challenging questions. We want students to challenge their own positions on politics, public health, and policy. Every classroom is a learning environment for both students and faculty. The University of New Hampshire (UNH) MPH Health Policy class in the spring of 2022 provided feedback on the beginning political chapters. Special thanks to Grace Roy and Marciana Johnson for their assistance with updating Breakout Boxes, for research on policy and data science, and for sharing additional student perspectives.

We appreciate the support and encouragement for a second edition by Springer Publishing Company, notably David D'Addona and Hannah Grace Greco. We received anonymous advice from reviewers at the proposal stage, which was encouraging and helpful in moving forward. We very much appreciate the assistance of Randolph Brown at UNH for his technical support.

Finally, this work would not be possible without the support of our respective families, who have put up with lost evenings and weekends and even made useful comments on chapters.

Instructor Resources

 A robust set of instructor resources designed to supplement this text is located at http://connect.springerpub.com/content/book/978-0-8261-8543-3. Qualifying instructors may request access by emailing textbook@springerpub.com.

- **Instructor Manual** containing learning objectives, media and resources, active learning exercises, essay questions, and more.
- **Test Bank** with over 160 multiple-choice questions. All questions include answers with full rationales and are available on Respondus®.
- **Instructor Chapter PowerPoints** with presenter notes.

CHAPTER 1

PERSPECTIVES FOR PUBLIC HEALTH POLICY ANALYSIS

This chapter provides an overview of public health perspectives for policy analysis. Health policy shapes the social, environmental, economic, and planetary determinants that affect our daily lives. Policy and political and systems are essential aspects of public health, locally and globally. We explore how policies can simultaneously be viewed as contributors to public health problems and also how they are critical to creating solutions.

LEARNING·OBJECTIVES

Be able to:

- Explain the social, political, environmental, and planetary determinants of health.
- Describe the exposome.
- Define health equity.
- Discuss an example of a health disparity.
- Explain how policy relates to the core functions of public health.
- List the five key elements of Health in All Policies.

DETERMINANTS OF PUBLIC HEALTH

Public health policy is a key determinant of population health status. The political structures and processes determine access to resources, infrastructure, and services that contribute to health outcomes, quality of life, and health disparities observed across the globe. These disparities are evidenced in the rate of the uninsured in several countries, notably the United States, and the divergence of life expectancies. In 2020, a child born in Norway is expected to reach 82.4 years while a child born in the Central African Republic will barely reach 53, and a child born in some lower-income U.S. communities may not live beyond age 65 (NYU

FIGURE 1.1 Determinants of health.

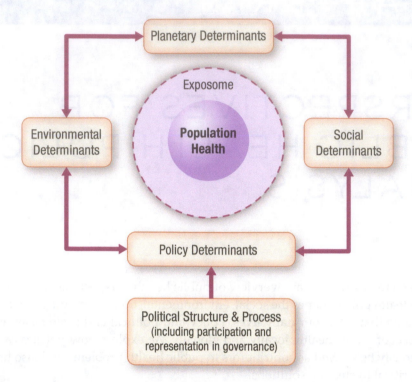

Langone Health, 2022; Tejada-Vera et al., 2020; United Nations, 2022). These disparities continue to persist despite the continual advances in medical care and medical technology. In fact, health policy shapes the social, environmental, and planetary determinants of health that frame the *exposome* (Juarez et al., 2014)—the cumulative exposures (both positive and negative) that affect health behavior and health status across the life course. See **Figure 1.1** and **Breakout Box 1.1**.

DETERMINANTS OF HEALTH

The evolving public health perspective recognizes many different determinants of health, including social, environmental, economic, policy, and planetary determinants. As shown in **Figure 1.1**, we posit that policy mediates the social, environmental, and planetary determinants of health that frame the *exposome*—the cumulative exposures (both positive and negative) that affect health behavior and health status across the life course (Juarez et al., 2014). We provide working definitions for the determinants of health as follows:

Social Determinants—The social determinants of health refer to the conditions under which people are born, grow, live, work, play, and age that affect a wide range of population health outcomes (Centers for Disease Control and Prevention [CDC], n.d.). Social determinants include access to education, employment, housing, food, and safe spaces for physical activity/recreation as well as access to medical and social services and supportive social networks. Research has demonstrated that social determinants of health play a greater role in overall population health than genetics and medical care, determining over 75% of population health status. Social determinants are influenced by policies, rules, and regulations that are constructed through deliberate actions by political actors in both public and private institutional arenas.

Environmental Determinants—Environmental determinants of health refer to factors such as access to clean air, water, and soil; sanitation services; natural resources; and safe workplaces (Gibson, 2018; World Health Organization [WHO], 2013). Environmental determinants can also refer to the built environment, which includes transportation systems, housing, buildings, parks, and other infrastructure that supports health.

Political Determinants—The political determinants of health mediate resource allocation for key systems and services that support health, globally and locally (Dawes & Williams, 2020; Kickbusch, 2005; Mishori, 2019). These include the institutions and decision-making arenas, including formal and informal rules, laws, organizational norms, and processes that shape social and environmental conditions. Political determinants of health also include the power dynamics and social structures that determine who has access to the political process, and whose interests are represented by the decisions that are made. Dawes and Williams (2020) define the political determinants of health as *"the systematic process of structuring relationships, distributing resources, and administering power, operating simultaneously in ways that mutually reinforce or influence one another to shape opportunities that either advance health equity or exacerbate health inequities"* (p. 1).

Planetary Determinants—Planetary determinants of health include the combined factors and conditions that affect "the health of human civilization and the natural systems on which it depends" (Whitmee et al., 2015, p. 1978). Planetary health encompasses a solutions-oriented, transdisciplinary social movement that began with the 2015 release of the Rockefeller Foundation–Lancet Commission's report entitled "Safeguarding Human Health in the Anthropocene Epoch." The Commission described planetary health as "the achievement of the highest attainable standard of health, wellbeing, and equity worldwide through judicious attention to the human systems—political, economic, and social—that shape the future of humanity and the Earth's natural systems that define the safe environmental limits within which humanity can flourish" (Whitmee et al., 2015, p. 1978). Redvers et al. (2021) provide an Indigenous view of planetary health which emphasizes ten interconnected determinants. Planetary health takes a reciprocal, ecocentric perspective in order to frame the planet itself as a focal point when considering determinants of health. This lens includes factors such as Indigenous land rights, global governance structures, and threat multipliers such as climate change. It also attends to specific economic structures, regional and international politics, sustainable development, and decolonial issues (Planetary Health Alliance, n.d.).

Changes to ecological support systems or ecosystem services (such as air, water, soil, and climate) are already significantly impacting human health, and these impacts are projected to drive the majority of the global burden of disease over the coming century, disproportionately impacting the most vulnerable populations and future generations.

References

Centers for Disease Control and Prevention. (n.d.). *About CDC: Social determinants of health at CDC.* U.S. Department of Health and Human Services. https://www.cdc.gov/socialdeterminants/index.htm

Dawes, D. E., & Williams, D. R. (2020). *The political determinants of health.* Johns Hopkins University Press.

Gibson, J. M. (2018). Environmental determinants of health. In T. P. Daaleman & M. R. Helton (Eds.), *Chronic illness care: Principles and practice* (pp. 451–467). Springer. https://doi.org/10.1007/978-3-319-71812-5_37

Juarez, P., Matthews-Juarez, P., Hood, D., Im, W., Levine, R., Kilbourne, B., Langston, M., Al-Hamdan, M., Crosson, W., Estes, M., Estes, S., Agboto, V., Robinson, P., Wilson, S., & Lichtveld, M. (2014). The public health exposome: A population-based, exposure science approach to health disparities Research. *International Journal of Environmental Research and Public Health, 11*(12), 12866–12895. https://doi.org/10.3390/ijerph111212866

Kickbusch, I. (2005). Tackling the political determinants of global health. *BMJ, 331*(7511), 246–247. https://doi.org/10.1136/bmj.331.7511.246

Mishori, R. (2019). The social determinants of health? Time to focus on the political determinants of health! *Medical Care, 57*(7), 491–493. https://doi.org/10.1097/mlr.0000000000001131

Planetary Health Alliance. (n.d.). *Planetary health.* https://www.planetaryhealthalliance.org/planetary-health

Redvers, N. (2021). The determinants of planetary health. *The Lancet Planetary Health, 5*(3), e111–e112. https://doi.org/10.1016/s2542-5196(21)00008-5

Whitmee, S., Haines, A., Beyrer, C., Boltz, F., Capon, A. G., de Souza Dias, B. F., Ezeh, A., Frumkin, H., Gong, P., Head, P., Horton, R., Mace, G. M., Marten, R., Myers, S. S., Nishtar, S., Osofsky, S. A., Pattanayak, S. K., Pongsiri, M. J., Romanelli, C., ... Yach, D. (2015). Safeguarding human health in the Anthropocene Epoch: Report of the Rockefeller Foundation–Lancet Commission on planetary health. *The Lancet, 386*(10007), 1973–2028. https://doi.org/10.1016/s0140-6736(15)60901-1

World Health Organization. (2013). *Social and environmental determinants of health and health inequalities in Europe: Fact sheet.* https://www.euro.who.int/__data/assets/pdf_file/0006/185217/Social-and-environmental-determinants-Fact-Sheet.pdf

CORE FUNCTIONS OF PUBLIC HEALTH

Because it plays such an important role, policy development is recognized as one of the three core functions of public health. See Breakout Box 1.2. Policy also influences the other core functions of public health (assessment and assurance) in myriad ways.

The policy process reflects the values of a society, which we discuss in more detail in Chapter 2. Some countries, like the United States, have political cultures that align with more individualistic values, and others have more collective values (Hofstede, 2021; Levitsky & Way, 2022). We discuss the political culture further in Chapter 6. Importantly, public policy determines the allocation of resources that support health, and the political system is the social construct that distributes those resources. Thus, discussions about health policy are inherently connected to discussions of equity and justice. Philosophers from the Enlightenment period

Breakout Box 1.2

PANDEMICS AND THE CORE FUNCTIONS OF PUBLIC HEALTH

Assessment refers to the capacity to track the health status of the population and identify emerging diseases. This includes monitoring a community's health status by collecting and analyzing information about health problems. It also includes diagnosing and investigating health issues and health hazards in the community (CDC, n.d.).

Key to the assessment function is data capacity, public health surveillance systems, and health data analytics. The COVID-19 pandemic has revealed how the political policies have led to disinvestment in public health preparedness for surveillance, data infrastructure, human resources, and public health literacy. These problems included insufficient capacity for testing when the pandemic began, a lack of sensitive surveillance methods, and insufficient capability to carry out case investigations and rapid scientific study. Many current public health surveillance systems lack the capacity to fully utilize contemporary data science methods, and concerns about personal privacy (which ironically are not concerns with respect to how for-profit corporations collect, use, and sell personal data) and data governance pose further barriers to robust public health surveillance.

Policy development refers to developing policies and plans that support individual and community health efforts, as well as the capacity to mobilize community partnerships to address health problems. This includes the ability to consult with stakeholders, to weigh available information, to inform decisions about which interventions are most appropriate to optimize public health and safety, and to educate and empower people about health issues.

As described by Brownson et al., "[p]olicy development during the COVID-19 pandemic has been a patchwork; the lack of credible national leadership taking evidence-based approaches has left state and local public health agencies to deal with their epidemics without coordinated planning and optimized resource management. Even in the context of the stresses this pandemic has caused, the gaps have been evident in the lack of integration across public health agencies and in the lack of channels between the siloed realms of public health and health care" (2020, p. 1606).

For example, manual contact tracing is labor intensive and relies on self-reported knowledge of the interpersonal networks of physical interactions. Other countries had policies that immediately employed modern data science methods to assist with contact tracing. They also already had the data technology (e.g., mobile phone applications and spatial network analysis), governance structures, and a political culture to enable this.

Brownson et al. also describe how COVID-19 pulled back the curtain on "the consequences of long-standing and growing inequalities in the United States and the more recently soaring 'deaths of despair' (i.e., suicide, chronic liver disease, and fatal drug and alcohol and fatal drug and alcohol poisoning)" (2020, p. 1606; Brownson, 2020).

Assurance refers to promoting and protecting public interests through programs, events, campaigns, regulations, and other strategies, and ensuring that necessary services are provided to reach agreed-upon goals. This includes enforcing laws and regulations that protect public health (policy implementation). It also includes linking people to needed personal health services, assuring the provision of healthcare, and assuring a competent public health and personal healthcare workforce. Lastly, the assurance function includes a key aspect of policy analysis—the capacity to evaluate the effectiveness, accessibility, and quality of personal and population-based health services (CDC, n.d.).

Political culture also affects the assurance function. For example, public health scholars have called for attending to the determinants of health (from social determinants to planetary determinants; Institute of Medicine, Committee for the Study of the Future of Public Health, 1988; Jayasinghe, 2015; Knapp et al., 2019; Salerno & Bogard, 2019) and addressing the root causes of structural inequities that result in health disparities. This entails potentially shifting the allocation of power and resources, which are deeply entrenched in the U.S. political culture and its structure and processes. As stated by Brownson et al., "[a] greater emphasis is needed on a systems approach for addressing social determinants of health that more fully considers the interconnections between risk factors, the environment, and social and economic factors" (2020, p. 1608).

References

Brownson, R. (2020, July 9). *Dr. Ross Brownson—evidence based public health.* YouTube. https://www.youtube.com/watch?v=IBOX716TbTY

Brownson, R. C., Burke, T. A., Colditz, G. A., & Samet, J. M. (2020). Reimagining public health in the aftermath of a pandemic. *American Journal of Public Health, 110*(11), 1605–1610. https://doi.org/10.2105/ajph.2020.305861

Centers for Disease Control and Prevention. (n.d.). *The public health system and the 10 essential public health services.* https://www.cdc.gov/publichealthgateway/zz -sddev/essentialhealthservices.html

Institute of Medicine, Committee for the Study of the Future of Public Health. (1988). *The future of public health.* National Academies Press. https://www.ncbi.nlm.nih .gov/books/NBK218218

Jayasinghe, S. (2015). Social determinants of health inequalities: Towards a theoretical perspective using systems science. *International Journal for Equity in Health, 14,* Article 71. https://doi.org/10.1186/s12939-015-0205-8

Knapp, E. A., Bilal, U., Dean, L. T., Lazo, M., & Celentano, D. D. (2019). Economic insecurity and deaths of despair in U.S. counties. *American Journal of Epidemiology, 188*(12), 2131–2139. https://doi.org/10.1093/aje/kwz103

Salerno, J., & Bogard, K. (2019). What do social determinants of health determine? *Journal of Urban Health: Bulletin of the New York Academy of Medicine, 96*(6), 793–794. https://doi.org/10.1007/s11524-019-00402-z

(1685–1815), such as John Locke and Thomas Hobbes, are frequently discussed in relation to the values and perspectives underpinning public health (Hobbes, 1640; Locke, 1690/1796). These philosophers contend that society and politics should be based on values such as reason and the right to free speech. They also believed that government derived its legitimacy from a social contract between the people, rather than from divine rights of a monarchy. John Locke's historical writings about equality resonate with contemporary public health professionals' focus on equity, and with perspectives of freedom that include the rights of all persons to live free from preventable harm (Galea, 2022).

Justice has also been defined in different ways according to various sociocultural perspectives that are grounded in different political and economic theories (Aristotle, 1994; McCartney et al., 2019; Nussbaum, 1992; Wiesner et al., 2018). One conceptualization of justice relates to the fair and equitable allocation of resources that have moral importance (Aristotle, 1987). Defining moral importance is at the center of much historical and present-day debate. For example, Aristotle argued that health is foundational to a successful life and the ability for human beings to flourish (Nussbaum, 1992). More recently, in *A Theory of Justice*, John Rawls is largely silent on the topic of health and healthcare, but instead focuses on the foundations of the societal supports themselves (Rawls, 1971). These societal supports align with the social determinants of health in today's public health lexicon. In today's world, particularly in the United States, the debate continues as to whether health is a foundational social good or a good that is conditional on preference and privilege (Gwynne & Cairnduff, 2017; Jayasinghe, 2015; Kania & Kramer, 2011; Knapp et al., 2019; Nussbaum, 1998).

From a public health perspective, we consider policy as a mediator of the social, environmental, economic, and planetary determinants of health (Figure 1.1). Conceptual models of health, such as the socio-ecological model, posit that health is influenced by interrelated factors at the individual (e.g., genomic, physiologic, psychosocial), interpersonal, community/organizational, environmental, and policy levels (CDC, n.d.-c; Golden et al., 2015; Stokols, 1992). We use the term *healthcare* to refer to the constellation of medical, social, and ecosystem services that support healthy communities, with the understanding that public health is concerned with all these components. Put simply, from a public health perspective, health policy is concerned with everyone's health.

This is important when considering the values framework for this text. As Dr. Ruger (2004) thoughtfully considers:

[H]ealth and its determinants must be valued against other social ends in a broader public exercise of policy priorities. This exercise should be inclusive and democratic and should represent a process of public reasoning about the ends and means of public policy more broadly and about health policy specifically. (p. 1076)

The determinants of health are also intrinsically linked to notions of "health equity" (Harvey, 2020; Salerno & Bogard, 2019). As defined by the CDC, health equity is "the state in which everyone has a fair and just opportunity to attain their highest level of health. Achieving this requires focused and ongoing societal efforts to address historical and contemporary injustices; overcome economic, social, and other obstacles to health and health care; and eliminate health disparities" (CDC, n.d.-d, para. 1).

Many theorists have recognized that achieving health equity necessitates addressing the myriad determinants of health and committing to planetary health (Myers & Frumkin, 2020; Salerno & Bogard, 2019; The Lancet Public Health, 2022). Others view this as more aspirational than achievable, given the entrenched nature of inequities in society. However, moving toward health equity is an important goal of public health policy. This view is ethically aligned with ideas of environmental justice (Levy et al., 2022), distributive justice (Braveman & Gruskin, 2003), and the professional value sets espoused by the Hippocratic Oath, the Adelaide

Statement on Health in All Policies (WHO, 2010), and related calls to action in clinical and public health practice (Mahmood, 2022; Wabnitz et al., 2020).

HEALTH IN ALL POLICIES

Promoting a culture of health and equity requires engaging multisectoral stakeholders, including public policy makers as well as those in the private sector. This notion of Health in All Policies (HiAP) has become foundational in the field of public health for policy conceptualization (Brownson, 2020; Rigby & Hatch, 2016). HiAP is defined as, "a collaborative approach that integrates and articulates health considerations into policymaking across sectors to improve the health of all communities and people. HiAP recognizes that health is created by a multitude of factors beyond healthcare and, in many cases, beyond the scope of traditional public health activities" (CDC, n.d.-a, para. 1). HiAP is supported by several organizations including the American Public Health Association (n.d.), WHO (2019), the CDC (n.d.-a), and many others. HiAP considers five key areas for guiding policies. See **Breakout Box 1.3**.

Breakout Box 1.3

FIVE KEY ELEMENTS OF HEALTH IN ALL POLICIES (AMERICAN PUBLIC HEALTH ASSOCIATION, N.D.)

1. Promote health, equity, and sustainability
Health in All Policies promotes health, equity, and sustainability through two avenues: (1) incorporating health, equity, and sustainability into specific policies, programs, and processes, and (2) embedding health, equity, and sustainability considerations into government decision-making processes so that healthy public policy becomes the normal way of doing business.

For example, embedding health considerations into land use and transportation policies can support urban design and infrastructure that enable walking, biking, taking public transportation, and/or safely using a wheelchair or mobility device to get to destinations. This can help to create walkable commercial spaces, parks, greenspace, and community gardens.

2. Support intersectoral collaboration
Health in All Policies brings together partners from the many sectors that play major roles in shaping the economic, physical, and social environments in which people live, and therefore have important roles to play in promoting health, equity, and sustainability. A Health in All Policies approach focuses on deep and ongoing collaboration.

For example, transdisciplinary collaboration with civil engineering, business, urban planning, parks and recreation, food and agriculture, economics, political science, disability studies, justice studies, social work, psychology, and the arts, as well as medicine, nursing, and other clinical professions, is needed to create a culture of health.

3. Benefit multiple partners
Health in All Policies values cobenefits and win-wins. Health in All Policies initiatives endeavor to simultaneously address the policy and

programmatic goals of both public health and other agencies by finding and implementing strategies that benefit multiple partners.

For example, multisolving refers to developing solutions that address climate change while also improving health, well-being, and economic vitality (Sawin, 2018). Using green infrastructure to promote walkable communities and promoting urban agriculture are two examples of multisolving. Additional examples of multisolving can be found at: https://ssir.org/articles/entry/the_magic_of_multisolving and www .multisolving.org/about-us.

4. Engage stakeholders

Health in All Policies engages many stakeholders, including community members, policy experts, advocates, the private sector, and funders, to ensure that work is responsive to community needs and to identify policy and systems changes necessary to create meaningful and impactful health improvements.

For example, approaches like Collective Impact can be used to engage stakeholders around a common agenda, shared measurement systems, mutually reinforcing activities, and open communication (Gwynne & Cairnduff, 2017; Kania & Kramer, 2011).

The LA Promise Zone involves nearly 50 local institutions and nonprofit and community organizations that are working together to combat poverty in specific neighborhoods of Central Los Angeles (LAPromiseZone.org, n.d.). The network focuses on six major areas: education, civic participation, legal resources, health and wellness, economic development, and safe affordable housing (LAPromiseZone.org, n.d.; CDC, n.d.). The work of the LA Promise Zone is overseen by a leadership council and carried out by five working groups. The Los Angeles Department of Public Health played a key role in this council by addressing issues related to public safety, food security, access to housing, and access to services.

Also in Los Angeles is the Healthy Design Workgroup, created in 2012 by the Los Angeles County Board of Supervisors and involving 11 different city offices, including Parks and Recreation, Arts Commission, Community Development Commission, and more. The Healthy Design Workgroup focuses on policies that encourage safe outdoor activity, such as walking, biking, and visiting community gardens or farmers' markets (Wernham & Teutsch, 2015).

Other approaches to stakeholder engagement are being developed to be more responsive to the needs of Indigenous stakeholders and groups that have traditionally been underrepresented.

5. Create structural or process change

Over time, Health in All Policies work leads to institutionalizing a Health in All Policies approach throughout the whole of government. This involves permanent changes in how agencies relate to each other and how government decisions are made, structures for intersectoral collaboration, and mechanisms to ensure a health lens in decision-making processes.

For example, in 2012, an Australian nonprofit organization called Collaboration for Impact (CFI) began to convene stakeholders to directly address power dynamics for scaling collective impact in Australia. CFI incorporated

First Nations perspectives and leadership in their work. CFI reports that "Systemic collaboration in Australia necessitates working with the long tail of our colonial origins and our relationship with authority ... . The nation, which began as a penal colony and a process of forced removal from the United Kingdom, in turn forcibly removed Indigenous people from their land. Abuse of power and authority lingers and has been repeated over time and culture. In order to apply the collective impact framework, collaboratives must understand this context and navigate the dynamics of how formal and informal power enables and hinders collaboration.

Community members and leaders have had to undertake significant work to understand and step into their personal, cultural, and collective power. Backbone organizations and other intermediaries, dedicated to aligning and coordinating the work of a collaborative, need skills to help collaborations surface and navigate entrenched power dynamics to transform how both formal and informal power are either enabling or hindering their shared agenda. Governments and philanthropists must also acquire a greater level of power awareness to negotiate dialogues on power sharing and enable community decision-making over policy and allocation of funding" (Graham et al., 2021, para. 1–3).

References

American Public Health Association. (n.d.). *An introduction to Health in All Policies: A guide for state and local governments.* https://www.apha.org/-/media/files/pdf/factsheets/hiapguide_4pager_final.ashx

Becker, A. (2022). *The LA promise zone: Promise zones first round urban designees.* HUD Exchange. https://www.hudexchange.info/programs/promise-zones/promise-zones-urban-designees/#los-angeles

Centers for Disease Control and Prevention. (n.d.). *Childhood lead poisoning prevention: Los Angeles.* U.S. Department of Health & Human Services. https://www.cdc.gov/nceh/lead/programs/losangeles.htm

Graham, K., Skelton, L., & Paulson, M. Y. (2021, December 20). Power and collective impact in Australia. *Stanford Social Innovation Review.* https://doi.org/10.48558/xms6-6k45

Gwynne, K., & Cairnduff, A. (2017). Applying collective impact to wicked problems in Aboriginal health. *Metropolitan Universities Journal, 28*(4), 115–130. https://doi.org/10.18060/21740

Kania, J., & Kramer, M. (2011). Collective impact. *Stanford Social Innovation Review, 9*(1), 36–41. https://doi.org/10.48558/5900-KN19

LAPromiseZone.org. (n.d.). *Our partners.* LAPromiseZone.org. https://www.lapromisezone.org/partners

Sawin, E. (2018, July 16). The magic of "multisolving." *Stanford Social Innovation Review.* https://ssir.org/articles/entry/the_magic_of_multisolving#

Wernham, A., & Teutsch, S. M. (2015). Health in All Policies for big cities. *Journal of Public Health Management and Practice, 21*(Suppl 1), S56–S65. https://doi.org/10.1097/PHH.0000000000000130

Throughout this text, we align with the values of the public health profession (CDC, n.d.-b; Lee & Zarowsky, 2015), which view the remediation of health disparities as necessary and in the best interest of society. This perspective also aligns with population health management (PHM; Caron, 2014, 2017; Farmanova et al., 2019) and integrative healthcare system approaches that aim to improve the health of the communities they serve (see **Breakout Box 1.4**).

Breakout Box 1.4

POPULATION HEALTH AND PUBLIC HEALTH

The CDC (2020) defines population health as "an interdisciplinary, customizable approach that allows health departments to connect practice to policy for change to happen locally. This approach utilizes non-traditional partnerships among different sectors of the community—public health, industry, academia, health care, local government entities, etc.—to achieve positive health outcomes. Population health 'brings significant health concerns into focus and addresses ways that resources can be allocated to overcome the problems that drive poor health conditions in the population'" (para. 1).

Examples of strategies developed by the CDC to address population health include:

- The CDC's 6|18 initiative for healthcare purchasers, payers, and providers. In this initiative, the CDC is collaborating with healthcare providers, public health workers, insurers, and employers who purchase insurance to improve health and control healthcare costs through a variety of strategies. These strategies include providing partners with evidence about high-burden health conditions and related interventions, highlighting disease-prevention interventions to increase their use, and aligning proven preventive practices with value-based payment reforms. The aim is to enable partners to use this information to make decisions that improve health and help to control costs (see www.cdc.gov/sixeighteen/index.html).

- The Health Impact in 5 Years (HI-5) initiative focuses on community-level changes that can be achieved in 5 years. One example is the Earned Income Tax Credit (EITC), which helps eligible low- to moderate-income working people keep more of the money they earn by reducing the taxes they owe.

Other examples include multicomponent worksite obesity prevention programs and school violence prevention programs. Examples can be found at www.cdc.gov/policy/hst/hi5/publichealthinnovators/index.html and www.cdc.gov/policy/hst/hi5/index.html#:~:text=The%20Health%20Impact%20in%205,of%20the%20population%20or%20earlier.

How Does Population Health Complement Public Health?

As described by the Institute of Medicine, public health can be defined as what "we as a society do collectively to assure the conditions in which people can be healthy" (Institute of Medicine, Committee on Assuring the Health of the Public in the 21st Century, 2002, p. xi).

Population health complements public health by providing opportunities for healthcare systems, agencies, and other organizations to work together in order to improve the health outcomes of the communities they serve (Caron, 2017, 2022). From a population health management

(PHM) perspective, the geographic focus and scale of the exposome (**Figure 1.1**) may be more focused on the catchment area served by a healthcare system or hospital.

The definitions may differ slightly in their emphasis on equity. While addressing equity and eliminating health disparities is a main focus of public health, it may or may not be an explicit focus in population health, depending on how health outcomes are defined and prioritized in a particular context and which subpopulations are at risk. In countries such as the United States, population health is more closely aligned with payment reform, financial incentives, quality metrics, and reimbursement mechanisms within the healthcare delivery system.

Population Health Management

PHM has been defined as "a tool used to describe a variety of approaches developed to foster health and quality of care improvements while managing costs" (Caron, 2014, p. 698; Caron, 2017; McAlearney, 2003). The overall goal of PHM is to keep populations healthy via an integrative, prevention-oriented approach that can be embraced by clinical and public health professionals alike. PHM considers the determinants that most significantly affect the health of a health system's target population, such as employees or diabetes patients within a specific geographic area. PHM emphasizes community engagement and collaboration with clinicians and multisectoral professionals to address community health needs. Furthermore, PHM has the potential to contribute to the evaluation of the effectiveness of health policy interventions (Rimmasch, 2018).

References

Caron, R. (2014). Population health management. *Academic Medicine, 89*(5), 698. https://doi.org/10.1097/acm.0000000000000227

Caron, R. (2017). *Population health: Principles and applications for management.* Health Administration Press.

Caron, R. (2022). *Population health, epidemiology, and public health: Management skills for creating healthy communities.* Foundation of the American College of Healthcare Executives.

Centers for Disease Control and Prevention. (2020, October 6). *Population health training: What is population health?* https://www.cdc.gov/pophealthtraining/whatis.html

Institute of Medicine, Committee on Assuring the Health of the Public in the 21st Century. (2002). *The future of the public's health in the 21st century.* National Academies Press. https://www.ncbi.nlm.nih.gov/books/NBK221233

McAlearney, A. S. (2003). *Population health management: Strategies to improve outcomes.* Health Administration Press.

Rimmasch, H. (2018). *Four population health management strategies that help organizations improve outcomes.* Healthcare Catalyst. https://www.healthcatalyst.com/insights/4-population-health-strategies-drive-improvement

SUMMARY

Policy underpins many important determinants of health and is a key mechanism for addressing health disparities. Understanding the perspectives and values inherent in policy dialogues will allow you to clarify your position and intentionally craft the components of your policy analysis, which we will describe in subsequent chapters. This book will provide you with practical tools that enable you to become a "thoughtful policy analyst"—one that can contribute to the core functions of public health.

DISCUSSION QUESTIONS

Scenario: Consider a hypothetical case of Susan, a 35-year-old woman who lives in a lower income rural community. She suffers from diabetes, obesity, osteoarthritis, and depression. The closest grocery store is 20 miles away, and there are few parks, sidewalks, or bike paths in the community. There is a ski area that is open in the wintertime, but the prices of lift tickets are so high that local people can't afford it. Most people drive many miles each day to get to work, and sometimes they exceed the speed limit because they are worried about being late. If one loses one's job, there are very few options to get another one. Additionally, home prices and mortgages having been rising very quickly as the area is becoming attractive to people from the city looking to purchase second homes. Susan takes care of her wife, who has a hard time finding work and suffers from chronic pain due to an accident several years ago. Susan works at a chicken-processing factory, where she makes a little too much money to qualify for Medicaid. She worries constantly about being able to afford the rising premiums for her employer's health insurance plan. She often skips meals and forgoes her medication to save money for rent and her wife's treatments. There is a small local hospital that is affiliated with a larger urban medical center, but it is chronically understaffed. There are few medical providers in the area, and even fewer mental healthcare providers. When Susan called to try to find a therapist for her depression, she was told that the waiting list was over 6 months long.

- How might social, political, and environmental determinants of health contribute to the chronic diseases that Susan suffers from?
- Discuss examples of policy changes that might enable Susan to better manage her chronic health conditions.
- Discuss how political determinants of health may be contributing to health disparities in this scenario.
- Discuss how the core functions of public health could be leveraged to improve health for people like Susan.
- Discuss how different values (i.e., individual vs. collective) might lead to different perspectives about the "causes" of Susan's health conditions and the "solutions" that are warranted.

KEY TERMS

core functions of public health	health disparities
determinants of health	health equity
(social, environmental,	Health in All Policies
political, and planetary)	socio-ecological model
exposome	population health management

 SPRINGER PUBLISHING **CONNECT™**

A robust set of instructor resources designed to supplement this text is located at http://connect.springerpub.com/content/book/978-0-8261-8543-3. Qualifying instructors may request access by emailing textbook@springerpub.com.

REFERENCES

American Public Health Association. (n.d.). *An introduction to Health in All Policies: A guide for state and local governments.* https://www.apha.org/-/media/files/pdf/factsheets/hiapguide_4pager_final.ashx

Aristotle. (1987). *The nicomachean ethics.* (J. E. C. Weldon, Trans.). Prometheus Books.

Aristotle. (1994). *The politics.* (C. Lord, Trans.). University of Chicago Press.

Braveman, P., & Gruskin, S. (2003). Poverty, equity, human rights and health. *Bulletin of the World Health Organization, 81*(7), 539–545. https://doi.org/10.1590/S0042-96862003000700013

Brownson, R. (2020, July 9). *Dr. Ross Brownson—Evidence based public health* [Video]. YouTube. https://www.youtube.com/watch?v=IBOX716TbTY

Caron, R. (2014). Population health management. *Academic Medicine, 89*(5), 698. https://doi.org/10.1097/acm.0000000000000227

Caron, R. (2017). *Population health: Principles and applications for management.* Health Administration Press.

Caron, R. (2022). *Population health, epidemiology, and public health: Management skills for creating healthy communities.* Foundation of the American College of Healthcare Executives.

Centers for Disease Control and Prevention. (n.d.-a). *Office of the Associate Director for Policy and Strategy: Health in All Policies.* U.S. Department of Health and Human Services. https://www.cdc.gov/policy/hiap/index.html

Centers for Disease Control and Prevention. (n.d.-b). *Population health training: What is population health?* U.S. Department of Health and Human Services. https://www.cdc.gov/pophealthtraining/whatis.html

Centers for Disease Control and Prevention. (n.d.-c). *Violence prevention: The social-ecological model: A framework for prevention.* U.S. Department of Health and Human Services. https://www.cdc.gov/violenceprevention/about/social-ecologicalmodel.html

Centers for Disease Control and Prevention. (n.d.-d). *What is health equity?* U.S. Department of Health and Human Services. https://www.cdc.gov/healthequity/index.html

Farmanova, E., Baker, G. R., & Cohen, D. (2019). Combining integration of care and a population health approach: A scoping review of redesign strategies and interventions, and their impact. *International Journal of Integrated Care, 19*(2), Article 5. https://doi.org/10.5334/ijic.4197

Galea, S. (2022). *The values that bind us.* Boston University School of Public Health. https://www.bu.edu/sph/news/articles/2022/the-values-that-bind-us

Golden, S. D., McLeroy, K. R., Green, L. W., Earp, J. A., & Lieberman, L. D. (2015). Upending the social ecological model to guide health promotion efforts toward policy and environmental change. *Health Education & Behavior, 42*(Suppl. 1), 8S–14S. https://doi.org/10.1177/1090198115575098

Gwynne, K., & Cairnduff, A. (2017). Applying collective impact to wicked problems in aboriginal health. *Metropolitan Universities Journal, 28*(4), 115–130. https://doi.org/10.18060/21740

Harvey, M. (2020). How do we explain the social, political, and economic determinants of health? A call for the inclusion of social theories of health inequality within U.S.-based public health pedagogy. *Pedagogy in Health Promotion, 6*(4), 246–252. https://doi.org/10.1177/2373379920937719

Hobbes, T. (1640). The elements of law. In J. C. A. Gaskin (Ed.), *The elements of law, natural and politic* (p. 1990). Oxford University Press.

Hofstede, G. (2021, February 20). *The 6-D model of national culture.* Geert Hofstede. https://geerthofstede.com/culture-geert-hofstede-gert-jan-hofstede/6d-model-of-national-culture

Jayasinghe, S. (2015). Social determinants of health inequalities: Towards a theoretical perspective using systems science. *International Journal for Equity in Health, 14*(1), 71. https://doi.org/10.1186/s12939-015-0205-8

Juarez, P., Matthews-Juarez, P., Hood, D., Im, W., Levine, R., Kilbourne, B., Langston, M., Al-Hamdan, M., Crosson, W., Estes, M., Estes, S., Agboto, V., Robinson, P., Wilson, S., & Lichtveld, M. (2014). The public health exposome: A population-based, exposure science approach to health disparities research. *International Journal of Environmental Research and Public Health, 11*(12), 12866–12895. https://doi.org/10.3390/ijerph111212866

Kania, J., & Kramer, M. (2011). Collective impact. *Stanford Social Innovation Review, 9*(1), 36–41. https://doi.org/10.48558/5900-KN19

Knapp, E. A., Bilal, U., Dean, L. T., Lazo, M., & Celentano, D. D. (2019). Economic insecurity and deaths of despair in US counties. *American Journal of Epidemiology, 188*(12), 2131–2139. https://doi.org/10.1093/aje/kwz103

The Lancet Public Health. (2022). No public health without planetary health. *The Lancet Public Health, 7*(4), e291. https://doi.org/10.1016/s2468-2667(22)00068-8

Lee, L. M., & Zarowsky, C. (2015). Foundational values for public health. *Public Health Reviews, 36*(1), 2. https://doi.org/10.1186/s40985-015-0004-1

Levitsky, S., & Way, L. (2022, January 20). America's coming age of instability: Why constitutional crises and political violence could soon be the norm. *Foreign Affairs.* https://www.foreignaffairs.com/articles/united-states/2022-01-20/americas-coming-age-instability

Levy, C. R., Phillips, L. M., Murray, C. J., Tallon, L. A., & Caron, R. M. (2022). Addressing gaps in public health education to advance environmental justice: Time for action. *American Journal of Public Health, 112*(1), 69–74. https://doi.org/10.2105/ajph.2021.306560

Locke, J. (1796). *A letter concerning toleration* (W. Popple, Trans.). J. Brook. (Original work published 1690) http://onlinebooks.library.upenn.edu/webbin/book/search?amode=start&author=Locke,%20John

Mahmood, J. (2022). Beyond the hippocratic oath: A planetary health pledge for the Malaysian medical community. *Malaysian Journal of Medical Sciences, 29*(1), 1–3. https://doi.org/10.21315/mjms2022.29.1.1

McAlearney, A. S. (2003). *Population health management: Strategies to improve outcomes.* Health Administration Press.

McCartney, G., Hearty, W., Arnot, J., Popham, F., Cumbers, A., & McMaster, R. (2019). Impact of political economy on population health: A systematic review of reviews. *American Journal of Public Health, 109*(6), e1–e12. https://doi.org/10.2105/ajph.2019.305001

Myers, S., & Frumkin, H. (2020). *In planetary health: Protecting nature to protect ourselves.* Island Press.

Nussbaum, M. C. (1992). Human functioning and social justice: In defense of Aristotelian essentialism. *Political Theory, 20*(2), 202–246. https://doi.org/10.1177/0090591792020002002

Nussbaum, M. C. (1998). The good as discipline, the good as freedom. In D. A. Crocker & T. Linden (Eds.), *Ethics of consumption: The good life, justice, and global stewardship* (pp. 312–341). Rowman & Littlefield.

NYU Langone Health. (2022, July 21). *Explore health in your city.* City Health Dashboard. https://www.cityhealthdashboard.com

Rawls, J. (1971). *A theory of justice.* Harvard University Press.

Rigby, E., & Hatch, M. E. (2016). Incorporating economic policy into a 'health-in-all-policies' agenda. *Health Affairs, 35*(11), 2044–2052. https://doi.org/10.1377/hlthaff.2016.0710

Ruger J. P. (2004). Health and social justice. *Lancet, 364*(9439), 1075–1080. https://doi.org/10.1016/S0140-6736(04)17064-5

Salerno, J., & Bogard, K. (2019). What do social determinants of health determine? *Journal of Urban Health: Bulletin of the New York Academy of Medicine, 96*(6), 793–794. https://doi.org/10.1007/s11524-019-00402-z

Stokols, D. (1992). Establishing and maintaining healthy environments: Toward a social ecology of health promotion. *American Psychologist, 47*(1), 6–22. https://doi.org/10.1037/0003-066X.47.1.6

Tejada-Vera, B., Bastian, B., Arias, E., Escobedo, L., & Salant, B. (2020, March 9). *Life expectancy estimates by U.S. Census tract, 2010–2015.* National Center for Health Statistics. https://www.cdc.gov/nchs/data-visualization/life-expectancy/index.html

United Nations Development Programme. (2022, July 28). *Human development data.* Human Development Reports. https://hdr.undp.org/data-center

Wabnitz, K.-J., Gabrysch, S., Guinto, R., Haines, A., Herrmann, M., Howard, C., Potter, T., Prescott, S. L., & Redvers, N. (2020). A pledge for planetary health to unite health professionals in the anthropocene. *The Lancet, 396*(10261), 1471–1473. https://doi.org/10.1016/s0140-6736(20)32039-0

Wiesner, K., Birdi, A., Eliassi-Rad, T., Farrell, H., Garcia, D., Lewandowsky, S., Palacios, P., Ross, D., Sornette, D., & Thébault, K. (2018). Stability of democracies: A complex systems perspective. *European Journal of Physics, 40*(1), Article 014002. https://doi.org/10.1088/1361-6404/aaeb4d

World Health Organization. (2010, April 13). *Adelaide statement on Health in All Policies: Moving towards a shared governance for health and well-being.* World Health Organization & Government of South Australia. https://apps.who.int/iris/handle/10665/44365

World Health Organization. (2019, March 5). *Adelaide statement II on Health in All Policies: Implementing the sustainable development agenda through good governance for health and well-being: Building on the experience of health in all policies.* Author. https://www.who.int/publications-detail-redirect/adelaide-statement-ii-on-health-in-all-policies

CHAPTER 2

ELEMENTS AND HISTORY OF THE U.S. POLITICAL STRUCTURE

This chapter provides an overview of general elements of political and economic structures. Chapter 3 offers a more detailed explanation of the U.S. political structure. It takes multiple courses in political science and economics to fully understand these two social constructs. We encourage you to take advantage of courses in political science and economics. This is especially true if you are interested in one aspect of the political process such as Congress or the judiciary or wish to focus on consumer behavior or market concentration. Since political and economic systems are both social constructs, you should familiarize yourself with how other countries have designed their political and economic systems and how those different structural elements have influenced their medical and public health systems. We also encourage readers to explore Indigenous, decolonial, and other epistemologies that are relevant to the public health policy discourse (Carroll et al., 2022; Prescod-Weinstein, 2020; Redvers et al., 2022).

LEARNING OBJECTIVES

Be able to:

- Explain the need for the social construct of a political system.
- Analyze the meaning of authoritative allocation of values as it applies to the political system.
- Describe the tragedy of the commons and its implications for public health policy.
- Discuss the meaning of freedom in a political context.
- Explain the difference between policy and law.
- Discuss the importance of the separation of powers in the development of policy.

(continued)

- Explain the importance of federalism in the development of health policy for the United States.

- Explain the general difference between delegated and implied powers and the difference between those concepts at the federal, state, and local levels.

THE NEED FOR POLITICAL STRUCTURE

There are multiple definitions of politics, but perhaps the one that captures the essence of politics best is the authoritative allocation of values of society (Easton, 1953). A country's political system is the social construct created to carry out this task. *Values* are central to any political system. Note that *"values"* is plural. Individuals and societies have multiple values. When one takes any one value to the extreme or makes it the ultimate value, it will quickly conflict with another value that is also held dear. For example, most people can agree that not taking another human's life should be a social value, perhaps even the ultimate. However, if taken as the ultimate value, it would limit self-defense and allow the domination of any person or group that does not equally value human life. As a result, the word *allocation* is also important in this definition. We and society balance the value of not taking a life with self-defense, protection of the homeland, compassionate end-of-life decisions, the control of one's body, and so forth. Exactly where the balance lies between multiple values results in a conflict within us as well as within society. If all individuals were allowed to act on their own set of values, society would be in turmoil. To quote the English philosopher and political theorist Thomas Hobbes, life would be a war of all against all and be "solitary poore, nasty, brutish, and short" (Tuck, 1991, p. 62). Thus, social order becomes a value in itself. This is where the word *authoritative* becomes key in the definition.

Authoritative does not imply that a decision made by the political system is right, rational, or moral. Nation states may, and indeed do, enact laws (e.g., the legalization of slavery, denying women the right to vote) that are opposed by some of its population and/or seen as immoral from a historical perspective. Decisions by the political system can be amended or repealed for any number of reasons. *Authoritative* only means that the "police powers" of the state (its enforcement mechanisms such as Homeland Security, police, and the judicial system) will be used to enforce the political system's value decisions. If individuals violate these societal decisions as reflected by the "laws of the land," they may face fines, imprisonment, loss of life, and so forth. If conflicting laws exist, those must be resolved or adjudicated. Usually, they are resolved by some form of a judiciary with variable degrees of independence. The political system is the social construct charged with the authoritative allocation of values for a society (Easton, 1953).

As an example, the U.S. Supreme Court (USSC) case of *Dobbs v. Jackson* declared that the previously declared right to obtain an abortion with restriction was not a guaranteed constitutional right and the various states could regulate abortion (*Dobbs v. Jackson Women's Health Organization*, 2022). This case will be discussed in further detail in Chapter 5. Some states had trigger laws that automatically made abortion illegal; other states had previously passed state laws making abortion legal with various degrees of restrictions. Which of these laws is right, rational, or moral? The use of *authoritative* in the definition of a political system does not affirm that any of these laws are right, rational, or moral; they are merely the laws that will be enforced within that political jurisdiction.

Every nation state develops its own value priorities. What is legal in one's home country has no relevance when you are physically present in another country. One must legally abide by that nation's value priorities as reflected by its laws or face potential penalties. One nation state may look askance at another nation state's authoritative allocation of values.

Public policy reflects the values of society. Consequently, one way to understand the values of any nation state is to examine its laws and regulations. Some nation states might place a higher value on individual freedom while others might place a higher value on the general welfare. An even quicker way to examine a society's value system is to analyze its public budget. The public's budget is the monitary conversion of a society's priorities and values. How much of the public's money is spent on public education? How much is spent on public health as opposed to medical care? How much is spent on threats to the homeland for military weapons versus climate change? How much is spent on childcare versus elder care? How much is spent on highways versus public transit? How much is spent of public parks versus the industrialization of natural resources? The public budget is a shorthand for the political system's ranking of values.

Another aspect of values that needs to be acknowledged is that *facts* and *values* operate on different levels of cognition and that the two frequently collide. Certain facts may fit comfortably or uncomfortably within a cluster of social values. As we experience today, there may be a multitude of scientifically proven facts favoring the mandatory vaccination of people against COVID-19. Historically in the United States, the political system has mandated vaccinations and such actions have been upheld by the USSC.[1] Given the value of the public welfare or commonweal, the scientific facts of vaccination fit comfortably with a state vaccination mandate. However, given a heightened value for individual freedom, those scientific facts might be dismissed. The disagreement comes less over the validity of the facts than the difference in the weighting of two values, the common good and individual freedom. It becomes difficult to argue facts in the absence of a shared set of values. To use a quote from James Morone:

[M]edical science seeks objective answers to questions about health and health care. It documents, for example, the dangers of smoking, obesity, stress, unsafe sex, and delayed medical care. The surgeon general, the Institute of Medicine, and the Centers for Disease Control and Prevention might issue warnings based on good science. However, any effort to act on those findings simply triggers the politics of self-interest. No cultural mores penalize such a reaction: in politics, economic self-interest is every bit as legitimate as medical science.

The result appears to pose a conflict between medicine and politics. No matter how robust the scientific findings, political interests routinely mobilize and often delay or derail action. The politics of individualism offers health-minded reformers unambiguous advice:

---

1 *Jacobson v. Massachusetts* (1905) held that a state may require members of its population to obtain the smallpox vaccination. This was recently upheld when the Supreme Court refused to review the Seventh Circuit's decision in *Klaassen v. Trustees of Indiana University* (2021) that found Indiana University could issue a vaccine policy requiring all students, faculty, and staff members to be fully vaccinated against COVID-19 prior to returning to campus.

use your scientific findings to mobilize your own side. In the political arena, your science is only as strong as your political coalition. (Morone, 2005, pp. 14–15)

In the debate over vaccination and the loss of individual freedom, it is important to recognize different definitions of *freedom*. Fromm (1941) argues that freedom can be defined in two ways, *freedom from* and *freedom to*. The burden of losing individual freedom due to being forced to undergo a vaccination also results in the freedom to be able to socialize or work without the fear of getting a potentially fatal disease or infecting loved ones. The denial of a child's freedom for 12 years due to mandatory public education provides the freedom to acquire skills and knowledge for individual advancement and the freedom to become a scientist, lawyer, healthcare provider, and so forth. In the United States, we tend to define freedom as "freedom from" rather than "freedom to." Other countries tend focus more on "freedom to." Requiring health insurance through a national healthcare system or individual mandate frees one from the potential of medical care bankruptcy or the fear of not receiving needed medical services and provides a healthier workforce for the country. Restricting individual freedom can provide other freedoms and benefits for both the individual and society.

There will always be differences in values within society. That is indeed what the political system attempts to resolve. These value conflicts, however, must be held in check. In their argument for deliberative democracy, Gutmann and Thompson provide the following warning:

In politics, disagreements often run deep. If they did not, there would be no need for argument. But if they ran too deep, there would be no point in argument. Deliberative disagreements lie in the depths between simple misunderstandings and immutable irreconcilability. (Gutmann & Thompson, 1996, p. 16)

As a result, there needs to be a level of toleration of civic differences in the weighting of values.

When norms of mutual toleration are weak, democracy is hard to sustain. If we view our rivals as a dangerous threat, we have much to fear if they are elected. We may decide to employ any means necessary to defeat them—and therein lies a justification for authoritarian measures. (Levitsky & Ziblatt, 2018, p. 104)

When the accommodation of widely held values becomes irreconcilable and when those values become more important than holding civil society together, the political system and the structure of the nation state are threatened. When the perceived unfairness of taxes became irreconcilable with obedience to king or the moral stain of slavery became irreconcilable with the economic retention of slavery, our national government faced dissolution. In any given year, there are multiple coups and civil wars occurring around the world, all involving a perceived irreconcilable clash of social values. Some believe that the level of value disagreement in the United States today is at a precarious level.

Each society makes its own decisions as to how to operationalize and structure its political system that will make these value decisions. Some nation states might believe in "the divine right of kings," meaning that a particular family or group has received divine guidance as to how society's values should be balanced. Some nation states might believe that might (money, military power, etc.) makes right and that those with the most power should dictate what values are important for its people. Some might believe that the power comes from the "people" and establish some type of a republic with a governance structure that reflects the "will of the people." Typically, the latter create some form of a democratic infrastructure, which can range from a pure democracy (majority rule) or a representative democracy with some type of protection for individual "natural rights" and the rights of minorities.

Natural rights were recognized by our Founding Fathers as rights coming from nature or God. Those natural rights cannot be denied by governments or other humans:

We hold these truths to be self-evident, that all men are created equal, that they are endowed by their Creator with certain unalienable Rights, that among these are Life, Liberty, and the pursuit of Happiness. That to secure these rights, Governments are instituted among Men, deriving their powers from the consent of the governed. That whenever any Form of Government becomes destructive of these ends, it is the Right of the People to alter or abolish it, and to institute new Government, laying its foundation on such principles and organizing its powers in such form, as to them shall seem most likely to effect their Safety and Happiness. (Jefferson, 1776, para. 2)[2]

In the U.S. political system, natural rights can be claimed in a court of law. In contrast, legal rights such as the freedom of the press are those rights granted by governments. Unlike natural rights, legal rights can be taken away by the same government that gave them.

The Economic System and Market Failure

One of the major decisions made by the political system is the establishment of another social construct, the economic system. One aspect of this economic system involves the balance between individual rights and the social good or the commonweal. Some nation states value the social unit over the individual and some value the individual over the social unit; there are all types of gradations in between both ends of the spectrum. Capitalism is one type of economic system that tends to place a high value on individual freedom. One of the basic principles of capitalism is that if an individual acts in their own self-interest, they will produce goods desired by society at a price that will be fair. Otherwise, a competitor will enter the market and produce a better product or the same product at cheaper price.

Therefore, according to capitalism, society will be better off having free market competition among providers of goods and services. Self-interest (maximizing profits) and competition are seen as the key values promoting the social good (O'Rourke, 2007). On the other hand, others believe that the commonweal should control or guide what individuals should be allowed to do within the economic sector. Thus, there is a continuum of economic systems within democratic countries placing a higher value on the individual (e.g., the United States) and those placing a higher value on the social good, various forms of democratic socialism

---

2 The English philosopher John Locke, who was a major intellectual foundation for the Founding Fathers, defined natural rights as "life, liberty and property" in *Two Treatises of Government* in 1690.

(e.g., Scandinavian countries). In contrast, communism is an economic system by which all means of production are owned by the state with limited private ownership. It is important to remember that each nation's economic system is on a continuum attempting to balance the interests of the commonweal with private interests.

One of the problems with the theory of pure capitalism is what has been called the *tragedy of the commons* made popular by Garrett Hardin (Frischmann et al., 2019; Hardin, 1968). He uses the analogy of the town commons (a legacy of our English heritage) and its free use by all citizens for grazing their cows. One of the important aspects of the commons is that it has a specific carrying capacity, meaning it can sustain a certain number of cows year after year thus producing the maximum amount of milk for society. Too few cows will reduce the amount of milk for the population and too many cows will begin to destroy the grass resulting in less milk for society. According to pure capitalism, each acting in their own self-interest will lead to the betterment of society. In fairness each family might be allocated the same number of cows, or each family unit can have the number of cows based upon the size of the family. What is critical is that the total carrying capacity is not to be exceeded so that the grass returns with abundance year after year.

Such an arrangement works well for the first year until Farmer A believes he and his family will be better off with one additional cow. By adding a cow, all cows now have access to less grass due to the existence of the additional cow. However, since Farmer A now has one more cow, he has more milk than before. By these actions, Farmer A has internalized the benefits of having 11 cows (gained more milk) and externalized the costs (reduced the amount of grass per cow) of that extra cow to the other farmers. However, the consequence of Farmer A's actions means that the carrying capacity of the commons has been exceeded and the grass the following year is not as plentiful. At first the other farmers may not notice the impact of one additional cow because the externalized cost of one additional cow has been spread among all the farmers. Knowing that he has gained more milk by adding an additional cow, Farmer A acting in his own self-interest decides to add another cow the following year to make up for the decline in the production per cow. He now has two extra cows and even more milk, however, total milk production for society has been reduced and the other farmers' incomes have been reduced. Because externalized costs to other farmers have now increased, they might notice a more significant decline in their amount of milk (income).

Noticing the amount of milk that Farmer A is now selling, Farmer B acting in his own self-interest adds a cow. Now the external costs of Farmers A and B are larger and more noticeable. Farmers C, D, and so forth notice what has been happening and acting in their own self-interest add their own cows. The result is that each person acting in their own self-interest and shifting external costs to society leads to the destruction of the commons and society becomes worse off. One solution to the tragedy of the commons is for the political system to enact a regulation limiting the number of cows or imposing fines for those who violate the commons. It is a tragedy as in a classical Greek tragic play since the destruction of the commons is the result of human failings. Nobel Prize winner Elinor Ostrom developed alternative theories of how common goods, or "common pool resources," could be allocated among small, self-organized groups. Ostrom's theories and perspectives of institutional design are often covered in courses of political economy, which may complement public health policy (Ostrom, 1990).

A modern-day tragedy of the commons plays out with pollution and public health. It is to every manufacturer's self-interest to maximizing profits by pouring industrial waste into the air, river, or ocean (the commons). From the producer's perspective, the pollutant "goes away" with little expense. However, since there is no "away," neighbors downstream or downwind bear the costs of polluted drinking water and cancer-causing chemicals in the air. In the meantime, the owners of the manufacturing plant save money; the cost of pollution has been externalized. At first the neighbors may not notice; diseases may take years to develop. The externalized costs keep growing as other producers see the benefit of externalizing the cost of their industrial waste. Eventually neighbors may start to notice that the local carrying capacity of the environment to cleanse itself has been exceeded. Taller smokestacks merely carry the pollution further "away" to unsuspecting people or other parts of the globe. The externalities of pollution increase lung disease and spread cancers downwind.

The tragedy could have been prevented through public regulation and forcing the costs of pollution to be borne by the producer and not externalized. When the externalized social costs become noticeable, the political system may or may not act to require an environmental clean-up. Even if the polluter pays for some of the clean-up, the polluter does not generally have to pay for the lives lost or the medical expenses incurred by the pollution unless there is a class action suit (another externalized cost), taking multiple years to adjudicate. Meanwhile, the original owners of the facility have sold their stake in the company, and the company has received bankruptcy protection or been forced to absorb some of the cost of the clean-up. Again, the solution to the tragedy is for the political system to prevent social externalities before they occur or alternatively to shift the cost of those externalities back to the producer (mandating chimney scrubbers, building holding tanks or treatment tanks, etc.). The penalty for externalizing pollution must be sufficiently large to incentivize the corporation (acting in their own self-interest) to reduce or eliminate the pollutant.

Another example of social externalities involves employee wages. It is to the advantage of a capitalist to pay as low a wage as possible to workers and thereby increase corporate profits. Tight labor markets might justify increasing wages. However, the practice of paying wages below a "livable wage" and forcing workers to have second jobs or a working spouse saves a corporation money but it also externalizes costs. There are many profitable corporations that pay their workers a legal minimum wage, making their employees eligible for food stamps, subsidized housing, Medicaid, subsidized childcare, and other social support mechanisms paid for by the commons. The impact of social externalities is a major argument for public health policy.

The tragedy of the commons is only one example of potential market failures that might occur within a capitalistic system. Others include the elimination of competition through market concentration or monopolies, the lack of lifesaving services to those for whom the market has little interest (i.e., those who cannot afford to enter the health insurance market), access to healthy air and water for all (public sanitation), protection of the public's health from dangerous products (tobacco, asbestos, lead, cocaine, etc.), assuring safe and sanitary market places (fire and health inspections), protection of irreplaceable natural resources (national parks), assessing the qualifications of those providing critical services (professional licensure), or preventing discrimination against certain groups for employment, housing, and so forth. There is also the generic problem of information asymmetries between the buyer and the seller so that the buyer is not able to make a rational choice. The political system is the major countervailing power to overcome market failures. Due to laws attempting to address some of these market failures, the United States is generally regarded as a modified capitalistic system.

However, it must be noted that public policy may not adequately overcome all market failures. The market does not control everything. Despite a conflict of values between individual freedom and social control, market failures may continue. There may be side effects of public actions that have unintended detrimental consequences that cause a reevaluation of the social cost and benefits of any policy. In addition, it is important to remember that one person's perception of a market failure is another person's perception of the market working perfectly well. Farmer A was pleased by the nonregulation of the commons.

POLICY AND LAW

Public policy reflects the value commitments of society. While this is frequently interpreted to mean the laws that are passed by the government, public policy is broader than merely the accumulation of laws. Policy has many sources. As we will see later, public policy comes from the Constitution, common law, statutes, popular initiatives and referendums, rules and regulations, executive orders, executive signing statements, the budget, judicial case law, and treaties. The judiciary frequently and correctly points out that it is not their job to make the law. While it is true that the judiciary does not "make" laws, it does prevent certain laws from being implemented and shapes policy by interpreting the language of legislation duly passed by the other two branches.

Kenneth Prewitt defined policy as "a standing decision characterized by behavioral consistency and repetitiveness on the part of those who make it and those who abide by it" (Eulau & Prewitt, 1973, p. 465). While a motorist may view the statutory speed limit of 65 miles per hour on hundreds of highway signs, both the motorist and the police assigned to enforce the law have mutually recognized that the real speed limit on that highway is actually 70 or even 74 miles per hour. In some states even driving the posted speed limit can result in a traffic violation given special road or weather conditions. The law is one thing and policy is another. To avoid a traffic violation, one needs to understand the variation in traffic policies within each jurisdiction. How a simple health code is interpreted by a health inspector and a restaurant owner is governed by mutual consistency and repetitiveness regarding the interpretation of the law. A change in health inspectors may result in a significant change in the enforcement of the health code. A tragic incident (such as a fire) may indeed result in a change in policy as to how an existing health code is to be enforced. Policy may change even when the law remains the same.

It is also important to distinguish between various types of laws. Within the United States, there is natural law, common law, constitutional law, and statutory law made by national, state and local governments. One element that we inherited from the British system of government was the inclusion of common law. Today the only state that does not have common law is Louisiana, due to its early Spanish control. Legislation cannot cover all facets of a civil society. To make up for that, common law is composed of precedents established over time by the judiciary ruling on individual cases. The purpose of common law is to add a degree of predictability as to how the courts would rule given similar cases. This legal principle is called *stare decisis,* following rules or principles laid down in previous judicial decisions unless they contravene principles of justice. *Stare decisis* is followed by federal and state court systems. A *writ of habeas corpus,* a *writ of mandamus,* and a common law marriage are examples of common law that date from Anglo-Saxon times in Great Britain. A *writ of habeas corpus* prohibits inappropriate detention or imprisonment by the government. A *writ of mandamus* is a judicial order to a government official to carry out their responsibilities as required by the law.

Another common law principle that is important for public health is the notion that governments can take actions against individuals if those individuals endanger the health of other people. Colonial governments (local and state) used quarantine to separate those who endangered the public's health. Islands (not masks) were used to isolate the infectious. Obviously sick residents were forcibly placed in specialty hospitals until they were either cured or dead. Ships from foreign ports were frequently subject to quarantines. Today, legislative statutes have been passed to further define the application of this common law principle. With the impact of the COVID-19 pandemic, federal, state, and local governments are reevaluating where the balance between common law and public health rests. Common law is one of the foundations of public health.

Constitutional law, which we will discuss in some detail in this chapter, sets out the basic framework as to the governmental units (legislative, executive, and judicial branches) authorized to pass statutory laws governing the behavior of individuals. In addition, constitutional law can impose certain restrictions on what those units of government can do. In the United States, constitutional law is supreme over federal statutory law and federal laws are supreme over state laws. Most countries, with the major exception of Great Britain, have a constitution. Statutory laws are those enacted by the units of government so empowered by the Constitution. These laws make up a large part of what is regarded as public policy. Most statutory law is enacted by the legislative branch, but some states in the United States allow popular initiatives and referendums that bypass the legislature. Budgets are also a source of policy. Laws can be enacted with no or little money to implement them, thus making them ineffective. Sometimes, laws are passed but the funding for their implementation is passed along to another political jurisdiction, "unfunded mandates." A change in policy regarding an issue may require only a change in the budget rather than a new statute. Eliminating or cutting a budget substantially can cripple the implementation of a statute. It is important to remember that there are multiple sources of public policy.

AMERICAN HISTORICAL PERSPECTIVES

It is important to recognize that before the United States and before the English colonies there were probably more people in the Americas than in Europe and that there were relatively large Indigenous communities throughout what is now the United States (Mann, 2005). There were hundreds of different Indigenous Peoples with their own sets of values, governance structures, and political and economic alliances. As a result of multiple early contacts with European fisherman, trappers, and explorers, the Native Americans in the country contracted diseases such as smallpox, scarlet fever, and influenza, which decimated their populations.

Initially the United States recognized Native American Peoples as independent nations and had agreements with them by means of treaties. The Indian Appropriations Act of 1871 prohibited additional treaties with Native Americans. The United States recognizes some Indigenous Peoples as "domestic dependent nations" and maintains a government-to-government relationship with them. There are currently 574 Tribes recognized by the Bureau of Indian Affairs; there are additional Indigenous groups recognized by state governments. Some recognized Indigenous Peoples cross state boundaries. Some Indigenous Peoples are not recognized by either federal or state governments in the United States. There are Indigenous constitutions recognizing membership as well as governance on the reservations. There are currently 326 Native American Reservations in the United States. There are also state-recognized reservations that lack federal recognition. Indigenous governments have their own court systems, which have been the subject of multiple USSC cases involving their jurisdiction. In 2022 the USSC ruled that the federal government and the state have concurrent jurisdiction to prosecute crimes committed by non-Indians against Indians in Indian country (*Oklahoma v. Castro-Huerta*, 2022).[3] In doing so it upended Native American sovereignty as well as federal preemption, giving states enforcement powers within Indigenous Peoples' territory. It will take years for this to play out in the future. The USSC is also involved with a number of religious liberty cases involving Native Americans.

The Native American reservations are important areas for public health. Because Native Americans had their own traditional medicine, the Indian Health Service (IHS) within the U.S. Department of Health and Human Services recognizes traditional medicine as well as providing Western medicine and public health to the federally recognized Native American Peoples. The IHS provides healthcare and public health in 37 states.

Since we are focusing on the current U.S. political system, we need to remember that the federal system evolved from the British political system. For over 150 years the original 13 colonies were controlled by the United Kingdom with a monarch, an evolving parliament, and a judiciary. Each of the original 13 colonies had their own appointed royal governor, a legislative body, and a judiciary. They fought a costly war against the British government over taxation and other perceived abuses as delineated in the Declaration of Independence. The other 37 states composing the present United States developed politically with very different historical influences. Today's state governments tend to reflect those various historical differences. As we will see, some of the Western and Midwestern states that became part of the United States when popular democracy was an ascending value have political characteristics that reflect that influence. However, the

---

3 *Oklahoma v. Castro-Huerta* (2022) was a 5-4 decision of the Court with Justice Kavanaugh writing the majority decision in favor of the state of Oklahoma. Justice Gorsuch wrote the dissent. The case involved a non-Indian (Castro-Huerta) convicted in state court with child neglect (his Indian stepdaughter) and sentenced to 35 years in prison. He was later tried in federal court, which traditionally has preemptive jurisdiction in tribal territory along with tribal courts. In federal court, he accepted a 7-year sentence in addition to deportation from the United States. The Supreme Court found in favor of the state's jurisdiction. This case followed an earlier Court case of *McGirt v. Oklahoma* (2020) in which the Court ruled that the tribal territory of Eastern Oklahoma had not been properly set and that it (including Tulsa) remained tribal territory making state/federal jurisdiction a major issue.

establishment of our federal government was heavily influenced by the experiences of the original 13 colonies with Great Britain.

The Articles of Confederation and the Constitution

During the American Revolution, the Founding Fathers created a political structure under the Articles of Confederation. The Articles of Confederation were approved on November 15, 1777, after considerable debate during the Second Continental Congress. They went into effect on March 1, 1781, after unanimous ratification by the 13 states. One of the major values behind that structure was the sovereignty of the 13 states. As indicated by its name, it was more a league of friendship or a confederation than a solidified nation state. It had one branch, the Congress of Confederation (Continental Congress) that was given extensive powers but had no enforcement mechanism. There was no executive branch or judiciary. Members of the Continental Congress were appointed by state legislatures, not elected by the people. While each state had multiple members based on population size, each state had only one vote in the Continental Congress. During the Revolutionary War, General Washington made executive wartime decisions. That worked sufficiently since the initial job for the Continental Congress was fighting a war. However, after the war, experience quickly demonstrated that this structure was inadequate for making and enforcing its decisions. That led to a movement in 1787 to reform the Articles of Confederation. The appointed delegates to the Philadelphia Convention of 1787 decided rather than reform the Articles, they would propose a whole new system of government. As a result, the Philadelphia Convention of 1787 was the real American revolution.

During the debate regarding the adoption of the Constitution there was a series of published newspaper articles written individually by Alexander Hamilton, James Madison, and John Jay that laid out the principles upon which the proposed new government was to be based. The articles were designed to convince people of the logic for a new political system and to advocate for its adoption by the individual states. *The Federalist Papers* remains the main source of insight into the thinking of the Founding Fathers and it is frequently cited in Supreme Court decisions, especially by conservative justices using an originalist interpretation of the Constitution (Hamilton et al., 1961).

The Founding Fathers were quick to recognize their first failure (the Continental Congress) to enact a workable governmental structure. Even this second political structure was seen by its authors as a hopeful experiment rather than a divinely inspired document. As expressed by Benjamin Franklin,

I confess that I do not entirely approve this Constitution at present; but sir, I am not sure I shall never approve it: For having lived long, I have experienced many instances of being obliged by better information, or fuller consideration, to change opinions even on important subjects, which I once thought right, but found to be otherwise. ... the older I grow, the more apt I am to doubt my own judgment and pay more respect to the judgment of others. ... I doubt too whether any other Convention we can obtain, may be able to make a better Constitution; for when you assemble a number of men, to have the advantage of their joint wisdom, you inevitably assemble with those men, all their prejudices, their passions, their errors of opinion, their local interests, and their selfish views. From such an assembly can a perfect production be expected? ... Thus I consent,

Sir, to this Constitution because I expect no better, and because I am not sure, that it is not the best. (Isaacson, 2003, pp. 457–458)

He then made the motion for the Convention to unanimously adopt the Constitution and refer it to the states for ratification.

GENERAL STRUCTURAL PRINCIPLES
Separation of Powers

There are several principles that are necessary to explain to understand the structure of the U.S. government. One is the separation of powers. This is built upon a basic distrust of human nature. As explained by James Madison, "ambition must be made to counter ambition" (Hamilton et al., 1961, p. 322).[4] According to this belief, the political system must be constructed to separate decision-making power between national government and the states (federalism). Moreover, they designed a national government where there would be a separation of power between the executive and legislative branches. Even within a branch such as the legislative branch, there would be further division of power between two distinctly different bodies, the House of Representatives and the Senate. Prior experience demonstrated that political power could easily be abused; countervailing centers of decision-making were the best protection of liberty. Today many people complain how difficult it is for our government to act. To the Founding Fathers, that was the whole point. The U.S. government was never designed to be a speedy decision-making body; a dictator can make decisions quickly. Liberty and not speed was the dominate value. The Framers of the Constitution did their best to set up a political structure that had multiple checks and balances to make political decision-making a difficult path to navigate; to most political observers of the U.S. political system, they were successful.

Federalism

A complementary concept that is important in our political system is federalism. Federalism is a political structure in which political power is divided between a central government and geographic subunits (states/provinces) with each having their own as well as shared or complementary powers. Some powers or policy areas may be delegated exclusively to the central government (foreign policy), some predominantly to the states (education), and some may be shared (public health). Not all nation states are federalist states; France and England are examples of nonfederalist nation states while Canada and Germany are other federalist nations. Given the emergence of the 13 sovereign states and the precedent set by the Articles of Confederation, a federal system was an essential compromise needed to create the United States.

Citizens within a federal political system are subject to the authority of both levels of government. Depending on the nation state, states/provinces may have different degrees of independence or shared jurisdiction. Generally, there is a provision that if there is a conflict between state laws and those of the federal

---

4 See also *Federalist Papers* #47 and #48 (Hamilton et al., 1961, pp. 300–313).

government, the latter prevails.[5] Being subject to both governments implies that there may be different values and rights under each one. There were states in which slavery was legal and those in which it was illegal. Before the 14th Amendment, the Bill of Rights (freedom of religion, speech, assembly, etc.) only applied to the federal government. It was legal for states to adopt a state religion or restrict other religions. As a result of the adoption of the 14th Amendment after the Civil War, there was a guarantee that certain rights applied to all Americans and that states (not just the federal government) were prohibited from violating those rights.[6] The 14th Amendment is sometimes referred to as the federalization of the Bill of Rights.

It is important for health policy analysts to realize that there are both federal laws and state laws as well as state and federal court systems that control public health policies. The COVID-19 pandemic has made these conflicts between the federal and state governments more visible. However, these conflicts have been there all along.

With the Great Depression in the 1930s and World War II, federalism in the United States was reshaped. There was an increase in the number federal laws, which had major implications for all states and citizens. Social Security, unemployment benefits, and other social safety net programs were created for all Americans and were administered nationally. In the 1960s and 1970s with civil rights and poverty concerns not being met by state governments, there was again an increase in federal legislation passed to solve those problems. These problems were perceived as being national problems rather than state problems and therefore required national policies.

As a result, federal grant programs were developed to provide money to state and local governments as well as local nonprofit organizations to tackle specific social, health, and economic problems. These grants had specific federal guidelines as to what was to be done with the federal money; since these were federal funds, fiscal accountability warranted federal oversight. State/local violations of the federal guidelines could mean the potential withdrawal of federal funds. For example, federally funded neighborhood health centers were established, and health planning agencies were established for the coordination and development of private medical care. With increased pollution and the recognition that pollution did not recognize state boundaries, landmark federal environmental laws promoting clean air and water were also passed by the Nixon administration during the 1970s.

However, by the late 1970s and early1980s, there was a political backlash to extensive national legislation. The existence of federal funding for local nonprofit agencies that was seen as bypassing state governments. There was a perception that state governments had evolved and become more responsive. As a result, states' rights and New Federalism became more popular. While the federal government

---

5 The Supremacy Clause in the Constitution states: "This Constitution, and the Laws of the United States which shall be made in Pursuance thereof; and all Treaties made, or which shall be made, under the Authority of the United States, shall be the supreme Law of the Land; and the Judges in every State shall be bound thereby, anything in the Constitution or Laws of any State to the Contrary notwithstanding" (U.S. Const. art. VI, § 2).

6 The 14th Amendment, Section 1, states "No State shall make or enforce any law which shall abridge the privileges or immunities of citizens of the United States; nor shall any State deprive any person of life, liberty, or property, without due process of law; nor deny to any person within its jurisdiction the equal protection of the laws" (U.S. Const. amend. XIV, § 1).

still provided the money, under New Federalism money was to go through the states and allow them greater flexibility to shape those programs to meet their perceived local needs. The argument was that what worked in New York did not necessarily work in Texas. Under New Federalism states were to be given block grants that allowed each state greater discretion as to how and where to spend the federal money. The initial block grants included the Community Development Block Grant, the Partnership for Health Act, the Omnibus Crime Control and Safe Streets Act, the Comprehensive Employment and Training Act, and Title XX of the Social Security Act. Title XX of the Social Security Act gives states money to provide childcare for working parents, establishes rehabilitation centers for the disabled, and provides assistance to the older adults living alone. Under block grants states are still required to spend the money for a particular generic purpose but they have greater flexibility in how to address local needs.

While the term New Federalism is not generally used today, states' rights and the use of block grants are widely accepted today. There remains a perennial debate within our political system as to the appropriate balance between the powers of the federal government and those of the states. The states' rights advocates argue that each state's unique circumstances justify differences in the application of federal laws and money. On the other hand, federalists tend to argue that the United States is one national economy (due to such things as technology, transportation, online shopping, and supply chains as well as a common ecosystem). Therefore, to effectively solve national problems (pollution, pandemics, drug addiction, hunger etc.), national policies and programs are required. Since federal funds are being used to implement such policies, fiscal accountability must be assured. In addition, federalists tend to argue that federal programs or protections should be equally available to all U.S. citizens regardless of their geographic location. Federalism raises the question, "What does it mean to be a citizen of the United States and what does it mean to be a citizen of South Carolina or California?" The political balance between the roles of federal and state governments remains an ongoing debate.

Medicare/Medicaid and Affordable Healthcare

This tension regarding federalism is demonstrated in the passage of Medicare and Medicaid in 1965 as well as the 2010 Patient Protection and Affordable Care Act (PPACA; Health Care & Education Reconciliation Act, 2010; PPACA, 2010; Social Security Amendments, 1965). Medicare and Medicaid were passed during President Lyndon Johnson's administration at the height of increased federalization of policy, for example, the passage of federal civil rights and the War on Poverty legislation. In contrast, the PPACA was passed during President Barack Obama's administration and a period of increased focus on states' rights.

Medicare is an example of a federal program that is federally funded and administered. All U.S. citizens 65 years and older who are U.S. citizens or legal residents for 5 years are eligible to be covered by Medicare. In addition, patients with certain disabilities can also qualify. Beneficiary contributions, benefit coverage, and reimbursement payments to healthcare providers are all nationally determined. A Medicare recipient can move to any state without impacting their Medicare costs or benefits. A valuable by-product of Medicare being a national program with uniform policies is that it has a public national data set on patients and providers.

As a result, Medicare's public data set is frequently used for academic research to examine diseases, treatments, and the impact of various public policies despite the fact that it consists of a skewed subset of the population (generally those over 65 years old).

Medicaid, passed under the same 1965 Amendments to the Social Security Act, is a federal- and state-funded program that is administered by each state or territory. While there are some minimum federal Medicaid guidelines, the determination of eligibility, coverage, costs, and reimbursement rates is left up to each state. A person may be eligible for Medicaid in one state but not in another. A disease may be covered in one state and not in another. Rates of provider reimbursement may be dramatically different between adjacent states, which may impact the availability of services to a state's Medicaid population. State borders can become critical medical barriers for Medicaid eligibles. State variation in policies may be the difference between life and death, restorative healthcare, or a lifetime disability. From a policy analyst's perspective, knowing how a state's Medicaid program works means that you only understand one of 56 such programs existing in the 50 states, the District of Columbia, and five territories (American Samoa, Commonwealth of Northern Mariana Islands, Guam, Puerto Rico, and the U.S. Virgin Islands).

The passage of PPACA came during the Barack Obama administration (see Breakout Box 2.1). The health of the working population is key to having a healthy economy. At the time, approximately 51 million Americans (one out of five) were uninsured, and the number of employees covered by employer health insurance was dropping (DeNavas-Walt et al., 2010). While other nations have versions of a national healthcare system, the bulk of the U.S. healthcare insurance system (except for Medicare) is largely controlled by the states. While a few states like Massachusetts were experimenting with various health insurance frameworks to expand access to health insurance, the national picture for the uninsured kept getting worse. One of the intents of PPACA was to reduce the number of the uninsured population in the nation as a whole and to decrease the disparity in healthcare insurance among the various states. The legislative debate went back and forth between a national system or national support for state-run systems. In the end, there was a major political decision to drop the availability of a national public option plan to run alongside private health insurance options controlled at the state level.

Breakout Box 2.1

THE PASSAGE OF THE PATIENT PROTECTION AND AFFORDABLE CARE ACT

Healthcare reform had been an issue in the 2008 presidential election between Democrat Barack Obama and Republican John McCain. Obama was elected president and the Democrats gained eight seats in the Senate and 21 in the House to hold a majority in both houses. On March 5, 2009, President Obama held an invitational Health Care Summit in the East Room of the White House for 150 representatives from Republicans, Democrats, business, healthcare providers, insurance representatives, unions, and so forth. The purpose of the meeting was to create an atmosphere for all stakeholders to work together to achieve healthcare reform.

On June 19, 2009, three house committees (Ways and Means, Energy and Commerce, and Education and Labor) issued a report with a proposal to pass healthcare reform. Sponsored by Democrat Charles Rangel (D-NY-15) of the House Ways and Means Committee, H.R. 3590 was introduced to the House. On October 8, 2009, it was approved by the House and sent to the Senate.

During the summer of 2009 there were a series of town halls around the United States in which the rhetoric of death panels and socialized medicine raised the temperature of the political debate. There was debate as to whether there would be a public option in addition to options for private health insurance coverage.

Due to Senator Kennedy's death on August 25, 2009, there was a special election to fill his seat. On January 19, 2010, in an upset in traditionally Democratic Massachusetts, Republican Scott Brown defeated Martha Coakley. While the Democrats maintained their majority in the Senate, they no longer had the 60 votes to rebuff a filibuster. On December 24, 2009, prior to Senator Brown taking his seat, the Senate passed H.R. 3590, Patient Protection and Affordable Health Bill 60-39 with all Democrats voting for the bill and all Republican voting against, except for one Republican who did not vote. Since there were Senate changes to H.R. 3590 (e.g., excluding the public option), the bill had to be sent back to the House for its approval for the changes. On March 21, 2010, the House of Representatives agreed with the Senate changes and passed H.R. 3590. Although the House leadership was not in agreement with the Senate changes, to send it back to the Senate would have made the bill subject to a filibuster. The vote was 219-212 with all Republicans and 34 Democrats voting no. Unable to break a filibuster in the Senate, the Democrats combined PPACA with H.R. 4872, Health Care and Education Reconciliation Act of 2010. H.R. 4872 made some health-related financing changes to PPACA. Because this was now an Omnibus Budget Reconciliation Act, it was not subject to a Senate filibuster.

On March 23, 2010, the bill was signed by President Barack Obama in a White House ceremony. It was implemented in stages lasting several years. Republican opposition to the bill continued with multiple attempts to repeal the legislation and a series of court cases to invalidate the law. See https://UScode.house.gov/statutes/PL/111/148.pdf for the text of PPACA.

The resulting legislation signed into law on March 23, 2010, was a series of compromises despite the partisan nature of the votes in the House and the Senate for approval (see **Breakout Box 2.1**). Under the law the federal government was to provide insurance protections for people with preexisting conditions, provide financial assistance for people below 400% of the federal poverty level, and impose an individual and employer mandate among other provisions that provided additional money for public health. States, however, were able to maintain control of the individual, small group, and large group insurance markets; retain their own Medicaid programs; create their own Basic Health Care Plan for people between 138% and 200% of the federal poverty level; establish risk adjustment and rate review programs; and make significant changes to the individual market through a state innovation waiver.

In 2012 the USSC upheld the legality of PPACA but also ruled that the requirement that states extend Medicaid to all adults below 138% of the federal poverty level must be optional and not mandatory.[7] During Donald Trump's presidency, several initiatives were undertaken to increase state flexibility, including reducing the penalty for not complying with the individual mandate to $0 (Collins & Lambrew, 2019). As a result, state implementation has resulted in substantial differences among the states as to the effectiveness of PPACA in reducing the number of uninsured both nationally and among the states. Thirty-nine states and the District of Columbia have now passed Medicaid expansion. In a review of the impact of PPACA, a Commonwealth Study concluded that those states not using the federal marketplace rules had higher insurance premiums and lower increased health insurance access. While PPACA reduced the number of uninsured by 20 million and narrowed geographic variation somewhat, geographic variation in the uninsured remains significant (Collins & Lambrew, 2019). Where you live in the United States still has a significant impact on your rights to gain health insurance, what type of insurance you can obtain at an affordable price, and how long you are likely to live.

Federalism is critical in other areas of public health as well. For example, laws and regulations (e.g., occupational health and environmental health) may be dramatically different depending upon the state. By law, states can have their own occupational health structure or adopt federal Occupational Safety and Health Administration (OSHA) standards and inspections (Clean Air Act, 1963). With the local political power of some high injury industries, this can have major consequences for employee safety.

Recognizing that pollution does not respect state boundaries, there are federal laws regarding air and water pollution. The Clean Air Act was initially enacted in 1963 at the height of the effort to enact national laws to address national issues. It has been amended many times. Republican President Richard M. Nixon established the Environmental Protection Agency (EPA). By an executive order, he reorganized various federal agencies into a single independent agency to work in conjunction with the states to solve air pollution problems across the nation (Reorganization Plan No. 3, 1970). States generally have their own agencies that receive EPA funds to deal with local issues that may have interstate implications. Since California had previously been more active in air pollution regulation, federal legislation grandfathered California's right to retain its ability to set its own automobile pollution standards. This provision has major economic and environmental consequences. Due to California's market size, automobile manufacturers build cars using the California air pollution standards rather than building two

---

7 *National Federation of Independent Business v. Sebelius*, 648 F.3d 1235 (2012), upheld PPACA by a vote of 5-4 and ruled by a 7-2 vote that the expansion of Medicaid requirement was optional.

models of the same car. In any public health issue, it is important to determine how the jurisdictional power is divided between the federal, state and local governments.

Delegated Powers

Another major principle of the political structure is that of delegated powers. According to the U.S. Constitution, the federal level of government is only authorized to have specific powers as described in the document, no more and no less. The 10th Amendment of the Constitution gives residual powers to the states or to the people.[8] The application of this amendment has, however, changed over time.

One of the powers delegated exclusively to the federal government is the regulation of interstate commerce. One of the major reasons for abandoning the Articles of Confederation was that states began using their boundaries to restrict the flow of goods from other states. One of the powers the Founding Fathers felt should be exclusive to the federal government was the regulation of interstate commerce (Hamilton et al., 1961). Consequently, one of the powers of the new government was to prevent states from instituting duties or tariffs that restricted commerce and to allow the federal government to build canals, roads, railroads, and so forth that would facilitate the transportation of goods across state lines.

With the passage of time and the growth of a national economy via an extensive interstate transportation system (rails and highways), almost all businesses need some goods or services that cross state lines. Therefore, today there is little business activity that has not been interpreted as impacting interstate commerce and in the past the courts have generally taken a broad interpretation of interstate commerce (*Wickard v. Filburn*, 1942). Using its exclusive ability to regulate interstate commerce, the influence of the federal government has increased substantially due to the interpretation of the Interstate Commerce Clause in the U.S. Constitution. For example, pharmaceuticals flow across state lines and, therefore, the safety of those drugs is regulated by the Food and Drug Administration (FDA) and not by state governments. However, despite that opioid drugs are approved by the FDA, and flow freely between states, the opioid epidemic remains a state problem. One of the reasons for this is that physicians, who are the prescribers of opiates, are licensed by the states. Similarly, if the opiates are being illegally manufactured, it remains a state policy enforcement issue, unless those illegal drugs are crossing state lines, which would then constitute a federal drug trafficking offense. While states through their own taxing powers and other regulations remain an important influence on the economic climate of each state, the federal government has become the major economic regulator.

At the state level, the principle of delegated powers takes on added significance. The original states came together as sovereign entities to establish a federal system of government. If states are sovereign, what powers do local governments have? The answer comes from a judicial decision by Judge Forest Dillon, Chief Justice of the Iowa Supreme Court in the mid-1880s that was widely adopted by other state supreme courts (Public Health Law Center, 2020). Known as Dillon's Rule, it declares that unless a local government has been specifically delegated a

8 "The powers not delegated to the United States by the Constitution, nor prohibited by it to the States, are reserved to the States respectively, or to the people" (U.S. Const. amend. X).

power by its state constitution, statutes, or regulations, the local government lacks the ability to pass local ordinances on that issue. Counties and municipalities are creatures of the state and have only those powers expressly delegated to them. In addition, localities can be specifically prevented by the state from acting in any particular policy area. In a conflict between municipal and state law, the municipal ordinances generally fail, unless some other state or federal right or law takes precedence.

One example where Dillion's Rule became a problem for public health was when some municipalities started to pass ordinances restricting smoking in public facilities, such as bars and restaurants. Those who opposed antismoking laws quickly went to state legislatures to prevent such local ordinances from being passed. This dilemma also arose with COVID-19 and mask mandates and other restrictions. Some states have given municipalities more leeway by enacting home rule. In home rule states, the state grants municipalities and/or counties the ability to pass laws to govern themselves as they see fit if those regulations or ordinances do not conflict with other state or federal laws. Those working in local public health agencies county or municipal governments need to be aware of what they are legally able to do, as well as the legacy of historical policies. An example of the latter is the legacy of redlining that resulted in long-term inequality at the local level. See **Breakout Boxes 2.2** and **2.3**.

Breakout Box 2.2

EXAMPLE OF LOCAL SUGAR ORDINANCES

Consumption of sugar-sweetened beverages (SSBs) has been associated with obesity, diabetes, and cardiovascular disease. Although SSB consumption has declined in recent years, children and adults in the United States still consume twice as many calories from SSBs compared to the amounts consumed 30 years ago.

Since 2015, SSB taxes have been implemented in eight local (municipal/county) jurisdictions in the United States (Albany, Berkeley, Oakland, and San Francisco, California; Boulder, Colorado; Cook County, Illinois; Philadelphia, Pennsylvania; and Seattle, Washington). One policy was eventually repealed (Cook County). Powell et al. (2021) reviewed the impact of these policies and found that, on average, following the implementation of local U.S. SSB taxes the demand for SSBs fell by approximately 20%. However, there was substantial heterogeneity across cities.

For example, in 2014, Berkeley, California, became the first U.S. municipality to pass an SSB excise tax for public health purposes. The city of Berkeley levied the $.01-per-ounce tax on distribution of SSBs, including soda; energy, sports, and fruit-flavored drinks; sweetened water, coffee, and tea; and syrups used to make SSBs (diet soda was not taxed). Falbe et al. (2016) compared changes in SSB consumption in low-income neighborhoods in Berkeley before and after implementation of the tax, versus trends observed in Oakland and San Francisco. The authors found that consumption of SSBs decreased 21% in Berkeley and increased 4% in the comparison cities ($P = .046$). Water consumption also increased more in Berkeley (+63%) than in comparison cities (+19%; $P < .01$). The authors concluded that Berkeley's excise tax helped to reduce SSB consumption in low-income neighborhoods.

In 2016, a team of researchers from Harvard University conducted a microsimulation analysis using data from 15 U.S. cities that had implemented excise taxes of $.01/ounce of SSBs. SSBs included all beverages with added caloric sweeteners (juice, milk products, and artificially sweetened beverages were not included; Gortmaker et al., 2016). The authors found that, on average, each 8.5-oz serving of SSBs/day increases the risk of diabetes by 18%. They estimated that the $.01/ounce SSB excise tax would lead to an average 6% reduction in diabetes incidence (preventing 325 cases of diabetes) over a 1-year period. They projected that municipal SSB excise taxes in the 15 cities would prevent 115,000 cases of childhood and adult obesity in 2025, increase healthy life years, and save more in future healthcare costs than the intervention costs to implement. Revenue from the tax could also be used to support education and health promotion efforts. The authors concluded that implementing SSB taxes could serve as a powerful social signal to help reduce sugar consumption in the United States.

Complementing the research on SSB policies in the United States, Andreyeva et al. (2022) conducted an international systematic review and meta-analysis of outcomes following implementation of SSB taxes in more than 45 countries. The authors found that SSB taxes were associated with higher prices of targeted beverages and 15% lower SSB sales. Importantly, no negative changes in employment were observed.

References

Andreyeva, T., Marple, K., Marinello, S., Moore, T. E., & Powell, L. M. (2022). Outcomes following taxation of sugar-sweetened beverages: A systematic review and meta-analysis. *JAMA Network Open, 5*(6), Article e2215276. https://doi.org/10.1001/jamanetworkopen.2022.15276

Falbe, J., Thompson, H. R., Becker, C. M., Rojas, N., McCulloch, C. E., & Madsen, K. A. (2016). Impact of the Berkeley excise tax on sugar-sweetened beverage consumption. *American Journal of Public Health, 106*(10), 1865–1871. https://doi.org/10.2105/ajph.2016.303362

Gortmaker, S. L., Long, M. W., Ward, Z. J., Giles, C. M., Barrett, J. L., Resch, S. C., Tao, H., & Cradock, A. L. (2016, December 12). *Cost-effectiveness of a sugar-sweetened beverage excise tax in 15 U.S. cities*. CHOICES Project. https://choicesproject.org/publications/brief-cost-effectiveness-sugar-sweetened-beverage-tax-15-cities

Powell, L. M., Marinello, S., Leider, J., & Andreyeva, T. (2021, August). A review and meta-analysis of the impact of local U.S. sugar-sweetened beverage taxes on demand. Policy, Practice, and Prevention Research Center. https://p3rc.uic.edu/wp-content/uploads/sites/561/2021/09/Rvw-Meta-Anal-Impct-Lcl-US-SSB-Taxes-Demand_Rsrch-Brf-No.-121_Aug-2021.pdf

Breakout Box 2.3

REDLINING

Redlining was a discriminatory practice in which financial and other services were withheld from potential clients who resided in neighborhoods classified as hazardous to investors; these neighborhoods often had high numbers of racial and ethnic minorities and lower-income residents. Redlining practices took hold in the 1920s to 1930s, with origins in sales and lending practices of the National Association of Real Estate Boards (Gabriel & Rosenthal, 1991).

The federal government became involved in redlining practices in 1934 with the National Housing Act and the establishment of the Federal Housing Administration (FHA). The FHA continued the redlining process as part of an initiative to develop the first underwriting criteria for home mortgages. The implementation of this federal policy accelerated racial segregation and disinvestment of minority inner-city neighborhoods through the withholding of mortgage capital.

In 1968, the Fair Housing Act was passed to fight the practice of redlining. The Fair Housing Act makes it unlawful to discriminate in the terms, conditions, or privileges of sale of a dwelling because of race or national origin.

However, echoes of redlining remain. Denial of healthcare and the development of food deserts in low-income, minority neighborhoods are contemporary examples that have also been attributed to the legacies of redlining. Examples of redlining maps can be found online (see www.npr.org/sections/thetwo-way/2016/10/19/498536077/interactive-redlining-map-zooms-in-on-americas-history-of-discrimination).

Reference

Gabriel, S. A., & Rosenthal, S. S. (1991). Credit rationing, race, and the mortgage market. *Journal of Urban Economics, 29*(3), 371–379. https://doi.org/10.1016/0094-1190(91)90007-t

Implied Powers

Another important concept that needs to be addressed is that of implied powers. Article 1, Section 8, Clause 18 of the U.S. Constitution is the "necessary and proper clause" or the "elastic clause."[9] Implied powers are those that reasonably flow from those powers that are expressly given. For example, if the government has the express power tax, it has the implied power to establish an agency to do so

---

9 "To make all Laws which shall be necessary and proper for carrying into Execution the foregoing Powers, and all other Powers vested by this Constitution in the Government of the United States, or in any Department or Officer thereof" (U.S. Const. art. I, § 8, clause 18).

(Internal Revenue Service and Custom Houses) and it also has the implied power to punish those who avoid paying their assessed tax. If the government has the express power to protect health and welfare of the population as well as tax people, it has the implied power to provide medical care (Medicare, Medicaid, National Health Insurance). If the federal government has the sole power to regulate interstate commerce, it can regulate the sale of cigarettes, guns, pharmaceuticals, and so forth that cross state lines. At the state level and given Dillion's Rule, the concept of implied powers is restricted for county and municipal governments.

SUMMARY

In this chapter we have introduced the importance of conflicting values for society and the need for a social construct such as the political system to resolve these conflicts. Its decisions regarding the authoritative allocation of values do not imply that these decisions are right, rational, or moral, only that the enforcement arms of the government will be used to enforce them. We also focused on the importance of these value conflicts to be moderated and the need for civic toleration of differences if the government is to remain. The economic system is a social construct created by the political system. One of the foundations for public health activities rests with the need to deal with the capitalistic market failures such as the tragedy of the commons for the protection of population health.

We examined the historical political experience prior of the enactment of the existing Constitution and then explored several key general principles of the U.S. political system, such as the separation of powers, federalism, the delegation of powers, and implied powers at the federal, state, and local levels. In the next chapter we will take a detailed look at the U.S. political structure as outlined by the U.S. Constitution.

DISCUSSION QUESTIONS

- Market failure is one justification for public health. How does one determine when market failure occurs?

- Given a specific public health policy issue of choice, how does the existence of federalism in the United States impact the substance of that policy?

- For vaccination policies, justify federal legislation, state sovereignty, or home rule as the best approach.

- Separation of powers is a key component of the American political system. What do you believe are the strengths and weakness of such a political structure?

- How did the political structure of the United States impact PPACA?

KEY TERMS

Articles of Confederation
authoritative allocation of values
block grants
constitutional law
delegated powers
Dillon's Rule
externalities
federalism
federalization of the Bill of Rights
freedom
implied powers
Interstate Commerce Clause

law
Medicaid
Medicare
natural rights
Patient Protection and Affordable Care Act (PPACA)
policy
redlining
separation of powers
states' rights
tragedy of the commons

A robust set of instructor resources designed to supplement this text is located at http://connect.springerpub.com/content/book/978-0-8261-8543-3. Qualifying instructors may request access by emailing textbook@springerpub.com.

REFERENCES

Carroll, S. R., Suina, M., Jäger, M. B., Black, J., Cornell, S., Gonzales, A. A., Jorgensen, M., Palmanteer-Holder, N. L., De La Rosa, J. S., & Teufel-Shone, N. I. (2022). Reclaiming Indigenous health in the US: Moving beyond the social determinants of health. *International Journal of Environmental Research and Public Health, 19*(12), Article 7495. https://doi.org/10.3390/ijerph19127495

Clean Air Act, 42 U.S.C. 85 (1963). https://www.govinfo.gov/app/details/USCODE-2010-title42/USCODE-2010-title42-chap85

Collins, S., & Lambrew, J. M. (2019, July 29). *Federalism: The Affordable Care Act, and health reform in the 2020 election.* Commonwealth Fund. https://www.commonwealthfund.org/publications/fund-reports/2019/jul/federalism-affordable-care-act-health-reform-2020-election

DeNavas-Walt, C., Proctor, B. D., & Smith, J. C. (2010, September). *Income, poverty, and health insurance coverage in the United States: 2009.* U.S. Census Bureau, U.S. Government Printing Office. https://www.census.gov/library/publications/2010/demo/p60-238.html

Dobbs v. Jackson Women's Health Organization, 597 U.S. ___ (2022). https://www.supremecourt.gov/opinions/21pdf/19-1392_6j37.pdf

Easton, D. (1953). *The political system: An inquiry into the state of political science.* Alfred A. Knopf.

Eulau, H., & Prewitt, D. (1973). *Labyrinths of democracy: Adaptations, linkages, representation, and policies in urban politics (the Urban Governors series).* Bobbs-Merrill.

Frischmann, B. M., Marciano, A., & Ramello, G. B. (2019). Retrospective: Tragedy of the commons after 50 years. *Journal of Economic Perspectives, 33*(4), 211–228. https://doi.org/10.2139/ssrn.3451688

Fromm, E. (1941). *Escape from freedom.* Farrar & Rinehart.

Gutmann, A., & Thompson, D. (1996). *Democracy and disagreement.* Harvard University Press.

Hamilton, A., Madison, J., & Jay, J. (1961). *The federalist papers* (C. Rossiter, Ed.). The New American Library of World Literature.

Hardin, G. (1968). The tragedy of the commons. *Science, 162*(3859), 1243–1248. https://doi.org/10.1126/science.162.3859.1243

Health Care and Education Reconciliation Act, Pub. L. No. 111-152, 124 Stat. 1029 (2010). https://www.govinfo.gov/content/pkg/PLAW-111publ152/pdf/PLAW-111publ152.pdf

Isaacson, W. (2003). *Benjamin Franklin: An American life.* Simon & Schuster.

Jacobson v. Massachusetts, 197 U.S. 11 (1905). https://supreme.justia.com/cases/federal/us/197/11

Jefferson, T. (1776). *U.S. Declaration of Independence.* National Archives. https://www.archives.gov/founding-docs/declaration-transcript

Levitsky, S., & Ziblatt, D. (2018). *How democracies die.* Broadway Books.

Mann, C. C. (2005). *1491: New revelations of the Americas before Columbus.* Alfred A. Knopf.

McGirt v. Oklahoma, 591 U. S. ___ (2020). https://www.supremecourt.gov/opinions/19pdf/18-9526_9okb.pdf

Morone, J. (2005). *Policy challenges in modern health care.* Rutgers University Press.

Oklahoma v. Castro-Huerta, 597 U.S. ___ (2022). https://www.supremecourt.gov/opinions/21pdf/21-429_8o6a.pdf

O'Rourke, P. J. (2007). *On the wealth of nations: Books that changed the world.* Atlantic Monthly Press.

Ostrom, E. (1990). *Governing the commons: The evolution of institutions for collective action (political economy of institutions and decisions).* Cambridge University Press.

Patient Protection and Affordable Care Act, Publ. L. No. 111-148, 124 Stat. 119 (2010). https://www.congress.gov/111/plaws/publ148/PLAW-111publ148.pdf

Prescod-Weinstein, C. (2020). Making Black women scientists under white empiricism: The racialization of epistemology in physics. *Signs: Journal of Women in Culture and Society, 45*(2), 421–447. https://doi.org/10.1086/704991

Public Health Law Center. (2020, November). *Dillon's Rule, home rule, and preemption.* https://www.publichealthlawcenter.org/resources/dillons-rule-home-rule-preemption-2020

Redvers, N., Celidwen, Y., Schultz, C., Horn, O., Githaiga, C., Vera, M., Perdrisat, M., Mad Plume, L., Kobei, D., Kain, M. C., Poelina, A., Rojas, J. N., & Blondin, B. (2022). The determinants of planetary health: An Indigenous consensus perspective. *The Lancet Planetary Health, 6*(2), e156–e163. https://doi.org/10.1016/s2542-5196(21)00354-5

Reorganization Plan No. 3, Pub. L. No. 98–80, 84 Stat. 2086 (1970). https://uscode.house.gov/view.xhtml?req=granuleid:USC-prelim-title5a-node84-leaf178&num=0&edition=prelim

Social Security Amendments. (1965). Pub. L. No. 89–97, 79 Stat. 286 (1965). https://www.archives.gov/milestone-documents/medicare-and-medicaid-act

Tuck, R. (Ed.). (1991). *Leviathan.* Cambridge University Press.

U.S. Constitution, amend. XIV, § I.

U.S. Constitution, amend. X.

U.S. Constitution, art. I, § 8, clause 18.

U.S. Constitution, art. VI, § 2.

Wickard v. Filburn, 317 U.S. 111 (1942). https://supreme.justia.com/cases/federal/us/317/111

CHAPTER 3

THE U.S. POLITICAL STRUCTURE

This chapter uses the Constitution of the United States to describe the skeletal outline of the structure of the federal government. We discuss the various powers of the three branches of the federal government and their role in policy making. We also describe some of the main similarities and differences between the federal governmental structure and the structures of the various states. However, it is important to remember that there is much more to the political system than the structure of the government. The next chapter focuses on the process used to make the structure perform their functions.

LEARNING OBJECTIVES

Be able to:

- Analyze the policy implications of having two different chambers performing the legislative function.
- Discuss the implications of the composition of the Senate for the passage of the Patient Protection and Affordable Care Act (PPACA).
- Discuss the importance of *Baker v. Carr* (1962) for state legislative districts and how that shapes policy today.
- Analyze the significance of the structural differences between the federal court system and state courts for policy.
- Explain the significance of the initiative and referendum provisions within various state constitutions.
- Discuss the relationship between the Bill of Rights and democracy.
- Analyze the policy significance of the 14th Amendment to the U.S. Constitution.
- Describe the power of the federal judiciary to make policy.

THE PREAMBLE

The Preamble to the Constitution sets out the basic purpose and philosophical principles for instituting a new government. It is both familiar and brief:

We the People of the United States, in Order to form a more perfect Union, establish Justice, insure domestic Tranquility, provide for the common defense, promote the general Welfare, and secure the Blessings of Liberty to ourselves and our Posterity, do ordain and establish this Constitution for the United States of America. (U.S. Const. pmbl.)

Although not referring to any powers or structures, U.S. courts frequently cite the Preamble to demonstrate the general purpose of what the Founding Fathers were attempting to achieve.

THE LEGISLATIVE BRANCH

Article I is the first and longest section of the Constitution. Article I describes the bicameral legislative branch with its general powers and responsibilities. While today both the House of Representatives and the Senate are elected, only the House was initially elected by a portion of the people. The House of Representatives consists of 435 members proportioned by each state's population with 2-year terms. With the expansion of who can vote, it remains directly elected by the people. The Senate, with longer terms (6-year terms with staggered elections), was intended to be a calming force compared to a potentially volatile House. Members of the Senate were initially appointed by each state's legislature and were generally viewed as people of note with previous political experience.[1] A number of the Founding Fathers were afraid that the populace would be an angry mob (Dahl, 2001). The number of each state's House members reflects the size of its population, but unlike under the Articles of Confederation, each member has their own vote. The Senate has two senators from each state with each having their own vote. The two different houses were seen as balance between a democracy (majority/plurality rule) and state sovereignty.

One of the consequences of the provision that each state has two senators is that a minority of the U.S. population can control a majority of the seats in the Senate. This provision favors smaller population states and disadvantages more populous states. The 26 states with the lowest populations control 52% of the Senate seats. Given the 2020 census, those 26 states contain less than 18% of the population in the United States but they can control the U.S. Senate. Since legislation must pass both chambers to become law, this provides smaller states a major advantage in the legislative process. In contrast, it takes only two states, California and Texas, to exceed the population of these 26 states (68,760,047 compared to 58,200,744). The nine most populous states account for 51.1% of the U.S. population but only have 18% of the votes of in the U.S. Senate (see Tables 3.1a and 3.1b). Alexander Hamilton warned about this in the *Federalist Papers* (Hamilton et al., 1961). Political scientist, Robert Dahl has asked the question, what additional rights do people in smaller population states have that are more significant than national majority? Indeed, is the federal government built for the states or for the people? What rights are protected by the overrepresentation of smaller population states, since fundamental protections are guaranteed to all by the 14th Amendment to the Constitution (Dahl, 2001)?

---

1 Although some states experimented with some form of popular input to the selection of U.S. senators, the 17th Amendment adopted in 1913 guaranteed that all states would hold popular elections for U.S. senators.

TABLE 3.1a STATE VERSUS POPULAR SOVEREIGNTY: 26 LEAST POPULOUS U.S. STATES

STATE	2020 POPULATION	SENATORS
Wyoming	577,719	2
Vermont	643,503	2
Alaska	736,081	2
North Dakota	779,702	2
South Dakota	887,770	2
Delaware	990,837	2
Montana	1,085,407	2
Rhode Island	1,098,163	2
Maine	1,363,582	2
New Hampshire	1,379,089	2
Hawaii	1,460,137	2
West Virginia	1,795,045	2
Idaho	1,841,377	2
Nebraska	1,963,333	2
New Mexico	2,120,220	2
Kansas	2,940,865	2
Mississippi	2,963,914	2
Arkansas	3,013,756	2
Nevada	3,108,462	2
Iowa	3,192,406	2
Utah	3,275,252	2
Connecticut	3,608,298	2
Oklahoma	3,963,516	2
Oregon	4,241,500	2
Kentucky	4,509,342	2
Louisiana	4,661,468	2
Total	**58,200,744 or 17.6% of the U.S. population**	**52 senators or 52% of the U.S. Senate**

Source: U.S. Department of Commerce & U.S. Census Bureau. (2021, April 26). 2020 Census apportionment results: Table 1. Apportionment population and number of representatives by state: 2020 Census. U.S. Department of Commerce & U.S. Census Bureau. https://www.census.gov/data/tables/2020/dec/2020-apportionment-data.html

TABLE 3.1b STATE VERSUS POPULAR SOVEREIGNTY: NINE MOST POPULOUS U.S. STATES

STATE	2020 POPULATION	SENATORS
California	39,576,757	2
Texas	29,183,290	2
Florida	21,570,527	2
New York	20,215,751	2
Pennsylvania	13,011,844	2
Illinois	12,822,739	2
Ohio	11,808,848	2
Georgia	10,725,274	2
North Carolina	10,453,948	2
Total	**169,368,978 or 51.1% of the U.S. population.**	**18 senators or 18% of the number of senators**

Source: U.S. Department of Commerce & U.S. Census Bureau. (2021, April 26). 2020 Census apportionment results: Table 1. Apportionment population and number of representatives by state: 2020 Census. U.S. Department of Commerce & U.S. Census Bureau. https://www.census.gov/data/tables/2020/dec/2020-apportionment-data.html

Article I Section 7 mandates that proposed legislation must pass both houses of Congress and be presented to the president for signature of approval. If the president does not approve, the proposed legislation is returned to Congress, which can then override the president's veto by a two-thirds vote in each chamber.

Article I Section 8 enumerates the 18 delegated powers of Congress (the ability to lay and collect taxes, coin money, declare war, establish courts below that of the Supreme Court, regulate interstate commerce, establish a navy, etc.). Article I Section 9 lists eight things that Congress cannot do: pass *ex post facto* laws; suspend the common law *writ of habeas corpus* unless in a state of rebellion or invasion for public safety; grant a title of nobility; and so forth.

One of the striking things about the Constitution's description of Congress is what is not mentioned. Other than age qualifications and a few powers delegated to one branch versus the other (spending bills must originate in the House and the Senate has the power of advice and consent of various executive appointments and treaties), there is little description as to how Congress is to function. There is no mention of political parties, legislative committees, seniority, legislative staff, party caucuses, the filibuster, investigative commissions, and so forth. All these policies are governed by the rules adopted by each of the two branches and are largely continued by tradition from one Congress to the next.

While not mentioned in the Constitution, these structures and procedures have a major impact on what policy can be passed in each house. For example, the role of the filibuster in the Senate has been debated for decades. The number of votes required to break a filibuster has changed over time and some pieces of legislation have been excluded from the filibuster (e.g., Omnibus Budget Reconciliation Act [OBRA]). However, the filibuster still presents a major barrier for proposed legislation.

State Legislatures

Even though the 50 U.S. states tend to generally reflect the basic structure of the federal government, some state constitutions predate the federal Constitution of 1787. New Hampshire's Provincial Congress adopted the first state constitution on January 5, 1776. Other states' constitutions, such as Hawaii's, did not go into effect until August 21, 1959, although it was written 20 years earlier. As a result, the environments in which state constitutions were enacted vary tremendously and those historical circumstances impact the provisions within their constitutions. The differences between state constitutions can differ in significant ways.

All states, except one, have a bicameral legislative branch. Nebraska is the only state that has only one legislative chamber. Historically, in creating their bicameral branches, some states might have given equal representation to counties in one branch (much as the Senate does for states at the federal level). This tended to favor rural areas within states and discriminate against urban areas. This became a major problem in the 1960s when urban areas were rapidly expanding/modernizing and needed additional state assistance but were blocked by rural dominated state legislatures.

Baker v. Carr (1962) was a U.S. Supreme Court (USSC) case originating from Tennessee that addressed different population sized electoral districts. The legislative districts for that state had not been adjusted for 60 years despite large population changes.[2] Consequently, a rural vote was worth more than an urban vote since it required far fewer voters to be elected in less populated districts. In *Baker v. Carr*, the USSC ruled that legislative redistricting based upon population was a justiciable question and that the 14th Amendment guaranteeing equal protection of the law could be applied. Two subsequent Supreme Court rulings decided in the same year established the principle of "one person, one vote." Beginning in 1964, all states were mandated to make legislative districts of roughly equal size to assure that each individual vote counted relatively the same. Now all state legislative districts and state districts for the U.S. House of Representatives must be of roughly equal population size based upon on the decennial U.S. Census.

While "one person, one vote" has become "settled law," states remain free to gerrymander legislative districts to favor one political party over the other. The USSC has determined that while gerrymandering may be antithetical to democratic principles, it is a "political question" and not a "justiciable question" and therefore cannot be addressed through the federal courts.[3] The legislative branch under control of a particular party can create districts of equal population size but design them to favor their own party's potential political success. For example, the dominant party may take an urban area controlled by the opposite party and divide it into several pieces and then join those pieces with outlying areas dominated by their political base. While not guaranteeing electoral success, such gerrymandered districts increase their chance of electing more candidates and therefore

---

2 *Baker v. Carr* (1962) was a landmark ruling by the Supreme Court that legislative redistricting was a judiciable and not a political issue and it began addressing the issue of legislative redistricting. After *Baker*, *Westbury v. Sanders* (1964) ruled that the districts established by the states for the U.S. House of Representatives had to be of roughly of equal population size. *Reynolds v. Sims* (1964) ruled that state legislative districts had to be of roughly equal population size.

3 *Rucho v. Common Cause* (2019) was a 5-4 decision that partisan gerrymandering was a nonjusticiable "political question." Chief Justice Roberts wrote the majority opinion. Justice Kagan wrote the dissent joined by Justices Ginsburg, Breyer, and Sotomayor.

keeping control of the state legislature. Although geographically contiguous, a district may stretch hundreds of miles. As a result, some electoral districts can have strange geographic configurations. Since redistricting occurs after the decennial U.S. census, gerrymandering gives the dominant political party an electoral advantage for the next 10 years. Both parties tend to do this when they can.

Another political consequence of gerrymandering is that electoral outcomes can be determined by the primary election in those states that have a dominant political party. Since primary elections tend to have lower voter participation, if there are multiple candidates, a small plurality of party voters can not only determine the winner of the primary election but be assured of winning the general election as well. This tends to favor small heavily organized factions within a state's dominant political party. As a result, some states have initiated a rule that if a primary victor does not have a majority of the primary voters, there is a runoff primary involving the top two candidates.

To minimize gerrymandering, some states have adopted the use of nonpartisan commissions and computer programs to design more impartial redistricting plans. Since redistricting occurs only every 10 years after the U.S. Census, redistricting has long-term implications for party control and policy development. That was why the perceived politicization of conducting the 2020 census became a major issue in 2019. After the U.S. Census was completed, state battles continued over proposed new legislative districts. As we will discuss later, the USSC will address gerrymandering and state legislative authority over elections in its 2022 term.

Another major difference between state constitutions and the federal structure is that some states wrote their constitutions during a national period of increased democratization. As a result, some states have constitutional provisions providing for direct popular action that is not available at the federal level. For example, nonelectoral removal from public office at the federal level is solely the prerogative of Congress through its power of impeachment. However, 19 states plus the District of Columbia have state constitutional provisions allowing recall elections. Sometimes recall provisions apply to all state elected officials or sometimes only to specific offices, most commonly the governor. A relatively high number of certified registered voters is typically needed to petition for a recall election so that recalls are used for extraordinary events and not used to merely have an election "re-do." Certification of voter signatures can be a very important function of the Secretary of State's office. What happens after the official is removed from office varies greatly from state to state. If there is a lieutenant governor, that person generally becomes the governor. If you are working at the state level, you need to determine what, if any, specific recall provisions operate within your state.[4]

Another major difference in state political systems is that some states allow for referendums to enact policies. While referendums are typically required for state constitutional amendments, they may also be used to adopt ordinary laws as well. Twenty-three states have provisions for referendums. A referendum allows a popular vote for approval or disapproval of a piece of legislation. Again, there will be specific state requirements (e.g., a certain percentage of registered voters) to have a referendum appear on the ballot. Sometimes the legislature will voluntarily place a controversial piece of legislation on a referendum.

---

4 See information from the National Conference of State Legislatures for the states having recall, referendum, or initiative provisions.

An initiative (or ballot initiative) is an actual piece of legislation that is authored and put forth by a certified number of voters and then voted upon by the population. States in the West and Midwest are more likely to have an initiative process, although Massachusetts and Maine do as well. Initiatives can be either direct or indirect. Direct initiatives go to a popular vote, thus totally bypassing the legislature and executive branches. Indirect initiative proposals are submitted to the legislature, which then can act on that proposed legislation. If the legislature rejects it, submits a different proposal, or takes no action, the initiative then goes on the ballot for a public vote. The specific wording of both referendums and initiative provisions are critical so that the population clearly understands both the intent and the specifics of the proposal.

In Maine, bipartisan legislation had passed the Maine legislature to take advantage of the passage of the Patient Protection and Affordable Care Act's (PPACA's) provision for the expansion of the state's Medicaid program, but those bills were repeatedly vetoed by the Republican Governor Paul LePage. In response, healthcare advocates collected more than 67,000 signatures to place the issue on the ballot. The Maine Secretary of State had to authenticate at least 61,123 signatures for it to appear on the ballot (Maine's People Alliance, 2017). The referendum appeared on the November 2017 ballot as Question 2 and passed by approximately 60% of the voters. This allowed approximately 80,000 Mainers to qualify for Medicaid. Maine became the 32nd state to approve Medicaid expansion under PPACA, but the first to do so by means of a referendum.

A thoughtful policy analyst should be aware of each state's provisions for recall, referendums, and initiatives. These forms of direct democracy provide the means for the popular majority to bypass a resistant legislature. However, these proposals can often have confusing language or provisions that need to be carefully explained for the populace to understand both the intended and unintended consequences of adopting the proposal. Sometimes the printed ballot contains brief, unbiased statements both for and against the proposal. Referendums and initiatives on controversial issues generally result in expensive public relations campaigns. The ability to raise money to support the public advocacy portion of the process can be a major obstacle. However, these processes provide alternative means of policy adoption.

THE EXECUTIVE BRANCH
The President

The authors of the Constitution were politically torn over Article II of the Constitution. Having just fought a war against a king, they were skeptical about a powerful executive. However, having experienced the Articles of Confederation without an executive, they knew that they needed one, but the executive had to be held in check.

Article II is relatively brief. The longest section of Article II is devoted to the electoral process. The president has always been indirectly elected by the people. The Electoral College elects the president of the United States. Each state has the number of electors equal to the number of their House and Senate members. Since all states have the same number of senators, this distribution of electoral votes advantages smaller states. Initially, the person with the highest number of Electoral College votes became president and the one with the second number of votes became the vice president. As a result, people of opposing political ideologies could fill the top two executive positions. This was changed in 1804 with the adoption of the 12th Amendment.

Voters in each state vote for a slate of electors pledged to support a specific presidential candidate in the Electoral College vote. In all but two states (Maine and Nebraska), the candidate winning the plurality of votes in the presidential election wins all that state's Electoral College votes (winner-take-all). Maine and Nebraska have procedures to proportionately distribute their Electoral College votes. In most states, a presidential candidate can win all of that state's electoral votes by winning by a single vote or by several million. States in which a dominant political party continually wins the presidential election will receive less candidate attention than key battleground states where the presidential election could be decided by a small number of popular votes but win the entire number of the state's electors. Due to the difference between a popular vote and the Electoral College vote, a person can be elected president with a majority of the Electoral College vote but not win a majority of the national popular vote. Presidents Adams (1824), Hayes (1876), Harrison (1888), Bush (2000), and Trump (2016) all lost the national popular vote but were elected president by their Electoral College votes.

Initially, there was no limit on presidential terms. The decision by George Washington not to seek a third term set a precedent for those who followed. President Franklin Delano Roosevelt's four terms during the Depression and World War II broke that precedent. Although seen as a special situation due to World War II, the 22nd Amendment was adopted in 1951, limiting the president to two successive 4-year terms. A president can serve multiple terms, just not more than two successive terms.

Section 2 is relatively brief and describes the president's role as commander in chief and the ability to make appointments with the "advice and consent" of the Senate and the sole ability to grant pardons. The role of the president as commander in chief and the ability of Congress to declare war have come into conflict. Senatorial approval or rejection of presidential appointments raises frequent controversies. The president's sole ability to grant pardons is also frequently debated. Section 3 says the president shall from time to time provide Congress with the "State of the Union," and has certain powers when Congress is not in session. The tradition of the State of the Union Address is typically used to present the administration's policy agenda.

One important portion of Section 3 states that the president "shall take Care that the Laws be faithfully executed." This is a power that is very expansive and gives the president great discretion as to how laws passed by Congress will be implemented.

Section 4 is a one sentence description of the process for impeachment. This process has been used for Presidents Andrew Johnson, Bill Clinton, and twice for Donald Trump. No president has been removed from office using this process.

The Federal Bureaucracy

As noted above, the president is the executive. How the president faithfully executes the laws of the land is not defined in the Constitution.

The Office of the President

The Executive Office of the President (EOP) was created in 1939 by President Franklin D. Roosevelt. See **Breakout Box 3.1**. There are approximately 1,800 people working in the EOP. Most of these positions do not require Senate approval, except

Breakout Box 3.1

EXECUTIVE OFFICE OF THE PRESIDENT

The EOP can vary by president but consists of the following:

- Personnel within the West Wing of the White House
- Council of Economic Advisors
- Council on Environmental Quality
- Domestic Policy Council
- Gender Policy Council
- National Security Council
- National Economic Council
- Office of Intergovernmental Affairs
- Office of Management and Budget
- Office of National Drug Control Policy
- Office of Public Engagement
- Office of Science and Technology Policy
- Office of the U.S. Trade Representative

for the head of the Office of Management and Budget, the Chair of the Council of Economic Advisors, and the U.S. Trade Representative. The EOP is managed by the president's chief of staff. Most of these people are housed in the Eisenhower Executive Office Building near the White House. The Eisenhower Executive Office Building also contains the office of the vice president.

The Cabinet

Cabinet appointments are political appointments made by the president and confirmed by the U.S. Senate. By custom, the president's choice is normally, but not always, accepted by the Senate. A nominee may sometimes withdraw their appointment to avoid a contentious confirmation hearing or a negative vote. They serve at the pleasure of the president and can be dismissed at any time for any reason. Typically, these presidential appointees have a letter of resignation prepared and ready to be dated and signed when asked. See Breakout Box 3.2.

Breakout Box 3.2

THE CABINET

The cabinet generally consists of the secretaries of

- Agriculture
- Commerce
- Defense
- Education

- Energy
- Health and Human Services
- Homeland Security
- Housing and Urban Development
- Interior
- Labor
- State
- Transportation
- Treasury
- Veterans Affairs
- Attorney General

In addition, the cabinet frequently includes:

- The White House Chief of Staff
- The U.S. Ambassador to the United Nations
- The Director of National Intelligence
- The U.S. Trade Representative
- The Environmental Protection Agency
- The Office of Management and Budget
- The Council of Economic Advisers
- Office of Science and Technology Policy
- Small Business Administration

The Civil Service

There are approximately 2 million positions in the federal government and an additional 500,000 postal workers that are protected by the 1883 Pendleton Act. That act provides that federal civil servants, including public health professionals, are to be hired by merit and competitive examination and not according to political affiliation. In addition, the act forbids the firing or demotion of civil servants based on their political affiliation.[5] These are the people who do the day-to-day tasks keeping the federal departments and agencies operating. Because they serve from one administration to the next, they develop expertise and provide historical memory on the operation of the government. In addition to these civil servants, there are approximately 4,000 presidential appointments within the bureaucracy of whom about 1,200 require Senate approval.

Within the executive branch is the U.S. Department of Health and Human Services (DHHS), which includes the major offices of public health, such as the Surgeon General, the Centers for Disease Control and Prevention, Food and Drug Administration, National Health Information Center, National Institutes of Health, and so forth. However, public health officials exist in other agencies as well, such

---

5 The Pendleton Civil Service Reform Act was passed by the 47th Congress and signed by President Chester A. Arthur on January 16, 1883. Previously appointments were based on "the spoils system" (i.e., to the victor go the spoils).

as the Department of Agriculture, Department of Labor, Department of Defense, Department of Education, and so forth.

States have various mixes of civil servants with civil service protections and political appointments within the administrative branch. Typically, but not always, political appointments terminate with the election of a new governor. You need to explore your own state's provisions.

State Executives

A state's executive function is held by the governor. Only some states have a lieutenant governor, although all states have some formal process for a successor in case of death, incapacity, impeachment, or recall. Many of the early states had gubernatorial terms of 2 years, reflecting a distrust of executive power. In addition, some states have an elected executive or governor's council (from colonial times) that provides advice to the governor or has authority to approve or block specific gubernatorial actions. During the 1960s and 1970s there was a nonpartisan effort to strengthen the powers of state governors. Many states, but not all, changed gubernatorial tenure to 4 years and eliminated governor's councils. Statutory term limits became popular in the 1980s. Some states impose a two-term limit, others have no limit, or have a limit imposed by tradition but not law. Some states favor term limits to make it difficult to become a "professional politician." However, rather than running for re-election, many politicians merely run for a different office. Other states oppose the concept of term limits, contending that they remove people with important political knowledge and substantive policy expertise that comes with experience.

Local governments vary considerably regarding the powers of an executive. Historically, local government consisted of an annual town meeting, with no executive. As town populations grew and became more complex, different types of local executive positions have been created. Elected mayors with various levels of executive decision-making authority and city councils became common. Smaller communities began to use professional trained managers to perform executive functions while maintaining some type of legislative body (city councils) to make policy decisions. The elected local representatives generally are either elected at-large or in city districts or some combination of both. These differences can be critical in terms of the policy process. District elections can allow specific economic, racial, or ethnic groups with geographic concentration to win elections while they might not be able to win in city-wide elections. The dynamics of local government can sometimes be turbulent, and an understanding of the local structural elements is important.

THE JUDICIAL BRANCH
The Federal Court System

Article III of the U.S. Constitution deals with the federal judiciary. This article is relatively brief. Section 1 establishes the USSC and makes provision for Congress to create inferior federal courts. All judges were given lifetime appointments contingent upon good behavior. Lifetime judicial appointments were seen as enabling judges to make difficult but unpopular decisions without fear of retribution. The size of the USSC changed seven times between 1800 and 1869 for political reasons

(Levitsky & Ziblatt, 2018). Section 2 covers the original and appellate jurisdictions of the federal courts. Section 2 is interesting in that it specifically states that Congress can alter the jurisdiction of the Supreme Court.[6] Congress could hypothetically enact a law removing USSC jurisdiction for cases involving firearms or cases involving personal medical care (patient-physician privacy). Section 3 deals with cases of treason.

The actual structure of the court system was left to Congress. The Judiciary Act of 1789, officially titled An Act to Establish the Judicial Courts of the United States, was signed into law by President George Washington on September 24, 1789. It established the structure and jurisdiction of the federal court system and created the position of Attorney General of the United States. Although it has been amended several times, the basic outline of the federal court system established by the First Congress remains largely intact. Notice that the Constitution says nothing about the ability of the USSC to declare federal or state laws to be unconstitutional. However, Alexander Hamilton in the *Federalist Papers* indicated that any law contrary to the Constitution must be invalid, and it is the province of the judiciary to determine what is contrary to the Constitution (Hamilton et al., 1961). The source of the USSC's ability to declare a law unconstitutional was implemented by itself in its decision of *Marbury v. Madison* (1803). By refusing to issue a *writ of mandamus* for what it considered to be an unconstitutional action, the USSC was able to enforce its own decision rather than rely on the president or Congress for enforcement. The power of the USSC to declare laws unconstitutional was established by its own ruling and *stare decisis* maintains it as precedent.

The judiciary likes to think of itself as a nonpartisan body that does not make law. While it is true that the judiciary cannot pass laws, they can and do invalidate laws. In addition, it is important to remember that laws are only one source of policy. Policy certainly flows from judicial decisions. In addition, as noted previously, some judges at the state level are elected in partisan elections. Justices of the USSC have attempted to deflect the notion that the Court is a partisan body. However, increased partisan nature of the Senate's approval process and multiple Court decisions have raised the question as to whether the USSC is just another partisan branch of government. Chief Justice John Roberts has in the past tried to protect the institution of the USSC from being characterized as being political. However, during the 2021 to 2022 term, the USSC decisions on abortion, school prayer, the Second Amendment, separation of church and state, and COVID-19 in the workplace were perceived by some as being politically decided. How the USSC will deal with the appearance of partisanship will test the legitimacy of USSC decisions in the years to come.

Supreme Court decisions have major policy implications at the state and federal levels, especially those that break *stare decisis*. As previously cited, *Baker v. Carr* (1962) had major policy implications for state and national electoral districts. The *Citizens United v. Federal Election Commission* (2010) decision that the Federal Election Campaign Act, by restricting the amount of money that people could contribute to federal election campaigns, was a violation of the First Amendment has made substantial differences in election financing. See **Breakout Box 3.3**.

---

6 "In all the other Cases before mentioned, the Supreme Court shall have appellate Jurisdiction, both as to Law and Fact, with such Exceptions, and under such Regulations as the Congress shall make" (U.S. Const. art. III, § 2).

Breakout Box 3.3

CITIZENS UNITED V. FEDERAL ELECTION COMMISSION

In January 2008, Citizens United, a conservative nonprofit corporation, released the film *Hillary: The Movie*, a political documentary about Hillary Clinton. The release was close to the presidential primaries in which she was a candidate. Because of the political nature of the film and its advocating the defeat of a candidate within 30 days of a primary election, the Federal Election Commission ruled that it violated the Federal Elections Campaign Law. Citizens United sought a declaratory judgment and injunctive relief in the Washington, DC district court. Citizens United argued that the ban on corporate electioneering communications in the Federal Elections Campaign Act was unconstitutional and that the disclosure and disclaimer requirements of the law were also unconstitutional. The district court declared a summary judgment for the Federal Election Commission and denied Citizen United's petition.

Due to a provision in the Bipartisan Campaign Reform Act of 2001, any court appeal went directly to the USSC. The USSC took oral arguments on March 24, 2009, asked for additional briefs on June 29, and heard oral arguments again on September 9. It issued its opinion on January 21, 2010. The 5-4 majority opinion was written by Justice Kennedy with Justices Roberts, Alito, Scalia, and Thomas joining the majority. Justice Stevens wrote a dissenting opinion with Justices Ginsburg, Breyer, and Sotomayor joining. There are a couple of interesting sidebars to the case. Chief Justice Roberts was the original author of the majority decision, but he withdrew his opinion in favor of Justice Kennedy's. Also, the person arguing for the government was Solicitor General Elena Kagan, soon to become a USSC Justice.

The landmark decision overturned previous decisions of the USSC. The majority opinion concluded that corporate election spending was free speech and due to the First Amendment "strict scrutiny" required that the government had to prove that it had a compelling interest to restrict free speech and that any such restriction had to be narrowly drawn. For more than 100 years, the courts agreed that the government could restrain political spending to prevent corruption in politics. In *Buckley v. Valeo* (1976), the USSC had ruled that the limitation of campaign expenditures was not a violation of free speech and that the government's anticorruption rationale for restrictions were sufficient to justify limitations on political contributions. In 1990 the USSC had ruled in *Austin v. Michigan State Chamber of Commerce* that the state of Michigan could prohibit corporations from using their funds to make expenditures for state elections. In *Austin* the compelling government's interest was to prevent "the corrosive and distorting effects of immense aggregations of wealth that are accumulated with the help of the corporate form and that have little or no correlation to the public's support for the corporation's political ideas." The *Citizens United* majority decision reversed *Austin* and found that corporate spending did not present a substantive threat to corruption if the spending was not coordinated with a candidate or political party. It also ruled that those within the organization who did not support the corporate expenditure for political action had corporate governance remedies. Finally, it ruled that the reporting requirements were valid. The *Citizens United* decision applies to both corporations and unions.

Justice Stevens wrote the dissent in which he argued in favor of not overturing USSC precedents and that the government had a valid anticorruption interest in regulating campaign finance. Stevens also argued that the appearance of corruption as well as the appearance of undue influence were important considerations and not just quid pro quo corruption.

As a result of *Citizens United*, there was an explosion of Political Action Committees (PACs and Super PACs) that fund candidate campaigns as well as policy referendums, initiatives, and recalls. Super PACs can accept money but are not required to disclose who donates to the PAC. As a result of *Citizens United*, corporations and unions can donate money to multiple PACs without being identified, thus the appearance of what has been termed "dark money." In addition, it has been difficult to prove what constitutes coordination with a candidate or political party when those policy positions are clearly and publicly pronounced.

References

Austin v. Michigan State Chamber of Commerce, 494 U.S. 652 (1990). https://supreme.justia.com/cases/federal/us/494/652
Bipartisan Campaign Reform Act, Pub. L. No. 107-155, 116 Stat. 81 (2002). https://www.congress.gov/107/plaws/publ155/PLAW-107publ155.pdf
Buckley v. Valeo, 424 U.S. 1 (1976). https://supreme.justia.com/cases/federal/us/424/1
Citizens United v. Federal Election Commission, 558 U.S. 310 (2010). https://supreme.justia.com/cases/federal/us/558/310

The State Court Systems

From a policy perspective one must remember that there are two separate judicial systems in the United States, one federal and then 56 at the state/territorial level court systems. According to the principles of federalism, citizens are subject to both court systems. Having rights under one system does not mean that the same rights exist under the other. The legal principle that citizens cannot be subjected to double jeopardy comes from common law (i.e., one cannot be charged for the same crime after previously found innocent). However, while double jeopardy is prohibited within each judicial system, it is not prohibited between federal and state systems. A person found innocent of a crime in a state court system can be tried in the federal court system for the very same offense (albeit as a violation of a federal law) and vice versa.

The federal judicial structure was built to mirror the existing state systems at the time. There are different levels of courts, one with jurisdiction to hear initial cases and then a level of appellate courts, and then a supreme court for final appeal. While one is entitled to appeal the decision of the initial court, the right to appeal to the state supreme court is generally restricted. While there are a few types of cases in which a state supreme court may have original jurisdiction, each supreme court can generally select those cases it wishes to hear by issuing a *writ of certiorari* that orders a lower court to deliver its record of the case so that the higher court may review it.

One of the major differences between federal and state courts is the method of appointment. All federal judges are appointed by the president and serve for life unless they are impeached or voluntarily retire. Generally, the older states have retained judicial nomination by the executive with some form of approval process for lifetime appointments. Typically, these states have a built-in screening process conducted by the state's bar association to evaluate the qualifications of people being nominated. Those reviews tend to merely grade a person on their judicial qualifications rather than result in approval or disapproval of nominees.

However, most states have adopted some form of popular judicial election. This raises the philosophical question as to what degree judges should be "independent" as opposed to being representative of the majority. Since the popular majority may be ill disposed to minority rights or unpopular views, state decisions regarding judicial selection procedures have significant policy implications. Some states include the election of most judges; some include only their supreme court judges. Some states have instituted generally "nonpartisan" elections of judges for fixed terms of office, and others have clearly partisan elections. Even if party affiliation is not be identified on the ballot, candidates can generally be identified as to their party affiliation by prior experience or reputation.

States also vary as to how often judges must undergo re-election. The length of judicial tenure attempts to balance providing independence for a judge to make unpopular but legally based judgments versus making them accountable to popular opinion. With state supreme courts making judicial decisions having major economic and/or political consequences, state judicial elections can become intense and costly. Some state judicial elections have even drawn national attention. Like other political candidates, candidates for judicial positions seek support from donors, including specific interest groups. This can create a conflict of interest or the appearance of one that may undermine the perceived legitimacy of court decisions. Judges under such an electoral system may also be subject to a potential recall election. Policy analysts must be aware of the judicial selection process for their state and how that may influence policy outcomes.

Remaining Constitutional Provisions

Article IV deals with certain interstate issues. States must give other states full faith and credit to their actions; that is, states must respect other state's laws, thus the extradition of citizens who violate another state's laws or the payment of motor vehicle violations in another state. According to Article IV, citizens from another state have the same privileges as those citizens of that state. This article also guarantees that the federal government will assure that states have a republican form of government and protect them from invasion or domestic violence.

Article V describes the constitutional amending process. The most common vehicle has been the adoption of a constitutional amendment by Congress and then the ratification of that amendment by three-fourths of the state legislatures. The last such amendment to pass was Amendment XXVII in 1992, prohibiting compensation for senators and representatives to change without an intervening election. The Equal Rights Amendment, stating that "[e]quality of rights under the law shall not be denied or abridged by the United States or by any state on account of sex," was approved by Congress on March 22, 1972. It needed 38 states to approve the amendment to pass. By 1977, 35 states had approved it and Congress extended the deadline for approval to June 30, 1982, but no further states have approved it.

Thirty-two states have passed state legislation calling for a new national constitutional convention. The advocates for a constitutional convention have generally been proponents for the adoption of a balanced budget amendment. However, three states have rescinded their call for such a convention, although one of those recissions is legally questionable. It would take two or five more states (depending on the legality of few state recissions) to convene a national constitutional convention. However, as demonstrated by the Constitutional Convention of 1787, if convened, such a convention could make other major changes as well.

Article VI also involves a historically controversial provision whereby the federal government assumed state debts arising from state actions prior to the Constitution's adoption. These included war debts, which varied from state to state. Another part of Article VI includes the statement that acts and treaties made by federal government "shall be the Supreme Law of the Land." This is an important principle when state and federal laws conflict. The third paragraph of that article requires all federal and state officials to take an oath of allegiance to support the U.S. Constitution.

Article VII, the final article, merely states that the Constitution will go into effect upon adoption by the ninth state. It did not take a unanimous vote to create the United States, although all 13 states eventually adopted the Constitution. The Constitution was not adopted by popular vote. Each state created a constitutional convention. Debate in each convention was intense and the assurance of the Constitution's approval was uncertain. Smaller states tended to be the first to approve it. Approval by the most politically and economically powerful states such as Massachusetts, Pennsylvania, New York, and Virginia was critical. The *Federalist Papers* were written to influence these state conventions. After much acrimonious debate, the Constitution of the United States was adopted when the ninth state, New Hampshire, ratified it on June 21, 1788. However, several large states had still not ratified it. Virginia was the 10th state to ratify the Constitution on June 26, 1788, with the major proviso that a bill of rights had to be adopted. On July 26, 1788, New York became the 11th state to adopt it. Its approval was critical due to its size as well as its geography, which created a contiguous geographic entity. The U.S. federal government officially began March 1, 1789, with a new executive (president), a bicameral legislative branch (the popularly elected House of Representatives and an appointed Senate), and a new federal judicial branch.

THE BILL OF RIGHTS

Even after adopting a totally new structure in 1789, the Constitution was changed in 1791 with the adoption of the first 10 amendments, the Bill of Rights. The promise of the passage of these amendments was critical to the Constitution's final adoption. See Breakout Box 3.4.

Breakout Box 3.4

THE FIRST TEN AMENDMENTS, THE BILL OF RIGHTS

- *First Amendment*—regarding freedom of religion, of speech, of press, of assembly, and to petition government
- *Second Amendment*—regarding the right to bear arms
- *Third Amendment*—regarding the quartering of troops
- *Fourth Amendment*—regarding search and seizure
- *Fifth Amendment*—regarding grand juries, double jeopardy, self-incrimination, and due process
- *Sixth Amendment*—regarding criminal prosecutions, trial by jury, the right to confront witnesses, and the right to counsel
- *Seventh Amendment*—regarding common law and jury trials
- *Eighth Amendment*—regarding excessive bail or fines and cruel and unusual punishment
- *Ninth Amendment*—regarding nonenumerated rights
- *Tenth Amendment*—regarding rights reserved to states or people

These amendments plus the 14th Amendment tend to be a major source of constitutional litigation. We will only deal with three of the amendments, although almost all of them (except for the Third Amendment) have important implications for public policy. Most people have a general sense of their First Amendment rights to freedom of religion, of speech, of press, of assembly, and to petition government.[7] As will be discussed later, the 14th Amendment made these provisions applicable to the states as well. However, these rights are not absolute since any right taken to an extreme will conflict with other rights. The Oliver Wendell Holmes famous example that freedom of speech does not include the right to yell "fire" in a crowded theater when no fire is present is but one example.[8] All constitutional rights have limits and may be taken away.

Freedom of Religion

In the past, courts have held in cases involving Christian Scientists that public health can take precedence in particular circumstances. Freedom of religion has become a hot topic lately regarding COVID-19, LBGTQ, and Native American issues. In 1971 the USSC decided in *Lemon v. Kurtzman* (1971) that there were three tests that needed to be passed for a law to pass constitutional muster regarding the freedom of religion: (1) it must have a nonreligious purpose (e.g., protecting public health); (2) it must not promote or favor any set of religious beliefs (e.g., favoring

---

7 "Congress shall make no law respecting an establishment of religion, or prohibiting the free exercise thereof; or abridging the freedom of speech, or of the press; or the right of the people peaceably to assemble, and to petition the government for a redress of grievances" (U.S. Const. amend. I).

8 *Schenck v. United States* (1919) lays out the clear and present danger test.

a Protestant religion over the Jewish religion); and (3) it must not overly involve the government with religion (e.g., subsidizing a religion). As such, public educational systems cannot teach religion while private educational schools can and do teach religion. Of course, what constitutes the teaching of religion or subsidizing religion can and has been debated. Some state and local laws have recently blurred the subsidization of private religious schools.

In 1993 the Religious Freedom Restoration Act (RFFA; Pub. L. No. 103–141) was overwhelmingly passed by both houses of Congress and signed by President Bill Clinton. The purpose of the legislation was to broadly protect religious freedom. In *City of Boerne v. Flores* (1997), the USSC ruled that the application of this law to the states was an unconstitutional application of its enforcement powers of the 14th Amendment but that the law did apply to the federal government. In response, almost half of the states have passed their own version of RFFA.

The application of RFFA to the federal government was extended by the USSC in decisions such as *Burwell v. Hobby Lobby Stores, Inc.* (2014), in which the Court ruled for the first time that a privately held corporation (like an individual) could invoke a religious conviction regarding a federal contraceptive coverage mandate. On July 8, 2020, in two related cases, the USSC upheld President Trump's administration's allowing organizations to prevent their employees or students from receiving contraceptive services based on moral or religious grounds.[9]

The application of RFFA is complicated further by other USSC cases. In the USSC landmark *Lyng* case, the Court ruled that the free exercise clause of the First Amendment does not prohibit the federal government from harvesting timber or constructing roads through a national forest that is considered a sacred religious site by three California Native American Tribes (*Lyng v. Northwest Indian Cemetery Protective Association*, 1988). Another USSC case held that the state could deny unemployment benefits to a person fired for violating a state prohibition on the use of peyote even though the use of the drug was part of a religious ritual (*Employment Division v. Smith*, 1990).

The traditional rulings on the separation of church and state were muddied further by the 6-3 decision of the USSC in *Carson v. Makin* (2022). In that case the Court ruled that Maine's educational voucher program could not refuse to fund religious schools. This was seen as an expansion in the Court's interpretation of religious freedom. The conflict between religious rights and public health will likely be contentious in the years ahead.

The Second Amendment

The Second Amendment is another contentious area given the number of deaths caused by firearms.[10] The Second Amendment has been debated for years and was traditionally dealt with cautiously by the courts to balance the control of deadly weapons for public safety and the use of weapons for hunting and recreation. The first phrase of the Second Amendment states that the purpose of the amendment

---

9 *Little Sisters of the Poor Saints Peter and Paul Home v. Pennsylvania*, 591 U.S. ___ (2020) and *Pennsylvania v. Trump* (October Term, 2019 Syllabus. (2020, July 8). SupremeCourt.Gov. https://www.supremecourt.gov/opinions/19pdf/19-431_5i36.pdf).

10 The Second Amendment reads as follows: "A well regulated Militia, being necessary to the security of a free State, the right of the people to keep and bear Arms, shall not be infringed" (U.S. Const. amend. II).

was to establish a "well regulated militia." When the Constitution was written, there was no standing army; the defense of the country depended on state militias being mobilized by the federal government, much as a state's national guard can be done today. Traditionally, the courts interpreted the Second Amendment right of the people to keep and bear arms as a collective right (to maintain a militia) and not an individual right. This was decided in the 1939 USSC case of *United States v. Miller* (1939), a case involving the National Firearms Act of 1934 designed to regulate sawed-off shotguns. This precedent lasted for about 74 years until the USSC ruled in *District of Columbia v. Heller* (2008) that Washington, DC's handgun ban, which had existed for 32 years, was unconstitutional based on an *individual right* to bear arms. In 2010, the Court strengthened the application of the individual right to own a handgun in *McDonald v. City of Chicago* (2010) by ruling that the 14th Amendment prohibited states from abridging the individual's freedom to bear arms.

The deaths of thousands by gun violence and suicide with access to high-caliber guns and munitions remains a contentious public health issue. Beginning with the 1997 Centers for Disease Control and Prevention (CDC) Appropriations bill, the Dickey Amendment of 1996 prevented the CDC from advocating or promoting gun control and it removed money that it had previously used for gun research. This was interpreted by the CDC to mean that no research could be sponsored or conducted. With federal funding gone, researchers stopped studying gun violence. However, after the 2012 Sandy Hook school shooting in Newtown, Connecticut, there was increased pressure on the federal government to do something. In January 2013 President Obama issued a Presidential Memorandum ending the freeze on gun violence research. In 2013 the Institute of Medicine (IOM) and the National Academies of Science, Engineering, and Medicine (NASEM) released a report to identify the most pressing research questions regarding gun violence (Leshner et al., 2013). Subsequently, the Violence Prevention branch of the CDC's Injury Section now issues millions of research dollars in gun violence studies (CDC, 2021).

As a result of additional mass casualty shootings in 2022, there was additional pressure on Congress to pass some new gun legislation. The Bipartisan Safer Communities Act (2022) was passed by Congress and signed by President Biden on June 25, 2022. That legislation strengthened background checks for those under 21 years of age, clarified federal firearms licensure requirements, provided funding incentives for state red flag laws, provided funding for mental health interventions, further criminalized arms trafficking and straw firearm purchases, and partially closed the boyfriend loophole—preventing those convicted of domestic abuse or stalking former or current intimate partners from obtaining firearms. The continuation of mass shootings in the United States will continue to make gun regulation a contentious policy area for years to come.

The Ninth Amendment

The Ninth Amendment is a source of great debate. It states that "[t]he enumeration in the Constitution, of certain rights, shall not be construed to deny or disparage others retained by the people" (U.S. Const. amend. IX). This was James Madison's assurance that the rights of citizens were not restricted to only those specified in the Bill of Rights. There were other rights that existed, un-enumerated rights. The right to privacy in the United States was first put forth in an 1890 article in the *Harvard*

Law Journal (Warren & Brandeis, 1890). At the time, the concern was over government invasion of privacy arising from new technology, the telephone. Although the right to privacy is implied in several of the Bill of Rights (e.g., freedom of religion, freedom from having to house soldiers, freedom from unreasonable searches and seizures, freedom from self-incrimination), it is not explicitly stated in the Constitution. Many federal and state laws and policies such as the Health Insurance Portability and Accountability Act of 1996 (HIPAA) are based on the un-enumerated right to privacy. The right to privacy has again become a heightened concern given increased technology such as drones and cybertechnology to impinge on privacy.

The USSC first addressed the right to privacy in *Griswold v. Connecticut* (1965). In this landmark USSC decision, the Court ruled that Connecticut's law prohibiting married couples from buying and/or using contraceptives violated marital privacy. This ruling was based on the Ninth Amendment as well as substantive and procedural rights protected by the 14th Amendment. Since *Griswold*, the right to privacy has been the basis for subsequent Supreme Court rulings based on the Due Process and Equal Protection clauses of the 14th Amendment for invalidating specific state laws. In *Loving v. Virginia* (1967), the USSC held that state laws banning interracial marriages violated the Constitution. In *Roe v. Wade* (1973), the USSC ruled that the right to privacy, the Due Process Clause, and the 14th Amendment protected a woman's ability to choose whether to have an abortion within certain restrictions according to the stage of pregnancy. In *Cruzan v. Director, Missouri Department of Health* (1990), the USSC ruled that individuals have the right to make their own decisions regarding terminating lifesaving medical treatments. In *Lawrence v. Texas* (2003), a Texas sodomy case was struck down. In *Obergefell v. Hodges* (2015), the USSC guaranteed same-sex couples the right to legally marry.

Justices holding a "strict constructionist" or "original intent" judicial philosophy (i.e., interpreting a constitutional provision narrowly and/or using the literal meaning of its words in their historical context) have called into question unremunerated constitutional rights. The consequences of the 2022 USSC decision in *Dobbs v. Jackson Women's Health Organization*, overturning the 50-year-old decision of *Roe v. Wade*, will take years to play out not only for abortion, but also for other unremunerated rights. See **Breakout Box 3.5**.

Breakout Box 3.5

DOBBS, STATE HEALTH OFFICER OF THE MISSISSIPPI DEPARTMENT OF HEALTH, ET AL. V. JACKSON WOMEN'S HEALTH ORGANIZATION, ET AL.

This landmark 5-4 decision by the USSC struck down the 50-year-old 7-2 precedent of *Roe v. Wade* (1973). In a 6-4 vote, the Court ruled that the Mississippi's ban on abortion after the 15th week (with exceptions for medical emergencies and severe fetal abnormalities but with no exceptions for rape or incest) was valid.

The majority opinion written by Justice Samuel Alito was substantially unchanged from the leaked draft except for an added section attacking the positions taken by the dissenting justices and Chief Justice Roberts's partial dissent. Justices Thomas, Gorsuch, Kavanaugh, and Barrett joined in the majority opinion. The majority based its decision first by dismissing *Roe*'s reliance on the First, Fourth, Fifth and Ninth Amendments for its constitutional basis. It then focused on the 14th Amendment since this case involved a state law. The USSC has ruled in the past that "liberty" in the 14th Amendment has had a substantive meaning (e.g., right to marry) as well as a procedural meaning (e.g., right to a fair trial). However, the majority opinion maintained that 14th Amendment substantive liberties must be based on our "deeply rooted history or tradition" or on our "national scheme of ordered liberty." The *Dobbs* majority opinion went through an historical analysis going back to the 12th century and concluded that there was no historical right to abortion nor was there a need for it based on a "national scheme of ordered liberty."

Dobbs stated that although *stare decisis* is important, it cannot go unexamined by the Court. Otherwise, segregation would still be legal in the United States. The majority opinion states that while it is important to have settled law, the majority places a higher value on that it be "settled right." It discussed five factors justifying *Roe v. Wade* be overturned: (1) nature of the Court's error, (2) quality of reasoning, (3) workability, (4) effect on other areas of law, and (5) reliance interests. It gives reasons in all five areas as to why *Roe* should be overturned. It states that *Roe v. Wade* was "egregiously wrong and deeply damaging" (*Dobbs v. Jackson Women's Health Organization*, 2022, p. 44) as was *Planned Parenthood of Southeastern Pennsylvania v. Casey* (1992), the 1992 5-4 USSC decision that reinforced *Roe v. Wade* as precedent. The majority opinion states that *Roe* and *Casey* have enflamed debate and deepened division. The majority decision determined that since there was no Constitutional right to an abortion, the USSC had to use the lower bar of judicial review as to whether the state of Mississippi had a rational basis for its law. Finding that the state had an interest in protecting the unborn, the majority ruled that the decision by the elected representatives in Mississippi held. The majority opinion states that other substantive 14th Amendment rights such the right to contraceptives (*Griswold v. Connecticut*), the right to same-sex intimacy (*Lawrence v. Texas*), and the right to same-sex marriage (*Obergefell v. Hodges*), are not at risk since they do not result in the loss of potential life.

There was a separate opinion by Chief Justice Roberts stating that while he supported the majority opinion regarding the Mississippi law, the decision by the majority to overrule *Roe v. Wade* as precedent was "a serious jolt to the legal system" (*Dobbs v. Jackson Women's Health Organization, Roberts concurring opinion*, 2022, p. 11), which he could not support. Instead, he reinforced the Court's historical rule of minimalism, not ruling more than is necessary.

There were two separate concurring opinions. Justice Kavanaugh indicated that the USSC was being neutral on the issue of abortion, making it neither legal or illegal, but merely leaving the question to the states. Justice Thomas's opinion made a more sweeping statement, saying that other substantive "liberty" rights under the 14th Amendment (namely, *Griswold, Lawrence,* and *Obergefell*) should be reexamined. His opinion was an invitation for such lawsuits to be brought to the USSC.

Justices Breyer, Sotomayor, and Kagan wrote a rare joint dissent. They stated that they believe "in a Constitution that puts some issues off limits to majority rule" (*Dobbs v. Jackson Women's Health Organization*, Breyer, Sotomayor, Kagen dissenting opinion, 2022, p. 7). They defended the 50-year-old precedent *Roe v. Wade* as reaffirmed by *Casey* as an attempt by the Court (by using the trimester system) to strike a balance on a very divisive issue. They criticized the majority decision for not considering the burdens that childbirth imposes on a woman and for deriding *Roe*'s attempt to strike a balance of interests. The dissent discussed the unequal impact of the majority's decision on poor women who are unable to afford to travel long distances to seek legal healthcare. The dissent also pointed to the unequal burdens that poor women face when forced to bear a child and, as stated in *Casey*, are not able to participate equally in the economic and social life of the nation. The dissent rejects Justice Kavanaugh's description of the USSC as being neutral regarding abortion when the majority's decision leaves a previous constitutional right up to majority rule in states that clearly oppose the right to an abortion. It pointed to past and current state efforts to enact severe restrictions on access and penalties on providers that were being proposed by states. They ask whether Kavanaugh would think the Court "scrupulously neutral" if the Court allowed New York or California to outlaw guns (*Dobbs v. Jackson Women's Health Organization*, Breyer, Sotomayor, Kagen dissenting opinion, 2022, p. 20). It also stated that the majority opinion does not prohibit any action taken by the states; for example, a state could force a woman impregnated by her father to have that child.

The dissent doubted the majority's statement that its ruling applies only to abortion and not to other substantive liberties as affirmed in *Griswold, Lawrence,* and *Obergefell.* The dissent points out that the latter rights rest on the same legal basis and the lack of historical tradition as *Roe*. "Either the majority does not really believe in its own reasoning. Or if it does, all rights that have no history stretching back to the mid-19th century are insecure. Either the mass of the majority's opinion is hypocrisy, or additional constitutional rights are under threat. It is one of the other" (*Dobbs v. Jackson Women's Health Organization*, Breyer, Sotomayor, Kagen dissenting opinion, 2022, p. 5). The dissent noted Justice Thomas's opinion inviting USSC challenges to "all of this Court's substantive due process precedents" (*Dobbs v. Jackson Women's Health Organization*, Breyer, Sotomayor, Kagen dissenting opinion, 2022, p. 26). Including *Griswold, Lawrence,* and *Obergefell* could apply to other substantive rights such as the right of interracial marriage (*Loving v. Virginia*, 1967) and the right not to be sterilized without consent (*Skinner v. Oklahoma ex rel. Williams*, 1942).

The dissent discussed the role of *stare decisis* and it states that nothing has changed in terms of circumstances or law to justify overruling a 50-year-old precedent. "The Court reverses course today for one reason and one reason only: because the composition of this Court has changed. *Stare decisis*, this Court has often said, 'contributes to the actual and perceived integrity of the judicial process' by ensuring that decisions are 'founded in the law rather than in the proclivities of individuals.' *Payne v. Tennessee,* 501 U. S. 808, 827 (1991); *Vasquez v. Hillery,* 474 U. S. 254, 265 (1986). Today, the proclivities of individuals rule. The Court departs from its obligation to faithfully and impartially apply the law. We dissent" (*Dobbs v. Jackson Women's Health Organization,* Breyer, Sotomayor, Kagen dissenting opinion, 2022, p. 6). The dissent concludes by referring to Justices Sandra Day O'Connor, Anthony Kennedy, and David Souter (justices deciding in the *Casey* decision) that constitutional rights should never hang by a thread with the threat of it being overturned by a new majority. The dissent noted that the majority decision threatens the perceived legitimacy of the Court. To highlight the tension in the USSC, the dissent omitted the word "respectfully," which is traditional within the closing line of a dissent.

Some public health policy issues raised by the *Dobbs* decision include:

- Can states that make abortion illegal penalize a woman seeking healthcare in another state that has statutes for legal abortions?
- Are multistate health organizations/providers subject to state penalties that make abortion illegal when that provider performs abortions in a state where it is legal?
- Can women in states banning abortions retain legal access to Food and Drug Administration (FDA) approved abortifacients?
- Can FDA-approved abortifacients be sold over the counter or be prescribed by additional healthcare providers?
- Can states force a woman to give birth that was caused by incest or rape?
- In a state where abortions are illegal, can a woman who has had a spontaneous abortion have remaining tissue removed?
- In those states allowing abortion only in the case of rape or incest, what level of proof of rape or incest protects the medical professional from prosecution?
- Can a state ban abortion even if it results in maternal death?
- If laws allow for protecting the health and life of the mother, who decides and how is that to be evaluated? Is a 30% risk of maternal death sufficient to allow an abortion and protect the provider from legal jeopardy?
- How can public health mitigate the impact of abortion bans on maternal health?
- Can states penalize business/insurance companies that provide transportation benefits to women for abortion?
- In states banning abortion, what public health activities can reduce maternal death rates?

References

Dobbs v. Jackson Women's Health Organization, 597 US___ (2022). https://www
.supremecourt.gov/opinions/21pdf/19-1392_6j37.pdf
Griswold v. Connecticut, 381 U.S. 479 (1965). https://supreme.justia.com/cases/
federal/us/381/479
Lawrence v. Texas, 539 U.S. 558 (2003). https://supreme.justia.com/cases/federal/
us/539/558
Loving v. Virginia, 388 U.S. 1 (1967). https://supreme.justia.com/cases/federal/
us/388/1
Obergefell v. Hodges, 576 U.S. 644 (2015). https://supreme.justia.com/cases/federal/
us/576/14-556
Payne v. Tennessee, 501 U.S. 808, 827 (1991). https://supreme.justia.com/cases/
federal/us/501/808
Planned Parenthood of Southeastern Pennsylvania v. Casey, 505 U.S. 833 (1992).
https://supreme.justia.com/cases/federal/us/505/833
Roe v. Wade, 410 U.S. 113 (1973). https://supreme.justia.com/cases/federal/us/410/113
Skinner v. Oklahoma ex rel. Williams, 316 U.S. 535 (1942). https://supreme.justia.com/
cases/federal/us/316/535
Vasquez v. Hillery, 474 U.S. 254, 265 (1986). https://supreme.justia.com/cases/federal/
us/474/254

SUMMARY

The description of the basic political principles and structures in this chapter outlines the basic framework of government and its decision-making processes. Details of how members of each house in Congress are elected have significant consequences for policy determination. Since the president and vice president are the only politicians that all citizens have an opportunity to vote for, the construction of the Electoral College plays a significant role as to whether the national majority is represented. The power of the judiciary and its construction as a nonpartisan or partisan branch of government is a critical structural element. Every structural element has a bias influencing the policy process. The Framers deliberately designed the structure to set ambition against ambition so that no one person or branch was dominant. There is a continual debate as to which branch has become stronger in the political process. There are certainly eras when different branches have tended to hold sway. However, structure alone is not the only definitive factor. Policy outcomes are determined by multiple factors. The political structure ignores much of the critical elements that make the system work. As we will discuss in the next chapter, *process* can be key.

DISCUSSION QUESTIONS

- Given what you currently know about the American political system, if you were asked to edit the *Federalist Papers*, what are two major changes you would recommend?

- The federal and state courts are radically different in the appointment of judges. Which do you perceive to be a better model for a fair judiciary? Justify your answer.

- Describe the significance of the 14th Amendment.

- What is the meaning of *stare decisis* given *Dobbs v. Jackson* (2022)?

KEY TERMS

Baker v. Carr (1962)

bicameral

Bill of Rights

Bipartisan Safer Communities Act (2022)

Burwell v. Hobby Lobby Stores, Inc. (2014)

Carson v. Makin (2022)

civil service

Citizens United v. Federal Election Commission (2010)

Cruzan v. Director, Missouri Department of Health (1990)

Dickey Amendment of 1996

District of Columbia v. Heller (2008)

Dobbs v. Jackson Women's Health Organization (2022)

Due Process Clause of the 14th Amendment

Electoral College

gerrymandering

Griswold v. Connecticut (1965)

initiatives

Judiciary Act of 1789

justiciable question

Lawrence v. Texas (2003)

Loving v. Virginia (1967)

Lyng v. Northwest Indian Cemetery Protection Association (1988)

Marbury v. Madison (1803)

McDonald v. City of Chicago (2010)

Obergefell v. Hodges (2015)

Office of the President

political question

recall

referendum

Religious Freedom Restoration Act (RFFA)

right to privacy

Roe v. Wade (1973)

Second Amendment

strict constructionist

term limits

United States v. Miller (1939)

REFERENCES

Baker v. Carr, 369 U.S. 186 (1962). https://supreme.justia.com/cases/federal/us/369/186

Bipartisan Safer Communities Act, Pub. L. No. 117-159, 116 Stat. 2135 (2022). https://www.govinfo.gov/app/details/PLAW-117publ159

Burwell v. Hobby Lobby Stores, Inc., 73 U.S. 682 (2014). https://supreme.justia.com/cases/federal/us/573/682

Carson v. Makin, 596 U.S. ___ (2022). https://supreme.justia.com/cases/federal/us/596/20-1088

Centers for Disease Control and Prevention. (n.d.). *Firearm violence prevention.* https://www.cdc.gov/violenceprevention/firearms/index.html

Citizens United v. Federal Election Commission, 558 U.S. 310 (2010). https://supreme.justia.com/cases/federal/us/558/310

City of Boerne v. Flores, 521 U.S. 507 (1997). https://supreme.justia.com/cases/federal/us/521/507

Cruzan v. Director, Missouri Department of Health, 497 U.S. 261 (1990). https://supreme.justia.com/cases/federal/us/497/261

Dahl, R. A. (2001). *How democratic is the American Constitution?* Yale University Press.

District of Columbia v. Heller, 554 U.S. 570 (2008). https://supreme.justia.com/cases/federal/us/554/570

Dobbs v. Jackson Women's Health Organization, 597 U.S. ___ (2022). https://www.supremecourt.gov/opinions/21pdf/19-1392_6j37.pdf

Employment Division Department of Human Resources of Oregon v. Smith, 494 U.S. 872 (1990). https://supreme.justia.com/cases/federal/us/494/872

Griswold v. Connecticut, 381 U.S. 479 (1965). https://supreme.justia.com/cases/federal/us/381/479

Hamilton, A., Madison, J., & Jay, J. (1961). *The federalist papers* (C. Rossiter, Ed.). The New American Library of World Literature.

Lawrence v. Texas, 539 U.S. 558 (2003). https://supreme.justia.com/cases/federal/us/539/558

Lemon v. Kurtzman, 403 U.S. 602 (1971). https://supreme.justia.com/cases/federal/us/403/602

Leshner, A. I., Altevogt, B. M., Lee, A. F., McCoy, M. A., & Kelley, P. W. (Eds.). (2013). *Priorities for research to reduce the threat of firearm-related violence.* National Academies Press. https://doi.org/10.17226/18319

Levitsky, S., & Ziblatt, D. (2018). *How democracies die.* Broadway Books.

Loving v. Virginia, 388 U.S. 1 (1967). https://supreme.justia.com/cases/federal/us/388/1

Lyng v. Northwest Indian Cemetery Protective Association, 485 U.S. 439 (1988). https://supreme.justia.com/cases/federal/us/485/439

Maine's People Alliance. (2017). *Mainers deliver signatures to launch health care referendum.* https://www.mainepeoplesalliance.org/content/mainers-deliver-signatures-launch-health-care-referendum

Marbury v. Madison, 5 U.S. 137 (1803). https://supreme.justia.com/cases/federal/us/5/137

McDonald v. Chicago, 561 U.S. 742 (2010). https://supreme.justia.com/cases/federal/us/561/742

Reynolds v. Sims, 377 U.S. 533 (1964). https://supreme.justia.com/cases/federal/us/377/533

Roe v. Wade, 410 U.S. 113 (1973). https://supreme.justia.com/cases/federal/us/410/113

Rucho v. Common Cause, 588 U.S. ___ (2019). https://www.supremecourt.gov/opinions/18pdf/18-422_9ol1.pdf

Schenck v. United States, 249 U.S. 47 (1919). https://supreme.justia.com/cases/federal/us/249/47

United States v. Miller, 307 U.S. 174 (1939). https://supreme.justia.com/cases/federal/us/307/174

U.S. Constitution, amend. I.

U.S. Constitution, amend. II.

U.S. Constitution, amend. IX.

U.S. Constitution, art. III, § 2.

U.S. Constitution, pmbl.

U.S. Department of Health & Human Services. (n.d.). HHS.gov. https://www.hhs.gov

Warren, S. D., & Brandeis, L. D. (1890). The right to privacy. *Harvard Law Review, 4*(5), 193–220. https://doi.org/10.2307/1321160

Westbury v. Sanders, 376 U.S. 1 (1964). https://supreme.justia.com/cases/federal/us/376/1

CHAPTER 4

THE POLITICAL PROCESS

We begin this chapter by first describing the iterative policy-making process and some general concepts not delineated in the Constitution such as political parties, lobbying, and other characteristics of our political process including our electoral system. We discuss the notions of democracy and democratic pluralism and then describe the political process in the United States. The next chapter walks you through the American political maze.

LEARNING OBJECTIVES

Be able to:

- Describe the iterative generic policy-making process.
- Delineate the difference between procedural democracy and constitutional democracy.
- Explain how the concept of democratic pluralism works.
- Explain the role of lobbyists within the policy-making process.
- Describe how scope and bias impact policy outcomes.
- Explain how the ability to block is facilitated in the U.S. political system.
- Define the U.S. political process.

THE POLICY-MAKING PROCESS

Policy operates in an iterative manner, much as a turning wheel (see **Figure 4.1**). In this text we focus primarily on the policy formulation phase. However, as we will see in Chapter 15, Recommendation and Strategies, we cannot overlook the policy adoption and implementation phases of this policy wheel. Policy can be created and analyzed anywhere on this wheel.

Policy making is a process that has been described in various ways within the political science literature. Theories and conceptual models from the literature

FIGURE 4.1 Policy wheel.

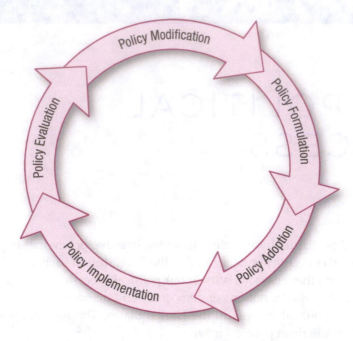

Source: Evenson, K., & Aytur, S. (2012). Policy for physical activity promotion. In B. E. Ainsworth & C. A. Macera (Eds.), *Physical activity and public health practice* (pp. 321–344). CRC Press.

can help us to better understand the policy process (Bacchi, 2016; Baumgartner & Jones, 1991; Coveney, 2008; Kingdon, 2003; Lasswell, 1971; Sabatier & Jenkins-Smith, 1993). For example, one commonly utilized model, proposed by Longest, has four general elements: (1) policy formulation; (2) policy implementation; (3) policy evaluation; and (4) policy modification (Longest, 1998).

Figure 4.1 provides a composite view of several different theories about the policy process. As illustrated by the circular nature of the diagram, these component parts of the process are quite iterative in practice. They do not always flow linearly from one to the other, nor do they have definitive boundaries. In some cases, the activities overlap. However, for descriptive purposes, we describe them generally here. The first step in the policy process is typically policy formulation (policy development). This includes identifying a problem or issue, considering value orientations, framing the issue, proposing one or multiple approaches to addressing the problem/issue, defining the policy objectives, estimating impacts, and then drafting the policy content and strategically moving the policy toward adoption.

However, this phase bridges with the other phases in the political process. It involves all the strategic alliances and negotiation points one must consider and engage in to get support for a formal piece of legislation. We focus on some of this in Chapter 15, Recommendation and Strategies. Once a policy has been legislatively passed into law and adopted, the policy implementation phase begins. This involves "who does what and when" to make the program operational. At times, this is distinct from the adoption phase, for example, creating a detailed blueprint for action and funding priorities. At other times, this phase overlaps with the adoption phase and the legislation prescribes specific implementation guidelines. For example, the adoption process could stipulate when various components of the law are to begin and allow time to build the capacity for implementation. In both cases, there should be clear goals and measures of success to evaluate outcomes. These are expanded upon in Chapter 13, Criteria for Success.

After some period of implementing programs/policy, progress toward the stated goals and outcomes must be measured. This is the policy evaluation phase. Here it is important that the previous phases be clear and explicit so that success (or lack thereof) can be empirically demonstrated. The final phase, policy modification, is the closing of the policy feedback loop where adjustments to a given policy are made if necessary. Here one might examine costs relative to benefits. Programs and policies are frequently modified due to changing needs and expectations as well as changes in the partisan control of the political system. There may also be calls to repeal the policy if outcomes are deemed negative or to expand the policy to other groups. The history of the Patient Protection and Affordable Care Act (PPACA) demonstrates the dramatic changes in legislation by various policy-making mechanisms. After passage of the law, the Obama Administration delayed implementing various portions of the bill such as the employer and Cadillac tax mandates. There have been repeated unsuccessful legislative attempts by Republicans in Congress to repeal and/or defund PPACA. As noted previously, the U.S. Supreme Court's (USSC's) decision in *National Federation of Independent Business v. Sebelius* (2012) upheld the PPACA's minimum coverage provision as an exercise of Congress's taxing power but repealed the PPACA's penalty for a state not expanding its Medicaid coverage. On January 28, 2021, President Biden signed Executive Order 14009 to strengthen access to the PPACA by, among other things, implementing a special enrollment period, increasing outreach efforts for PPACA enrollment, lowering the out-of-pocket costs by $400, and reducing application paperwork. In addition, the American Rescue Plan Act of 2021 (Pub. L. No. 117-2) made PPACA coverage more affordable and increased incentives for state Medicaid expansion. Adjustments are made continuously by various segments of the policy-making process.

PROCEDURAL DEMOCRACY AND CONSTITUTIONAL DEMOCRACY

If you ask most Americans what type of a political process we use, they will probably state that the United States is a democracy because that is what we have been taught since elementary school and what has been reinforced through repetition. However, it is more complicated than that. The Founding Fathers claimed that they established a republic where the ultimate authority rests with the people and not a monarch or other authoritarian person. They did not claim to establish a democracy.

While democracy is not a complicated concept, it can be complicated to implement. Since a procedural democracy works on the principle of majority/plurality rule, the first complication becomes a majority of whom? The Founding Fathers took the "who" to mean White male property owners, a clear minority of the entire population. Women and Indigenous persons were excluded; Black individuals were counted in a state's population total but only as three-fifths of a person and were not allowed to vote.[1] It is only relatively recently that the definition of "who" includes women, Black individuals, non–property owners,[2] and those 18 years and older. Those groups have been included by constitutional amendments.[3]

The next two major complications of democracy involve questions such as: "How will the majority make their voice known?" and "Are there any limits to majority rule?" This is where the term *constitutional democracy* becomes more appropriate for the United States. Such a political system establishes a constitution that creates the political structure that may be difficult for the majority to change and also restricts the majority from acting in specific areas. The Founding Fathers created multiple buffers to procedural democracy. The majority was to be represented through an electoral system with multiple different constituencies and terms of office. As discussed in Chapter 3, only members of the House of Representatives were elected directly by the people. As also noted in the previous chapter, the structure of the political system works against majority rule. One merely can compare the results of scientific polling on issues and passage of legislation to see significant gaps in the public opinion and adopted policy. The question in terms of the limits on the majority was answered by enacting the first 10 amendments, known as the Bill of Rights. For example, the First Amendment makes it clear that Congress shall pass no law restricting the freedom of religion, speech, press, or assembly, regardless of if a majority wants it.[4] Elements of procedural democracy have been gradually grafted onto a structure that was certainly suspicious of majority rule.

---

1   U.S. Constitution, Article 1, Section 2, "Representatives and direct Taxes shall be apportioned among the several States which may be included within this Union, according to their respective Numbers, which shall be determined by adding to the whole Number of free Persons, including those bound to Service for a Term of Years, and excluding Indians not taxed, three fifths of all other Persons."

2   The origins of the view that land is a private commodity (rather than a public good) can be traced back the Doctrine of Discovery of 1493 (The Gilder Lehman Institute of American History, n.d.). The Doctrine issued by Pope Alexander VI (Papal Bull "Inter Caetera") played a central role in Spain's conquest of the New World. It justified Spain's strategy to ensure its exclusive right to the lands discovered by Columbus the previous year. Many scholars view the Doctrine of Discovery as the foundation of colonialist justifications for taking land from people, and taking people from their land. In 2012, the United Nations (UN) concluded that "signs of such doctrines were still evident in indigenous communities, including in the areas of health; psychological and social well-being; conceptual and behavioral forms of violence against indigenous women; youth suicide; and the hopelessness that many indigenous peoples experience, in particular indigenous youth" (United Nations Department of Economic and Social Affairs, 2012, para. 3). The UN, along with contemporary public health scholars (Browne et al., 2016; Nguyen et al., 2020), emphasize the need for policies that support Indigenous peoples' right to their own culture and heritage.

3   Blacks were allowed to vote through the passage of the 15th Amendment in 1870: "The right of citizens of the United States to vote shall not be denied or abridged by the United States or by any State on account of race, color, or previous condition of servitude." Women were allowed to vote through the adoption of the 19th Amendment in 1920: "The right of citizens of the United States to vote shall not be denied or abridged by the United States or by any State on account of sex." And 18-year-olds were allowed to vote on adoption of the 26th Amendment in 1971: "The right of citizens of the United States, who are eighteen years of age or older, to vote shall not be denied or abridged by the United States or by any State on account of age."

4   First Amendment to the U.S. Constitution: "Congress shall make no law respecting an establishment of religion, or prohibiting the free exercise thereof; or abridging the freedom of speech, or of the press; or the right of the people peaceably to assemble, and to petition the Government for a redress of grievances."

DEMOCRACY AND DEMOCRATIC PLURALISM

How should we describe the policy process in the United States? As noted previously, the United States is more appropriately described as a constitutional democracy. However, the term *constitutional democracy* is so broad that all types of countries can fall under that category, and it does not really describe how the process of making laws and policies works in practice. As a result, political scientists have generally used another term for our political process. Robert Dahl was one of the first to coin the term *democratic pluralism* (Dahl, 1970). This is the theory that policy issues are resolved by the competition, accommodation, and alliance of issue-specific organized groups who have a concentrated interest in policy outcomes for that specific area. This theory relies on the concept of concentrated and diffused interests (factions). Concentrated interests (special interest groups) consist of those who feel sufficiently impacted by a particular public policy that they are willing to spend scarce resources (e.g., time, money, information) to both organize and attempt to influence political decisions regarding that issue. They have a concentrated interest in the price of wheat, automobile manufacturing, the exploration of various minerals, development of new technology, public education, weapons for national defense, the development of pharmaceuticals, public health, medical care, licensure of health professionals, and so forth. In contrast, diffused interests are those people who may be impacted by policies in those areas (consumers) but they are not sufficiently impacted that they are motivated to spend their own scarce resources to try to impact the outcome of the political process for that issue. Most people's interests are centered on their own needs based on Maslow's hierarchy of needs for food, shelter, security and safety, and so forth. They may have little free time to pay attention to the daily political activity. Perhaps they will vote in an occasional election, but they remain uninformed on specific policy issues. Membership in these concentrated interest groups may overlap, but in general they are composed of separate clusters of individuals and organizations depending upon the policy area. Families with young children may take an acute interest in their local schools, becoming members of the local Parent and Teachers Association or another group organized to influence public education. In so doing, they may become aware of state and federal policies that influence public education. Those without school-age children may be less willing to focus on educational issues but focus on national issues such as Social Security or medical care. There are significant costs involved in becoming knowledgeable about any area of public policy. Because most people and organizations have limited time, money, and resources, they might focus on one public health policy issue, ignore most other areas of public policy, or remain politically inactive.

For example, almost everyone is impacted by the price of pharmaceuticals in the United States since at one time or another, everyone will buy a pharmaceutical to supplement their health, alleviate symptoms, or provide a cure for a disease. U.S. residents spend two and half times more on prescription drugs than citizens in the 32 countries in the Organisation for Economic Co-operation and Development (OECD). Prescription drugs account for 10% of all healthcare spending and the cost of them has increased 76% between 2000 and 2017 (Mulcahy, 2021). So, everyone at one time or another is impacted. However, the impact is not uniformly felt among the population.

The Pharmaceutical Research and Manufacturers of America (PhRMA) is composed of the manufacturers of pharmaceuticals and has a concentrated interest in any proposed policies regarding the price of pharmaceuticals. Success of their business model is linked to their political involvement, especially in the United States. If the policy issue involves allowing additional healthcare providers to prescribe pharmaceuticals, the American Medical Association (AMA) would also have a concentrated interest since physicians would have more to lose if prescription privileges were to be expanded to other health professionals. Potentially, the American Association of Nurse Practitioners and the American Pharmacists Association, being potential beneficiaries of the expansion of prescription privileges, may also have a concentrated interest in that policy. The PhRMA may be interested in expanding prescription privileges due to it potentially increasing marketing costs, but that issue might not rate high on their policy wish list compared to pricing. However, if the issue is to increase the availability of generic drugs by shortening copyright privileges, PhRMA would become very active. Another faction such as the National Organization for Rare Disorders (NORD) would have a concentrated interest in any changes to the Orphan Drug Act of 1983. Of course, one organization that might be involved in each of these issues is the American Heart Association (AHA). However, it may not be as important as other public health issues such as COVID-19 or tobacco use. So, while everyone tends to disparage the power of interest groups, almost everyone is represented by one, whether it be a professional organization, a religious group, an industrial group, a union, or a lifestyle or recreational organization. Interest groups are ubiquitous. We like our interest group, but dislike others.

Some of these organizations might create temporary alliances with another interest group on one issue and then become opponents on other policy issues. For a policy topic such as a COVID-19 vaccine mandate, there will be a different but perhaps overlapping cluster of factions. Each group will determine what scope of decision-making is best for its desired outcome. In addition to public health organizations and pharmaceutical companies, major employer groups, unions, educational institutions, religious groups, public and private transportation providers, public health agencies, and so forth might decide that they have a concentrated interest in a COVID-19 policy.

Depending on the policy issue being discussed, there will be a defined set of interest groups that will organize to promote a certain policy outcome. Some of these groups will be permanent organizations and some may be temporary. The critical factor here is that they are organized. We will explore this further in Chapter 12, Stakeholder Analysis. These groups will conduct research and collect information supporting their policy position. They will create issue briefs for policy makers. You may be writing your public health policy analysis for one of these groups. They will develop a strategy to either broaden or restrict the scope of the conflict. They will hire a full-time or part-time lobbyist. If they have the monetary resources, they might pay for expensive media coverage or use available social media. Those with a diffused interest in that policy will not be active. However, even a diffused interest group might join a coalition of tangentially related organizations primarily to curry favor in the hope of receiving reciprocal support for their own policy priorities either now or in the future.

For medically related policies, there will be one cluster of concentrated interests. For public health, there will be another separate but overlapping cluster of concentrated interests. Due to the breadth of public health, all types of clusters of interest groups can be formed depending on the specific policy area, such as family violence, addiction, food safety, environmental pollution, and so forth. For most national defense policies, there will be a very different cluster of concentrated interests, except when it comes to medical care or public health for military personnel or veterans.

Of course, democratic pluralism has a bias. This process favors those who are better at gaining resources such as personnel, time, money, knowledge, and political connections to organize and participate in the public decision-making process. The organized beat the unorganized, and those that are better organized with more resources will typically beat those with fewer resources. To lobby legislators and administrators, conduct research, develop public relation materials for the news media or social media, or raise money for a political campaign fund or a Political Action Committee (PAC) takes valuable resources. Those who are not organized are at a disadvantage. Most of the population will remain on the sidelines concerning what is being debated while concentrated interest groups work with targeted policy makers. Concentrated interests know which policy makers are important for their issues and how to communicate with them.

FACTIONS

We must examine the role of factions because the Founding Fathers were very much aware of the political importance of factions. James Madison's famous *Federalist Paper* #10 is devoted to factions in which he states that they are "sown in the nature of man" (Hamilton et al., 1961, p. 79). He defines a faction as a group of people (either a minority or a majority of the whole) who are united and actuated by some common impulse of passion or interest that is averse to the rights of others or the community as a whole. Today he would include the modern political party, private interest groups, public interest groups, and so forth as factions. Madison maintained that the basic source of factions was the unequal distribution of property; thus, there were manufacturing interests, agricultural interests, debtor and loaner interests, and so forth. The existence of factions was not seen as a positive but as something that needed to be controlled. Majority as well as minority factions were both threats to individual liberty and both needed to be constrained.

SPECIAL INTEREST GROUPS AND LOBBYING

Lobbying is an activity a faction takes to influence public officials on a particular issue. Lobbying involves all sorts of activities. In the United States, lobbying is constitutionally protected by the First Amendment.[5] Any citizen can petition their congressional representatives or administrators within an executive department. Typically, lobbying implies something nefarious done by paid professionals with money and good political connections and a notion *of quid pro quo* ("I will do you a favor if you do a favor for me"), which is indeed illegal but may be difficult to prove. It is common

---

5 The First Amendment to the U.S. Constitution: "Congress shall make no law respecting an establishment of religion, or prohibiting the free exercise thereof; or abridging the freedom of speech, or of the press; or the right of the people peaceably to assemble, and to petition the Government for a redress of grievances."

for defeated/retired legislators, previous civil servants, or retired military personnel to become paid lobbyists since they have acquired close political contacts and/or substantive knowledge about a particular policy topic. Lobbying occurs at all levels of the policy process, not just in the formation of legislation in Congress. In Washington, DC, "K Street" has traditionally been synonymous with offices of well-paid lobbyists. As noted later, lobbying occurs within the executive branch as well. Foreign countries also hire lobbyists to represent their interests, whether it be for cultural exchanges, purchasing military hardware, getting favorable trade considerations, and so forth.

Of course, lobbying also occurs at the state and local levels as well. Factions representing companies, trade associations, educational institutions, public health, not-for-profit conservation groups, racial minority groups, and so forth all engage in lobbying activities. National lobbying groups frequently get involved in state policy processes to either promote or prevent a state policy that could be a model that other states might adopt.

While lobbying tends to have a negative connotation, it represents a valuable and important source of information during the policy process. By bringing substantive information and different perspectives from impacted groups, decision makers can gain insight on both intended and unintended consequences of that potential policy. While constitutionally protected, lobbying is regulated at both the federal and state levels. Lobbyists are normally required to register as a lobbyist and provide information as to whom they represent. There may be restrictions as to where lobbying can occur or limits on gifts, lunches, and so forth. In addition, there may be some distinguishing badge or identification to make everyone aware of who is a paid lobbyist in contrast to an average citizen seeking to talk with their representative.

Many large organizations may have their own in-house lobbyists, or they may use a large lobbying firm on either a full-time or part-time basis. Lobbyists may be hired by multipartnered law firms located in Washington, DC, or the state capital. Lobby firms have reputations as to their ability to gain access, the quality of the information they can provide, their area of expertise, and/or their partisan leanings. Policy makers may reach out to specific lobbyists to supply them with the information they need to support their own positions or to anticipate arguments countering their position. Because they represent a particular organization or groups of organizations, lobbyists have access to proprietary data and information that is not publicly available nor publicly scrutinized. While the information they provide is designed to make the best case possible for their client, lobbyists generally do not want to be labeled as providing misinformation.

Lobbyists attend fund-raising events and/or provide campaign donations for a legislator's primary, general, and re-election campaigns. Raising campaign money is a chief activity of politicians given the expense of election campaigns. With party control of Congress being decided every two years, it is important for lobbying firms to have good communications with members of both political parties. Receiving a return phone call from a legislator is the first step in making your case for a client.

SCOPE AND BIAS

One of the insightful classics in political science is the book *The Semisovereign People* by Schattschneider (1960). Schattschneider makes the case that the root of politics is conflict, and that the outcome of the conflict is greatly determined by the scope of that conflict, that is, the number of people or groups actively engaged. We learned this principle from childhood; when one parent said "no," we would try to involve the other parent to get the decision reversed or modified to our liking. Those involved in the political system consciously attempt to control who is involved in the decision-making process because the scope of the conflict influences who is likely to win. In some instances, those trying to influence the outcome of political decision-making will attempt to restrict the number of people involved if they feel it is advantageous to them. Those likely to lose with a few participants in the decision-making process will push to expand the number and types of participants to tip the balance in their favor. For example, a lobbyist for a particular cause might approach the chair of a legislative committee or a committee staff member to get a particular sentence included within a bill. The insertion of the sentence will probably not be noticed because its inclusion has been done quietly with limited participants. However, if the chair is opposed to the provision, the lobbyist will approach other majority or minority members of the committee in order to expand the scope of decision makers. The chair of the committee, however, will attempt to use their leverage to keep the scope contained. If expanding the scope fails at the committee level, the lobbyist might try to get the majority leader or members of one of the party's caucuses involved or contact bureaucrats from the impacted agency to testify on their behalf. Participants in the political process will strategically attempt to change the scope of the decision-making until they feel advantaged by the scope of decision-making. At this stage, "the people" are generally unaware of the political decisions being made.

However, one or more of the participants may decide to take the issue to the public arena. Advocates might contact allied groups or begin a public relations campaign to "Save Medicare," "Promote Good Government," "Save Our Environment," "Avoid Deficit Spending," and so forth to rally as many potential supporters as possible to their cause. Controlling the scope of decision-making creates a bias toward a desired outcome. As stated by long-time former Representative John D. Dingell, Jr., "I'll let you write the substance… you let me write procedure, and I'll screw you every time" (Feehery, 2019, para. 8).

A continuing example of scope and bias involves our election laws. It is not by accident that the traditional day for voting in the United States is Tuesday, a working day with a narrow window before and after the normal workday. This arrangement tends to advantage voters who are self-employed, professionals, or retired, as well as those able to access limited polling places with or without public transportation. It is also not by accident that one must register or reregister in person rather than have an automatic and permanent registration system as in other Western democracies. The 24th Amendment passed in 1964 forbids the use of a poll tax, and the 1965 Voting Rights Act forbids the use of literacy tests to suppress voter participation. The outcome of elections is tilted by provisions of whatever processes are used. Other countries tend to schedule national elections on weekends or declare a national holiday to encourage greater voter participation. Increased access to voting can be created using mail-in ballots and additional polling places where there is access by public transportation. Even the New England town meeting, the ultimate democratic policy body, has a bias since only certain people can afford to take a full day off from their work to attend. Every process has its bias and those engaged with the political system attempt to use process to their advantage.

Expanding or restricting scope does not guarantee a successful outcome; it merely biases it toward a desired outcome. For 30 years the voting age had been debated at the federal and state levels. In the late 1960s, this debate came to a head due to the war in Vietnam when 18-year-olds were drafted and died in the military but were not allowed to vote. Democrats felt that younger voters were more progressive and would favor them in future elections. The voting age was reduced to 18 nationally on July 1, 1971, with the ratification of the 26th Amendment. However, lowering the voting age failed to materialize in Democratic victories since younger voters have historically had a relatively low level of voting participation.

Manipulation of voting continues today. During the COVID-19 pandemic, many states made it easier for people to both register and vote without physical contact to contain the spread of COVID-19. However, Republicans perceived this as affecting the outcome of the 2020 elections. As a result, Republicans, especially at the state level, have passed restrictions on the ease of voter registration and voting (Brennan Center for Justice, 2021). Any change in the scope of decision-making sets up a different number of competitors and changes the nature of the competition between factions. As stated by Schattschneider, "every change in the scope of conflict has a bias" (1960, p. 4).

Schattschneider distinguishes between self-interest factions and public interest factions (Schattschneider, 1960). The former factions have major self-interest gains at stake (lowering specific taxes for their own benefit, increasing the public regulation on others, gaining an exemption, etc.). On the other hand, a public interest faction is one that promotes a public good (these factions tend to be not-for-profit institutions promoting environmental conservation, public health, etc.). Their policy outcomes are not intended to benefit themselves as individuals but rather the common good. However, the distinction between these two groups is not always clear cut. Since it may appear unseemly to be seen promoting one's self-interest, self-interest factions may attempt to publicly equate their self-interest with that of the public good, as for example, "Save Medicare," "Protect Our Children," or "Good Government Committee." Especially in public campaigns, private interests may fund separate public organizations to disguise their private interests. Here there is a common distinction between what is called a "grassroots" organization promoting a common good and an "AstroTurf" organization disguised as a grassroots organization but funded by a wealthy interest group.

The Ability to Block

We generally think of power as the ability to get things done. In the policy process, this frequently translates to being able to get a particular policy adopted. However, as pointed out by Bachrach and Baratz (1962), that is a short-sighted perception of power. The ability to block other people's policy agenda is just as important and frequently more important. One of the most politically powerful lobbying associations has been the nonprofit National Rifle Association (NRA). Its power comes not so much from getting legislation passed as preventing other groups from passing their legislation to restrict gun ownership, the use of firearms, access to ammunition, and so forth. Despite frequent mass shootings and the appearance of military-style guns and ammunition, the NRA has been remarkably successful in preventing legislation from passing at both federal and state levels.

Since the Founding Fathers wanted to divide political power, the ability to block is enhanced in the United States. It takes finding only one political leverage point to derail a policy proposal. Is there a committee chair who can block a bill? Is there a legislative procedure that can be used to block? Will the executive use multiple means to derail a policy? Can the courts be used to block? In contrast, as we will see in the next chapter, it requires a sustained effort of coalition building and overcoming multiple hurdles to enact a law. The U.S. political system's structure and processes facilitate the power to block.

POLITICAL PARTIES

Political parties are unique factions in that they are the only ones that can win elections and thereby organize a ruling government. The Founding Fathers did not particularly like political parties, but they emerged anyway. The U.S. winner-takes-all electoral system tends to favor a two-party system. It is interesting to note that none of the Western democracies created after the U.S. Constitution was signed in 1787 followed the U.S. example in terms of its structure. Instead, they established electoral systems favoring the existence of multiple parties and established a parliamentary form of government. Unlike our system in which anyone could declare themselves to be a Republican or Democrat and run for any office they wished using that label, they designed electoral systems in which political parties themselves selected who could run for which office representing their party. As a result, European political parties gained greater party loyalty and control over those being elected. In addition, the winner of an election is decided according to the proportion of the popular vote obtained by each party. The legislature is organized by the party gaining a majority within the legislature or the party that can cobble together a coalition with another party or parties to create a majority within the legislative branch. Party discipline provides greater assurance that the party's platform used for the election is likely to be enacted, since a defeat on any major piece of legislature might require a new national election. Since the national chief executive (prime minister) is selected by the majority party in the legislature, there is political party unity between the executive and legislative branches. A new national election means that executive and legislative branches both face potential defeat at the polls. Because one party (or party coalition) controls both the executive and legislative branches, there is no excuse for not implementing the policies that the majority political party advocated during the election. Rather than dividing power, parliamentary democracies made elections more consequential for policy adoption.

Our two-party system has evolved over time. Some parties have disappeared, some have changed philosophically, and new ones have emerged. While there are multiple U.S. parties at the national and state levels, the Republican and Democratic parties dominate due to the winner-take-all elections whereby the candidate winning a plurality is elected from an electoral district. Third-party candidates generally further divide the vote, allowing one of the dominant parties to win with a plurality. The Libertarian Party, Green Party, and Constitution Party are the best known of the minor political parties that run candidates for national, state, and local elections. However, not all states recognize them, while the Republican and Democratic parties are recognized in all states, the District of Columbia, the Commonwealth of Puerto Rico, and voting-eligible territories.

Each party will take positions on issues of the day that they perceive will gain them members/voters. Winning elections is a political party's primary focus. There are states where the same party wins consistently and states in which elections are highly contested with the winning party going back and forth between the two. Some state parties have runoff elections if a candidate does not gain a majority in the primary election. If a political party is not the dominant party, it may try to accommodate its positions to attract independent voters and/or a segment of the other political party. If it is the dominant political party, it has less of an incentive to accommodate other political opinions.

In conjunction with scope and bias, some parties will nominate their candidates by using a political convention or caucus and others might use a primary election or some combination. Some states may allow only voters registered as party members to vote in their primary. Others will allow nonaligned (Independent) voters to participate in their primary elections if they change their registration. After voting in the primary, the voter is then allowed to change their registration back to being an Independent or member of another party. Voters identifying with one political party may strategically change their party registrations for a primary election to vote for the other party's least electable candidate in the general election.

In the general election, some state electoral systems will make it either easy or difficult for a voter to cast a straight party line vote. Jurisdictions with a dominant political party may favor straight-line party voting, assuring that all their candidates down the ticket receive votes. Consequently, there may be one box or one lever to select all the candidates from that party for each political office. More contested states may require the voter to check each box or pull each lever to encourage voters to cross party lines. Some people disparage a straight party vote as not being an informed vote. However, unless the voter is knowledgeable about each individual candidate's qualifications and political positions on important issues, a straight-line party vote may be an intelligent vote, as long as the candidates share the same cluster of values as their political party. However, there is no guarantee that any candidate will agree with all or even major elements of the party's platform. Some party nominees may promote the fact that they will reach across party lines or be a maverick within their own party. Strict party loyalty is not always a positive for winning elections in the United States, especially when Independent voters are a significant part of the voting population.

During the late 19th century progressive era in American politics, there was a "good government movement" to encourage nonpartisan elections at the local level. This is reflected in the oft-quoted statement that "there is not a Republican or Democratic way to fix potholes." This push for nonpartisan election was part of a reaction to the rise of city bosses and party patronage. The good government movement also promoted an increase in the professionalization of local administration and civil service reforms. Even where elections are nonpartisan, most people running for local office have a history of political party involvement that can be easily identified or have held policy positions that cluster with one political party.

While there may be no Republican or Democratic way to fix potholes in the streets, the decisions to fix potholes versus investing in public transportation or to devote more resources to public education versus charter schools do indeed reflect value divisions along political party lines.

The federal electoral system in the United States is run by the states with some federal oversight. The Voting Rights Act of 1965 was an attempt to overcome legal barriers enacted by some state and local governments that made it difficult for African Americans to exercise their right to vote as guaranteed by the 15th Amendment.[6] In a 5-4 ideologically divided vote in *Shelby County v. Holder* (2013), the USSC ruled that Section 4(b) of the Voting Rights Act was unconstitutional; that section required that nine states and some counties and municipalities with historic discriminatory election laws had to receive court or U.S. Justice Department clearance for any changes to their election laws. The Court's majority opinion maintained that the country had changed since 1965 (noting the election of President Obama) and that if Congress wanted to regulate state election laws, it needed to use contemporary data. A deadlocked Congress meant no legislation would be forthcoming. The Voting Rights Act of 1965 was weakened further by another USSC decision in 2021 involving two Arizona election laws, one invalidating votes of ballots cast in the wrong voting precinct and another outlawing the collection of mail-in ballots (*Brnovich v. Democratic National Committee*, 2021). The issue involved whether these laws violated Section 2 of the Voting Rights Act of 1965. The court ruled that voter fraud was a legitimate state concern (the U.S. Court of Appeals ruled that there was no record of voter fraud in Arizona) and that the laws were not discriminatory (the U.S. Court of Appeals pointed to evidence that the two provisions would have a discriminatory impact on minorities).

The USSC case of *Moore v. Harper* (pending) is to be decided by the USSC in its 2022 to 2023 term. The case involves gerrymandering in the state of North Carolina. The North Carolina Supreme Court ruled that the Republican legislature's proposed election districts were unfairly gerrymandered based on the state's constitution. The issue before the Court is whether "the independent state legislature doctrine" (which has never been recognized by the USSC) should now be adopted. It would allow only state legislatures to have regulatory jurisdiction over federal elections. The USSC has already ruled that federal courts cannot regulate gerrymandering (*Rucho v. Common Cause*, 2019). This doctrine would prohibit any state court from reviewing the state legislature's regulation of elections even if it was authorized by the state's constitution. The debate over federal oversight of elections remains a contentious policy issue.

INCREMENTALISM

Another descriptor of our political process is incrementalism. *Incrementalism* refers to the tendency that public policy will change by small increments from the existing policy. Incrementalism is both descriptive of how things are done and prescriptive as to how policy making should be done. One makes step-by-step small

---

6 Amendment XV (1870): "The right of citizens of the United States to vote shall not be denied or abridged by the United States or by any State on account of race, color, or previous condition of servitude."

changes to improve policy outcomes rather than dramatic shifts. One advantage of incrementalism for a policy is that it can be more easily implemented since there has already been past agreement on it. One can use the existing bureaucratic structure to nudge the policy in one direction or another. Incrementalism is frequently used to describe how public budgets (the monetization of public values) are put together. Rather than calculating a budget from scratch each year (zero-based budgeting), incrementalism uses the existing budget and makes modest increases or decreases for various line items.

Incrementalism, of course, has its bias in terms of protecting the status quo, but it also provides stability and predictability. Another advantage of incrementalism is that if a policy turns out to be detrimental, it can be more easily reversed. If a policy is incremental, it is also less likely to create new or stimulate existing concentrated interests. However, incrementalism overlooks the fact that social problems may not increase incrementally, and a more drastic action may be needed to solve the problem rather than merely prolong the problem. Since incrementalism tends to reflect the status quo, correcting a past policy that may have imposed inequitable burdens on specific populations may warrant more drastic action. Over time, incrementalism might lead to excessive funding of unneeded programs that are being incrementally protected by the concentrated interests that benefit by its existence or expansion. Meanwhile, new problems not covered by past budgets (e.g., opioid addiction) may remain underfunded until a crisis emerges. Few political entities have a climate change budget item or have developed climate change policies that adequately address the threat to national, state, and community infrastructures. As we have experienced, an economic collapse or the spread of a pandemic may call for a drastic alteration of public policy and/or expenditures. Incrementalism remains a much-used descriptor of the American policy process at national, state, and local levels.

U.S. POLITICAL PROCESS DEFINED

So how should we describe the political process in the United States? Since there is a federal government, 50 states, the District of Columbia, and five territories, plus thousands of county and local governments, no one descriptor fits them all. Each of these political entities have their own institutional and policy process characteristics that make them unique. The one that we will use for the United States is that the *public policy process involves the strategic mobilization of organized factions competing for the authoritative allocation of values and resources of that society.* This incorporates the importance of multiple social values competing in different arenas such as schools, workplaces, various institutional arenas, municipal/state governments, and other organizational entities. While not all will agree with any given policy, there is the need for an authoritative decision to be made. Since a decision needs to be made, there will be a competition for one set of values to prevail over another. This description also refers to the importance of the ability of factions to organize and use critical resources to target the policy process as described by democratic pluralism. It reflects the importance of factions strategically leveraging scope and bias, organizational resources, and lobbying power to tilt the decision-making process in their favor. It indirectly implies that those that are not organized will be at a disadvantage in the policy-making process. We will examine these elements as we work through the paradigm of the policy process.

SUMMARY

In this chapter we have explored some general principles of the iterative political process. Most people refer to the United States as a democracy. However, it is important to distinguish between a procedural democracy (where the majority rules) and a constitutional democracy where the constitution places restraints on majority rule. The United States is a republic where the supreme power rests with the people and a constitutional democracy where there are limits on the majority rule. Through time, procedural democratic elements have been added to parts of the political process.

We noted the importance of the scope of decision-making as a means of gaining advantage by expanding or limiting scope. We discussed the importance of factions, how the two-party system evolved in the United States, and how the lack of party discipline and "winner-takes-all" elections impact the legislative process. We paid special attention to voting rights and the state legislatures' control of national elections. Finally, we discussed both incrementalism and democratic pluralism as important descriptors of the U.S. political process. We ended by describing the U.S. political process as involving the strategic mobilization of organized factions in competing for the authoritative allocation of values and resources of that society. The next chapter will walk you through the U.S. political maze.

DISCUSSION QUESTIONS

- What are the strengths and weaknesses of incrementalism?
- Given the First Amendment, to what extent and how should lobbying be regulated in the United States?
- Elections have become a controversial issue in American politics. Should there be modifications to the electoral system?
- What are the strengths and weaknesses of democratic pluralism?
- How much do Americans value democracy?

KEY TERMS

AstroTurf organizations
constitutional democracy
democratic pluralism
factions
incrementalism
lobbying
Moore v. Harper (pending)
policy wheel

procedural democracy
Rucho v. Common Cause (2019)
scope and bias
Shelby County v. Holder (2013)
U.S. political process
Voting Rights Act of 1965
winner-take-all elections

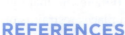

A robust set of instructor resources designed to supplement this text is located at http://connect.springerpub.com/content/book/978-0-8261-8543-3. Qualifying instructors may request access by emailing textbook@springerpub.com.

REFERENCES

Bacchi, C. (2016). Problematizations in health policy. *SAGE Open, 6*(2). https://doi.org/10.1177/2158244016653986

Bachrach, P., & Baratz, M. S. (1962). Two faces of power. *American Political Science Review, 56*(4), 947–952. https://doi.org/10.2307/1952796

Baumgartner, F. R., & Jones, B. D. (1991). Agenda dynamics and policy subsystems. *The Journal of Politics, 53*(4), 1044–1074. https://doi.org/10.2307/2131866

Brennan Center for Justice. (2021, October 4). *Voting laws roundup: October 2021.* https://www.brennancenter.org/our-work/research-reports/voting-laws-roundup-october-2021

Brnovich v. Democratic National Committee, 594 U.S. __ (2021). https://www.supremecourt.gov/opinions/20pdf/19-1257_g204.pdf

Browne, A. J., Varcoe, C., Lavoie, J., Smye, V., Wong, S. T., Krause, M., Tu, D., Godwin, O., Khan, K., & Fridkin, A. (2016). Enhancing health care equity with Indigenous populations: Evidence-based strategies from an ethnographic study. *BMC Health Services Research, 16*(1), Article 544. https://doi.org/10.1186/s12913-016-1707-9

Coveney, J. (2008). Analyzing public health policy: Three approaches. *Health Promotion Practice, 11*(4), 515–521. https://doi.org/10.1177/1524839908318831

Dahl, R. A. (1970). *Modern political analysis.* Prentice-Hall.

Feehery, J. (2019, February 11). *Feehery: Lessons learned from John Dingell.* The Hill. https://thehill.com/opinion/campaign/429509-feehery-lessons-learned-from-john-dingell

The Gilder Lehrman Institute of American History. (n.d.). *The doctrine of discovery, 1493.* https://www.gilderlehrman.org/history-resources/spotlight-primary-source/doctrine-discovery-1493

Hamilton, A., Madison, J., & Jay, J. (1961). *The federalist papers* (C. Rossiter, Ed.). The New American Library of World Literature.

Kingdon, J. W. (2003). *Agendas, alternatives, and public policies.* Longman.

Lasswell, H. (1971). Economies, political science, and law. *Annals of the New York Academy of Sciences, 184*(1), 329–348. https://doi.org/10.1111/j.1749-6632.1971.tb41336.x

Longest, B. B. (1998). *Health policymaking in the United States.* Health Administration Press.

Moore v. Harper, Docket 21–1271 (pending). https://www.supremecourt.gov/docket/docketfiles/html/public/21-1271.html

Mulcahy, A. W. (2021, January 28). *Prescription drug prices in the United States are 2.56 times those in other countries.* Rand Corporation. https://www.rand.org/news/press/2021/01/28.html

Nguyen, N. H., Subhan, F. B., Williams, K., & Chan, C. B. (2020). Barriers and mitigating strategies to healthcare access in Indigenous communities of Canada: A narrative review. *Healthcare, 8*(2), Article 112. https://doi.org/10.3390/healthcare8020112

Rucho v. Common Cause, 588 U.S. ___ (2019). https://www.supremecourt.gov/opinions/18pdf/18-422_9ol1.pdf

Sabatier, P. A., & Jenkins-Smith, H. C. (1993). *Policy change and learning: An advocacy coalition approach (theoretical lenses on public policy).* Westview Press.

Schattschneider, E. E. (1960). *The semisovereign people: A realist's view of democracy in America.* Holt, Rinehart, and Winston.

Shelby County v. Holder, 570 U.S. 529 (2013). https://supreme.justia.com/cases/federal/us/570/529

United Nations Department of Economic and Social Affairs. (2012, June 1). *Impact of the 'doctrine of discovery' on Indigenous peoples.* https://www.un.org/en/development/desa/newsletter/desanews/dialogue/2012/06/3801.html

CHAPTER 5

THE AMERICAN MAZE

This chapter walks you through the federal legislative process as to how a bill proposed by an individual member of Congress makes its way into becoming a law of the United States. We also cover critical elements of the policy process that follow the formal signature by the President. We describe how you can access various documents during this policy-making process. Next, we turn to the U.S. Supreme Court (USSC) and describe how cases come before the Court and the formal process used in reaching and announcing majority and minority decisions of the Court.

LEARNING OBJECTIVES

Be able to:

- Describe the importance of committees within the legislative process.
- Delineate the different roles of committees (e.g., Ways and Means and Rules) in the House of Representatives.
- Describe the differences between deliberations in the House of Representatives and the Senate.
- Describe the process one can use to obtain copies of committee reports, laws, and rules and regulations of the United States.
- Discuss the importance of the filibuster, cloture, and the Omnibus Budget Reconciliation Act.
- Delineate between the significance of executive orders and signing statements.
- Explain the importance of the Administrative Procedures Act and writing rules and regulations.
- Describe which federal cases make it to the USSC and the process used in deciding and announcing decisions of the Court.

THE LEGISLATIVE PROCESS

With few exceptions, the legislative process in the United States is primarily driven by rules and procedures developed by each branch of Congress and/or the two political parties. The party holding the majority of members in each chamber adopts rules and procedures that are continued by tradition from one Congress to the next. As indicated previously, there have been significant changes such as the Hastert Rule or the changes in the Senate's filibuster rules that have had major policy impacts. Some legislators learn the intricacies of these rules and become adept at using them to their advantage. Continually refer to **Figure 5.1** as we walk you through this process.

FIGURE 5.1 From bill to law: stages of the legislative process.

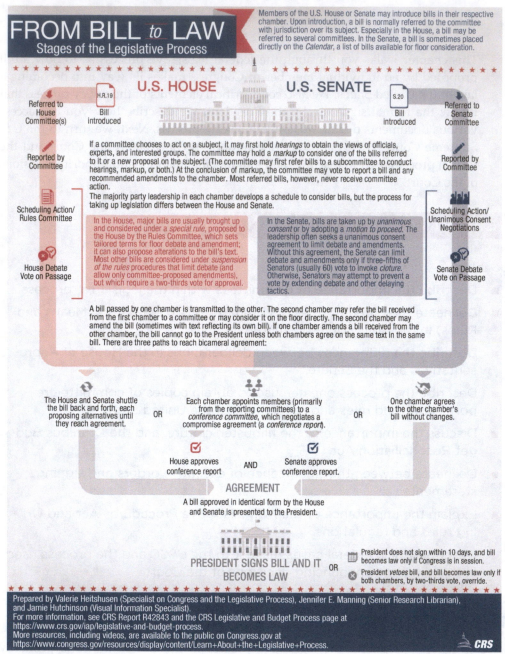

Source: Prepared by Heitshusen, V., Manning, J. E., & Hutchinson, J. *From bill to law: Stages of the legislative process.* https://www.crs.gov/iap/legislative-and-budget-process

Each party will caucus its members separately and select leaders to fill positions such as the Speaker of the House or the Majority Leader in the Senate. These are then voted upon respectively by their respective chamber along party lines. The President of the Senate is the Vice President of the United States, who normally does not attend meetings of the Senate. However, the Vice President can vote if there is a tie vote among the Senators. With the Senate of the 117th Congress split 50-50, the role of the Vice President's vote was critical for individual actions. Congresses are numbered consecutively from the First Congress in 1789; each Congress has two sessions (1st Session for the first year and 2nd Session for the second year). The Congress meeting in January 2022 following the 2021 election was the 118th Congress, 1st Session. The Speaker of the House is constitutionally third in line (following the Vice President of the United States) in succession should the president die or be declared incapacitated.[1]

Additional party leadership positions are selected by each party caucus. There are assistants to the respective leaders of both parties which are typically called whips since their primary function is to enforce party loyalty during votes on bills or procedures. Party leadership is also responsible for appointing their members to various House and Senate standing and special or select committees. By tradition, the names and jurisdictions of these standing committees continue from one Congress to the next. Although not common, committee names and/or jurisdictions can be altered by an incoming majority party. The political party holding a majority in each chamber holds a majority of seats on each of the standing committees of that chamber for the duration of that Congress.

All congressional committees are not perceived equally. Some committees have more national visibility or prestige while others are more desirable for a member of Congress due to its policy jurisdiction that is important for their congressional district. A member of Congress from a district with major military bases may try to position themselves on a Defense, Armed Services, or Appropriations Committee to support legislation favoring their district's constituents. A member of Congress from a rural district may try to get a seat on the Agriculture Committee to influence federal agricultural policy. Members of Congress serve on multiple committees. Those interested in running for president will typically attempt to gain a seat on a committee involving foreign relations or national security to bolster their perceived experience in foreign policy.

There are two generic types of legislative committees in both chambers: (1) Authorization committees deal with substance of bills, and (2) budget and appropriation committees allocate money to agencies and programs. Both are important for any substantive policy area. It is possible for an authorization bill to pass Congress and be signed by the president, but with no or insufficient money having been appropriated by the various appropriate or budget committees. Budget committees can also specify that an agency cannot spend its money on a particular activity. In requesting committee assignments, a member of Congress interested in public health may opt for an appointment on a health authorizing committee and/or an appropriations committee dealing with health. If there is no major piece of authorizing legislation expected during a particular Congress, it may be more important to be on a budget or appropriation committee than the authorizing

---

1 The 25th Amendment, which was adopted in 1967, describes the procedures to be used if the president is deemed to be incapacitated.

committee. However, both types of committees are critical for the implementation of any policy.

A Senator or member of the House of Representatives gains seniority based on the length of service in both Congress and on committees. Seniority in Congress and seniority on a particular committee are important (but not the sole) determinants of gaining desired committee assignments. Party leadership will attempt to balance the members' interests with the party's interests. Rewarding party loyalty or a member winning a critical state/house district may influence committee assignments. Members can request a move to other committees from one Congress to next, but they may drop in seniority on the new committee. Chairs or the ranking minority chairs (those who will become committee chairs with a change in that chamber's majority party) seldom give up their positions. The majority party's most senior member normally becomes the chair of that committee for the duration of that session of Congress, but there are exceptions.

Members who have been elected for multiple terms acquire substantive expertise on policy areas under the committee's jurisdiction. As a result, states that are traditionally one-party-dominated states tend to have representatives and/or senators with greater seniority and therefore tend to have greater policy influence. In running for re-election, members of Congress will frequently point to their seniority on a committee of importance to their district as an argument for their re-election. Losing a senior member on a critical committee can be a significant loss for a district or state. Some states have enacted term limits to discourage "professional politicians," but one of the costs of such a policy is the state's loss of the benefits of seniority.

Staff

The largest number of people within the U.S. Congress are nonelected staff. Members of the House and the Senate are each given money to hire multiple personal staff. A chief of staff will be named to hire and coordinate the other staff. Another significant role of the chief of staff is controlling access to that member of Congress. Personal congressional staff are generally divided into two groups. One set of personal staff is physically located in the multiple offices within that member's district or state. These staff workers deal with constituent services (e.g., helping a constituent receive a missing Social Security check, assisting in the appeal of a denial of benefits, helping a local business seek relief from a particular federal regulation, answering a constituent's letter about the Congress member's position on a piece of legislation, attending a ribbon-cutting ceremony or parade within the district in the absence of member of Congress, or attending a local political event along with the member of Congress). These constituent services are important for building a base of loyal voter support for re-election.

The second set of personal staff focuses on policy topics based on the congressional member's committee assignments. Some congressional members may want a staff person with expertise in public health, military hardware, public housing, agriculture, and so forth. These staff workers tend to be based in the member's office in Washington, DC, and come with some substantive policy background. Staff may move around depending on the time of year (election season) and some staff may move permanently from a district office to Washington, DC. Staff in

Washington, DC, will meet with constituents visiting the capital and provide a tour of the capitol or other assistance. While there are 535 members of Congress, there are approximately 11,000 staff workers for both the House and Senate members in Washington, DC, and scattered in district offices throughout the United States.

In addition, there is staff hired for each of the various congressional standing, joint, and special committees. The chair of a committee not only has available their personal staff but also the staff of the committee which they chair. These people tend to have substantive expertise in issues covered by the committee. Both parties will have committee staffs. There are approximately 2,500 committee staff employees. In addition, there are approximately 450 staff hired by the leadership of both parties for both houses. There are also approximately 1,400 staff workers who are officers of the House or Senate who perform functional duties for the daily operation of each chamber.

There are also special units within Congress that perform nonpartisan work. For example, the Government Accounting Office, the Congressional Research Office, the Congressional Budget Office, the Office of Technical Assessment, the Architect of the Capitol, and the U.S. Capitol Police make up an additional 7,000 people on the congressional payroll. Congress is not a small organization.

Some constituents seeking access to a member of Congress for the first time are frequently discouraged by being shuffled off to a staff member rather than meeting their elected representative or senator. However, what that constituent may not realize is that the person who probably knows the most about the topic or can make something happen is generally the staff member. Even if one does gain a meeting with the senator or representative, there is generally a staff member present who will follow up on any needed action. Congressional staff network with other staff in both legislative and administrative offices. A staff member can range from someone who has worked for multiple members of Congress over many years to a newly graduated college student who worked on the member's campaign. Members of Congress become known for the quality of their staff.

All staff quickly learn to network with other congressional staff and bureaucrats within numerous executive departments of interest to the member of Congress. They learn the idiosyncrasies of other senators and representatives as well as the likes and dislikes of their staffs. They learn who is married to whom and where spouses work within DC whether it be a law firm, a nonprofit interest group, defense contractor, and so forth. They learn who graduated from which schools and what alumni contacts might be useful. Any information about a person that can provide access or leverage becomes important. Receptions held in congressional office buildings become major points of contact, as well as free hors d'oeuvres for underpaid staff. Bars and restaurants around Washington, DC, as well as the recreational fields by the Potomac River are populated with staff members who are actively networking.

The staffs hired by the various standing committees of each chamber are critical in the legislative process. These staffs become highly specialized about a particular policy area such as Medicare, Patient Protection and Affordable Care Act (PPACA, 2010), public health, insurance, taxation, and so forth. They become the key players in policy development, because they are the ones who may write the legislation and negotiate compromises with other staff and lobbyists to gain support for its passage.

Experienced lobbyists work with the staff members who are critical for their employer's concerns. Staff members attend congressional committee hearings and provide support for their member of Congress. They generally sit directly behind their member of Congress during the hearings to provide them with any written or verbal information that may be needed. After spending years in Congress as a staff person engaged in writing legislation and negotiating with power brokers, these people can gain lucrative positions with consulting companies, think tanks, or lobbying firms.

At the state level, legislative staffing levels and expertise can vary greatly from state to state. During the 1960s and 1970s there was a national effort to increase the professionalization of state legislatures. A few large states such as California and New York may have full-time legislators with professional staff that somewhat mirror those of Congress. Other states rely upon part-time legislators (citizen legislators) with minimum staff assistance. For example, New Hampshire is famous for its House of Representatives which is composed of 400 members, each member representing around 3,300 citizens. Consequently, many communities will have multiple representatives. Other than a special license plate, the ability to go through state highway tolls for free, a salary of $200 for the biennium (set in 1889), and mileage for 145 legislative days, each legislator is pretty much on their own. New Hampshire legislative committees are assigned clerks and there is a legislative office to assist a member in writing legislation, but individual legislators have neither an office nor staff. This arrangement, of course, creates a bias in terms of who can afford to be a state legislator, the political influence of any one legislator, and the power of leadership. In contrast, New Hampshire's senate has 24 members, each receiving the same benefit package. Since bills must pass both houses, a lobbyist bent on defeating legislation can focus on 12 of the 24 senators and/or chairs of senate committees rather than the 400 members of the house.

A state capital may have one or two legal firms that have close political contacts and become the major source of lobbying. Since there may be no nonpartisan equivalent of the U.S. Government Accounting Office, the Congressional Research Office, or the Congressional Budget Office, lobbying becomes an important source of information. It is important for any policy analyst to understand the informal networks that exist and who is critical for building legislative support for any specific policy. These networks and people will vary depending upon the issue; a particular staff person, committee chair, or law firm may be critical for one issue but not another.

Legislative Committees

Not all congressional committees are equal. Standing committees tend to exist from one Congress to the next. Special or select committees tend to have a shorter duration. Revenue and expenditure committees generally are attractive committee assignment since the budget reflects the states' relative values and rewards certain factions over others. Gaining a seat on one of the appropriations committees can be important for supporting federal projects in one's district or getting increased price subsidies for farm products. This can be used to advantage for upcoming elections.

There are more committees in the House than in the Senate, and House committees tend to be larger due to the number of members of Congress that need to be accommodated. However, each house has one or more committees that cover any given policy area. See Table 5.1. Notice that there is no House standing committee

TABLE 5.1 CONGRESSIONAL COMMITTEES

HOUSE	SENATE
Agriculture	Agriculture, Nutrition, and Forestry
Appropriations	Appropriations
Armed Services	Armed Services
Budget	Banking, Housing, and Urban Affairs
Education and Labor	Budget
Energy and Commerce	Commerce, Science, and Transportation
Ethics	Energy and Natural Resources
Financial Services	Environment and Public Works
Foreign Affairs	Finance
Homeland Security	Foreign Relations
House Administration	Health, Education, Labor, and Pensions
Judiciary	Homeland Security and Governmental Affairs
Natural Resources	Judiciary
Oversight and Reform	Rules and Administration
Rules	Small Business and Entrepreneurship
Science, Space, and Technology	Veterans Affairs
Small Business	
Transportation and Infrastructure	
Veterans Affairs	
Ways and Means	

on either health or public health. Given the breadth of public health, there are several committees that have jurisdiction over certain aspects of public health. Since many major health/medical legislative bills involve amending the Social Security Act and/or taxes, the House Ways and Means Committee has traditionally taken jurisdiction of major health bills such as Medicare, PPACA, and so forth. Since public health is such a broad issue, committees with jurisdictions on agriculture, commerce, education, natural resources, science, technology, and Veteran Affairs policies also become important for public health. For a public health issue, it may be complicated to determine exactly which combination of committees, members of Congress, and staff are important.

Another important role for legislative committees is legislative oversight of the departments/agencies responsible for the executive's implementation of legislation under the committee's jurisdiction. Committees can call members of the president's cabinet and representatives from respective agencies as well as private concerns to testify before them as to how a law is being implemented and whether its implementation is in line with legislative intent or whether additional legislation is needed to fill gaps not covered by the original legislation. Depending upon which party controls each branch of the legislature and the Office of the President, these hearings can be used to either support additional efforts or attack the department/policy. Agencies understand that while oversight hearings cannot force them to make changes, the committee doing the oversight is the same committee from which they need support for additional legislation or future funding.

Introduction of a Policy Proposal

Only a member of Congress can introduce a bill. The Office of the President or a cabinet head must find a willing member of Congress to introduce a bill on its behalf. Since a bill must be approved by both the House and the Senate, sponsors of the bill will look for someone in the other chamber to submit the bill in that chamber. In the House, the member merely places the bill in the *hopper*, a wooden box adjacent to the rostrum on the House floor. The primary sponsor of the bill must officially sign the bill. There may be multiple cosponsors to indicate a broad level of support and potentially bipartisan support within that chamber. In the Senate, there are two ways to introduce legislation. The formal way is for a senator to gain recognition from the presiding officer and announce during the morning hour that they are introducing a bill and then provide a short explanation of its purpose. Since video recordings are now made of congressional sessions, these videos can be distributed to local news outlets for public relations purposes. The videos will focus on the member of Congress since the chamber will likely be relatively empty. However, if any senator objects, the introduction is postponed until the next day. An informal method to introduce legislation in the Senate is just to hand a proposed piece of legislation to one of the Senate clerks.

Once legislation is introduced, it is assigned a number in chronological order, H.R. 1 or S. 1. A low number may indicate that the legislation proposal is a priority of party leadership. Each bill is then assigned to one or more committees depending on the content of the bill. The committee assignment for legislation referral is normally routine and done by the House or Senate parliamentarian. The leadership of the majority party can assign controversial bills to either a favorable or unfavorable committee or split a bill and give it to multiple committees.

Once assigned to a committee, the chair of that committee can decide to assign it to a subcommittee or assign it to the whole committee. Committees and subcommittees can be jealous of their policy jurisdiction. If assigned to a subcommittee, the bill must come back to the full committee for a final vote. In the U.S. Congress, there is no requirement that once assigned to the committee, that the committee needs to do anything further with the bill. Committees become a burying ground for most bills. A bill can sit in a committee for the duration of that Congress and if not acted upon, the bill is dead. There are provisions for a discharge petition, forcing the bill out of committee, but it is a rare event due to the number of signatures required and because no member of Congress wants that done to their own committees. A bill blocked at the committee level can be reintroduced in the next Congress.

According to the Constitution all revenue bills must be first introduced in the House of Representatives. By tradition, appropriation bills are also first introduced into the House. Both then move to the Senate for its consideration.

Once in the committee or subcommittee, hearings may be called. A schedule of committee hearings is published in the daily *Congressional Record*. The committee or subcommittee chair is generally in charge of inviting people to testify in support or opposition to the bill. The committee will invite written and oral testimony from federal departments directly impacted by the legislation. Lobbyists will also attempt to submit both written and oral testimony as well as respond to questions from members of the committee. Testimony to the committee is generally stacked depending on the position of the majority party. Personal congressional staff or committee staff are involved in the development of questions asked by committee members. The written and oral testimonies of these meetings are available in public libraries that are designated as federal depository libraries. These 1,100 libraries in the United States have free copies of printings from the U.S. Government Printing Office and generally have a reference librarian who is familiar with the special cataloguing methodology used for government documents. The Hearing Record is a useful source of information regarding various perspectives and data for the proposed legislation and the type of input sought by the committee for its deliberations. You must remember that these hearings and presentations are biased in one way or another.

Once information has been gathered, the committee or subcommittee will hold a mark-up session in which members of the committee revise the bill. If there are substantial additions, the committee can create a "clean bill"; the old bill is then discarded and the bill is given a new number. If this is done at the subcommittee level, its recommendation must go to the full committee for another vote. Committee staff will write a summary of the bill and reasons for supporting it and any proposed amendments. The full committee will then vote on a motion for the bill to be "ordered to be reported." It is always positive to get members of the minority party to vote for the release of the bill. If the bill is contentious, there may be a minority report.

In the House of Representatives, all bills passed by a committee must next go to the House Rules Committee to be given a "rule." Because the House is large, the Rules Committee sets conditions for debate on the House floor. An *open rule* allows any germane amendment to be made by any House member. A *modified open rule* permits only amendments preprinted in the *Congressional Record* and/or puts a time cap on consideration of any proposed amendment. A *structured rule* limits the type of amendments that can be submitted. A *closed rule* limits time allowed for debate and specifies that no amendments can be introduced from the House floor. The type of rule that is assigned by the Rules Committee is likely to influence what the final bill might look like and whether it passes the House or not. The Speaker of the House wants to have a cooperative Rules Committee. Since by tradition the Senate has unfettered debate and amendment rules, it does not have an equivalent rules committee.

Since the exact same bill must pass both houses of Congress, the bill needs to be introduced in the other house, go through the committee process, and then be voted on by that chamber. The announcement in the press that a bill has passed the House, or the Senate should be taken with a grain of salt. Its initial passage by that chamber may be the one most likely to pass it and effective opposition to the law may exist in the other chamber. When one party controls one chamber and the other party controls the other chamber, passage in one may be more symbolic than an indication that the law will be passed by Congress.

After discharge from committees, bills in the House and the Senate are placed on the House Calendar or the Senate's Legislative Calendar. There are multiple calendars in each chamber. For example, the Senate's Executive Calendar schedules votes on presidential appointments and treaties, and so forth. These calendars are controlled in the House by the Speaker and the Majority Leader of the House and in the Senate by the Majority Leader. If the Speaker of the House wants the bill to be debated, it is placed on the Union Calendar of the Committee of the Whole (the entire House of Representatives). The House can then debate and amend it within the limits placed upon it by the Rules Committee. The debate on the floor of the House's Committee of the Whole is guided by the committee chair sponsoring the bill and time is divided equally between supporters and opponents. However, the Committee of the Whole cannot technically pass the bill. After, the Committee of the Whole votes, it reports the bill back to the House. It is then placed on the House Calendar for a formal vote. If it is then passed, it is forwarded to the Senate.

The Senate has a more open process in terms of debate and amendments. A senator can speak indefinitely, and any senator can offer multiple types of amendments. Originally, there was no cloture (ability to cut off debate); it was not introduced until 1917. Cloture is a rule of the Senate regarding debate in the Senate; it is not law. To pass legislation in the Senate it still requires at least a majority (51) of senators. However, to be able to get to vote on passage, debate must be cut off. That is where cloture comes into play. The filibuster is a continuing frustration for the majority party in the Senate since it currently requires 60 votes to break a filibuster by invoking cloture. While the majority party may have 54 senators, it is unusual for the majority party to have 60 or more senators. This gives a minority of senators (all from one party or a bipartisan group of senators) the ability to block legislation. Even if the majority party has the 60 seats, the lack of party discipline may not guarantee that each of its senators will support cloture for a particular bill.

Traditionally, the filibuster rules required that a senator had to physically talk continuously; as a result, it was not frequently used or filibusters that were held had a short duration. One of the most famous filibusters occurred in 1964 with Republican opposition to the Civil Rights Act of 1964. The filibuster on that bill began in April 1964. At that time, cloture required 67 votes and the cooperation of the Republican party. Senators slept on cots off the Senate chamber in case a quorum was called in the middle of the night. On June 10, 1964, Republican Senate Minority Leader Everett Dirksen agreed to help break the filibuster; he delivered 27 Republican votes to create a Democratic/Republican 71-vote majority for cloture. However, breaking the filibuster only meant that debate could continue over multiple amendments offered by senators opposed to the legislation. The Civil Rights Act was finally passed by the Senate on June 19, 1964; it was signed by President Johnson on July 2, 1964, more than 2 months after the filibuster had begun. It is reported that hours after he signed the Civil Rights Act, President

Johnson told his press aide, Bill Moyers, "I think we just delivered the South to the Republican Party for a long time to come" (Allen, 2014, para. 14).

Since then, the Senate cloture rule has been modified several times. The vote needed for cloture for legislation has been reduced from 67 to 60. In addition, the filibuster has also been modified regarding some presidential appointments. In 2013 the Democrats lowered the approval of most presidential appointees to 51 votes, but not for Supreme Court nominees. In 2017 Republicans lowered the approval of Supreme Court nominees to 51 votes. The 60-vote filibuster rule remains in the Senate for most legislation.

While the number of votes needed to break a filibuster has been lowered, the use of the filibuster has increased. As previously mentioned, tradition required that an actual person or persons had to physically speak. However, today the norm is that if any Senator merely announces that they will filibuster a piece of legislation, the bill is considered filibustered, thus requiring 60 votes for that legislation to get to a vote for passage. Now, the threat of a filibuster by one senator is all that it takes to potentially defeat a bill in the Senate. While most filibusters do not receive the same publicity as the 1964 filibuster, they remain effective in killing legislation. The filibuster is merely a rule of the Senate that can be changed by the majority party by 51 votes. However, both parties are cautious to change filibuster rules since each realizes that someday they will be the minority party and will want that ability to frustrate the majority party. In 2022, the Democrats in Congress considered changing the number of votes to pass voting rights legislation, but opposition by two Democratic senators prevented that from happening.

The Senate also has a tradition of using unanimous consent to expedite the normal noncontroversial business of the Senate. Unanimous consent does not mean that the Senate has unanimously agreed to something; it merely means that no senator has officially objected. The presiding officer generally will say, "Without objection, so ordered." The objection to unanimous consent is a tactic to slow things down. With the increase in partisan divide in the Senate, it takes only one senator's objection to delay moving forward.

Due to the importance of having a budget and the contentious nature of taxes, debt, and the federal budget, there is one bill that is exempt from a Senate filibuster. The Omnibus Budget Reconciliation Act (OBRA) is an optional procedure used by Congress to change current law to bring revenue and spending levels into conformity with the annual budget resolution passed by Congress. OBRA was created by the Congressional Budget and Impoundment Control Act, known as the Budget Act of 1974, and first used in 1980. It is not used every year. However, because it has expedited procedures in both the House and the Senate, it has become a major policy vehicle especially if a major proposal does not have the 60 votes for cloture. An OBRA bill can still be vetoed by the president. OBRA was used by Democrats to pass the PPACA in the Senate (see **Breakout Box 2.1**). Not every bill can be attached to OBRA legislation. The nonpartisan parliamentarian of the Senate must rule that the proposed legislation impacts the reconciliation of the budget. OBRA was also used to pass President Biden's *Inflation Reduction Act of 2022*, which included such public health provisions as allowing Medicare to negotiate on the price of certain drugs, cap insulin costs, expand PPACA, and invest in energy and climate change initiatives.

If one house passes a bill and the other fails to act or defeats the bill, the bill is dead. Both houses must pass identical versions of the same legislation; a single word, let alone a different provision, makes them different bills. If both houses pass different versions of the bill, a conference committee is appointed to attempt to resolve the differences. Members of the conference committee tend to be senior members of the House and Senate committees that sponsored the bill within their chamber. The committee members and staff work to resolve any differences. If the difference is over the amount of money to be authorized or appropriated, it is common that the conferees split the difference between the two amounts to get the legislation passed. Something is better than nothing and less is better than more. If the conference committee can reach an agreement on the language of the bill, staff members write a report which then goes back to their respective chambers. Each chamber must then approve the conference committee's report for the legislation to be passed.

If passed by both chambers, the legislation is then forwarded to the Office of the President for signature. The president has 10 days to sign it or allow it to become law without a signature. If Congress has adjourned before the 10 days have expired and the president has not signed it, it is called a pocket veto. The president can also veto the legislation and send it back to Congress with an explanation. If vetoed by the president, Congress can vote to override the veto with a two-thirds vote in each chamber for it to become law. If one chamber fails to override the veto, the legislation is dead. If the legislation is approved by both chambers and signed by the president, the policy process is far from over.

The president can also issue a signing statement, which has been used since the 19th century to comment on the legislation. It has become more frequent since President Ronald Reagan (Library of Congress, n.d.). Signing statements generally indicate how the executive branch interprets the legislation in the hope that the courts will reference the signing statement in any judicial decision regarding the law. Sometimes it indicates that the executive branch does not intend to execute certain provisions of the law. However, those statements do not undermine the validity of the law. The president must veto the legislation for that to happen. Objections have been raised to the increased presidential use of signing statements since they act like a line-item veto, which was ruled unconstitutional by the Supreme Court in *Clinton v. City of New York* (1998). Since 1986, signing statements have been published in *U.S. Code Congressional and Administrative News* (West Group).

RULES AND REGULATIONS

After a bill has been passed and signed into law by the president, it is incorporated into the laws of the United States and is given a new number, which refers to its passage by Congress. This number contains the number of the Congress and then a number indicating the order in which it was passed by that Congress. For example, the PPACA, is Public Law 111-148 because it was the 148th bill passed by the 111th Congress. Authorizing legislation is commonly referred to by its name, an abbreviated name, the major author of the legislation, or its public law number. There is no uniform protocol for naming a piece of legislation. Public Law 111-148 is generally referred to as the Affordable Care Act, PPACA, or Obamacare. Some laws are sometimes referred to solely by their public law number.

In addition, each of the law's various provisions are placed in specific sections of the *United States Code*. There are 59 different titles in the *U.S. Code*. Public health and welfare provisions are in Title 42, which has 151 different chapters within it. The requirement to maintain minimum health insurance coverage under PPACA is in 26 U.S. Code § 5000A. It is in Title 26 rather than Title 42 because this particular provision of PPACA deals with the tax provisions of PPACA. Title 26 of the *U.S. Code* contains laws concerning the Internal Revenue Service. Other provisions of PPACA are in different titles of the *U.S. Code*. The whole of PPACA is available by searching its public law number.

The executive branch is responsible for the administration of federal laws. Because laws tend to be written in broad strokes, the executive branch writes more specific guidance as to how the law will be implemented. Guidelines are issued by an agency of the federal government that provides instructions to people within the bureaucracy in Washington, DC, and the 10 federal regional offices as to how to interpret something or do something. This is done so that the law is interpreted and administered uniformly in each of the 10 federal regions across the country, whether it be in Region 1 serving New England or Region 7 serving Iowa, Kansas, Missouri, and Nebraska. Each region has its headquarters in one of the major cities within that region. All major regulatory and service agencies have offices in the regional headquarters to implement federal law regionally.

Federal agencies, such as the Food and Drug Administration (FDA), Environmental Protection Agency (EPA), Occupational Safety and Health Administration (OSHA), and approximately 50 other federal agencies are called *regulatory* agencies because they are empowered by law to create and enforce regulations. Regulations have the full force of law; a violation of a regulation is equivalent to a violation of the law and subjects violators to penalties such as fines, prohibitions, closures, and so forth. The development of regulations is major focus for lobbying because a change in one word in the regulation can have a major impact on how the law is interpreted and how it will be enforced.

The process of creating a regulation is itself governed by the Administrative Procedures Act (APA; 1946), which prescribes the process that a regulatory agency must follow in writing a regulation. If the regulatory agency deviates from the APA, that regulation can be challenged in court and determined to be invalid due to a violation of the process. Writing a regulation is not an easy task because it requires both an understanding of the substantive area being regulated (e.g., COVID-19, air or water quality, nutrition, pharmaceuticals) as well as an understanding of federal and perhaps state administrative structures that are involved in implementation. Under the APA any new rule must be published as a *proposed rule* in the *Federal Register* at least 30 days prior to it taking effect and provide a set period for interested parties to comment in opposition or support, or to propose changes to the new rule.[2] Depending on the authorizing legislation, some proposed regulations may require one or more public hearings. A notice of public hearings must then be published in the *Federal Register*. Comments can also be submitted in writing to the regulatory agency. After the established period for receiving comments, the agency usually responds to major comments by providing its rationale as to why it has accepted, rejected, or modified those suggestions. The

---

2 The *Federal Register* is published daily and is available in federal depository libraries as well as online at www.federalregister.gov.

regulatory agency then publishes the final rule in the *Federal Register*, in the the Code of Federal Regulations (CFR), and usually on its web page.[3]

There have been two major attempts to control federal regulations through the Congressional Review Act (CRA; 1996) and President Clinton's 1993 Executive Order (EO) No. 12866. The CRA provides a little used procedure by which Congress can overturn a final rule or regulation within 60 days of its enactment or for an incoming Congress to review regulations issued during the last 60 days of the previous Congress.[4] The CRA has mostly been used when there is a change of administrations, and control of Congress. Under EO 12866, all regulations must undergo a detailed cost-benefit analysis. In addition, any regulation with an estimated cost of $100 million or more must have a Regulatory Impact Analysis (RIA) that must be approved by the Office of Management and Budget (OMB) within the Office of the President. All of this takes time. If the administration is opposed to a law, the writing of rules and regulations can be dragged out. Even with the best of intentions, regulations may take months or years before the regulations are finalized and the law enforced.

EXECUTIVE ORDERS

EOs are issued from the Office of the President in the role of the chief executive officer of the federal government. An EO deals with the operation of the executive branch implementing the laws of the land. They are numbered consecutively and continue from one administration to the next unless they are reversed or amended by another EO. They are published in the *Federal Register* shortly after being signed by the president. EOs have the force of law and are codified under Title 3 of the CFR. EOs require no congressional approval, and they cannot be overturned by Congress. Congress can pass legislation to make it difficult to enforce an EO, but only a sitting president can reverse one. Presidential candidates frequently cite what they will do on day 1 of their administration; these actions generally involve issuing an EO since no further approval is required. Although they have the force of law and can have a major impact on how a policy is implemented, EOs are like regulations in that they are not "new law" but only how existing laws will be implemented.

One example that is particularly relevant for public health is the environmental justice EO (Exec. Order No. 12898, 1994) that was issued by President Clinton in 1994 (see **Breakout Box 5.1**). Environmental injustice (EJ) refers to the inequitable distribution of pollution and other environmental burdens on low-income communities and communities of color. EJ refers to: "the fair treatment and meaningful involvement of all people regardless of race, color, national origin, or income, with respect to the development, implementation, and enforcement of environmental laws, regulations, and policies" (U.S. EPA, 2022). Following a landmark report entitled *Toxic Wastes and Race in the United States* (Mascarenhas et al., 2021; United Church of Christ Commission for Racial Justice, 1987), more recent studies have documented that African Americans continued to be exposed to 38% more polluted air than White Americans and were 75% more likely to live in communities affected by noise, odors, traffic, and chemical emissions (Perls, 2020).

---

3 Code of Federal Regulations, www.govinfo.gov.
4 Federal regulatory agencies must submit a copy to both houses of Congress and the General Accounting Office before the rules can take effect.

Despite the signing of EO 12898, critics contend that it has been largely ineffective. This is because there is no actual federal law governing EJ, nor is there an agency such as the EPA that has the authority to mandate remedies addressing EJ concerns. President Biden has attempted to renew focus on EJ issues, as illustrated by actions taken during his first week in office. These actions included launching a "whole of government" effort to achieve environmental, public health, and climate goals. President Biden also signed several new EOs, including EO 13990 (2021), Protecting Public Health and the Environment and Restoring Science to Tackle the Climate Crisis (Public Health and the Environment EO) and EO 14008 (2021) on Tackling the Climate Crisis at Home and Abroad (Climate Crisis EO). President Biden began to integrate equity and racial justice concerns throughout the federal government (Exec. Order No. 13985, 2021), which ensures scientific integrity and science-based decision-making (Vizcarra & Perls, 2021). Despite these efforts, the concern remains that there is no federal EJ law. Notably, several states have passed their own EJ statutes (National Conference of State Legislatures, 2022).

Breakout Box 5.1

ENVIRONMENTAL JUSTICE EXECUTIVE ORDER

In 1994, President Clinton issued EO 12898—Federal Actions to Address EJ in Minority Populations and Low-Income Populations. The purpose of the EO was to focus federal attention on the environmental and public health effects of federal actions on minority and low-income populations with the goal of achieving environmental protection for all communities.

Specifically, the EPA states that EO 12898 directs federal agencies to:

- Identify and address the disproportionately high and adverse human health or environmental effects of their actions on minority and low-income populations, to the greatest extent practicable and permitted by law.
- Develop a strategy for implementing environmental justice.
- Promote nondiscrimination in federal programs that affect human health and the environment, as well as provide minority and low-income communities access to public information and public participation.

In addition, the EO established an Interagency Working Group (IWG) on EJ chaired by the EPA Administrator and comprised of the heads of 11 departments or agencies and several White House offices (U.S. EPA, 2021). Examples and resources pertaining to environmental justice can be found in the following references (Harvard Law School, n.d.; National Council of State Legislatures, n.d.; U.S. EPA, 2022).

References

Exec. Order No. 12898. 59 Fed. Reg. 7629 (February 16, 1994). https://www.archives.gov/files/federal-register/executive-orders/pdf/12898.pdf

Harvard Law School. (n.d.). *Federal environmental justice tracker*. https://eelp.law.harvard.edu/ejtracker

National Council of State Legislatures. (n.d.). *State and federal environmental justice efforts.* https://www.ncsl.org/research/environment-and-natural-resources/state-and-federal-efforts-to-advance-environmental-justice.aspx

U.S. Environmental Protection Agency. (2022, April 1). *EJScreen: Environmental justice screening and mapping tool.* https://www.epa.gov/ejscreen

U.S. Environmental Protection Agency. (2021, September 28). *Summary of Executive Order 12898—Federal actions to address environmental justice in minority populations and low-income populations.* https://www.epa.gov/laws-regulations/summary-executive-order-12898-federal-actions-address-environmental-justice

If you think that this political process is complicated and time consuming, you are right. However, you must remember that it was intended to be so. The Founding Fathers and subsequent politicians never intended to create a speedy decision-making machine. However, from an office holder's or policy advocates' perspective, the policy process can be frustrating in that from the time a bill is proposed to the time it is implemented to the time its impact can be observed, it is likely to take multiple years. In addition, a bill-signing ceremony does not end the policy process. Frequently, the politician originating the proposal may no longer be in office when the outcomes of the legislation become obvious. Indeed, a succeeding administration may take credit for what was passed before it came into office. Even politicians who voted in opposition to legislation such as PPACA may later take credit for the legislation's benefits to their constituents. Regulations issued by a subsequent administration can hobble or speed up the implementation of a previously passed law, and likewise, it takes time to reverse a previous administration's policies. Policy making is a long game.

THE JUDICIARY

The judiciary is an important aspect of the political structure. However, it is supposed to be nonpartisan in its interpretation of the law. While the courts cannot make law, they certainly make policy. As previously discussed, the USSC changed policy regarding the population size of the state's electoral districts by a series of judicial decisions. The USCC has allowed gerrymandering of legislative districts. *Rucho v. Common Cause* (2019) was a 5-4 USSC decision ruling that gerrymandering was a political and not a justiciable question and that unlike *Baker v. Carr* (1962), the Court could find no objective way to determine when a state had gone too far for redistricting to be gerrymandering.[5] Both those actions, one claiming judicial reviewability and one claiming nonjusticiability, have had a tremendous impact on election policy.

The judiciary has been an important resource for overturning both federal and state statues. The unanimous USSC decision in *Brown v. the Board of Education of Topeka* (1954) overturned a previous judicial policy of allowing "separate but

---

5 *Rucho v. Common Cause*: The decision was 5-4 with Chief Justice Roberts writing the majority decision with Justices Thomas, Alito, Gorsuch, and Kavanaugh joining. Justice Kagan wrote a dissenting opinion and was joined by Justices Ginsburg, Breyer, and Sotomayor. The suit arose from voters in both North Carolina and Maryland, reflecting perceived Republican and Democratic gerrymandering.

equal" services and thereby invalidated state racial segregation laws.[6] While this was followed by the Civil Rights Act of 1964, the USSC laid the foundation for a major change in U.S. public policy regarding the segregation of races. The same is true for the right to interracial marriage (*Loving v. Virginia*, 1967) and marriage for same-sex couples (*Obergefell v. Hodges*, 2015). The Court is also known for sometimes telegraphing potential congressional actions that it might consider to be appropriate to overcome legal difficulties.

The judicial branch is also an important source for a *writ of mandamus*, a court order forcing the government to perform a specific act which that body is obliged to do under the law. Lawsuits brought by nonprofit organizations or citizen groups in policy areas such as education, mental health, the environment, prisons, voting rights, and consumer rights have led to changes in policies or forced federal/state governments to implement laws differently. Suits filed in the 1960s claiming that states were unconstitutionally denying mentally ill patients humane treatment by institutionalizing them without appropriate therapy led to a wholesale redesign of the mental health infrastructure in the United States. Less use of institutionalization and increased use of outpatient and community-based mental health services were the results of such lawsuits. Civil lawsuits attempting to protect natural resources or endangered species by forcing governmental agencies such as the U.S. Forest Service to enforce existing laws designed to protect the environment or endangered species have also had major policy impacts.

It is important to remember that while citizens have access to both federal and state courts, these systems are separate, and litigants have different procedures and rights under each. Courts, especially the federal courts, have been critical in affirming civil rights for minority groups, Blacks, Hispanics, Asians, and LGBTQ+ populations in the United States. Some of these rulings that were initially contentious have gained popular support, while others remain contentious. Since courts tend to rely on *stare decisis*, making a change in policy through the courts may take many years and be very costly as cases work their way through the appellate courts.

Because most individuals cannot afford the expense of extensive litigation, policy groups with resources sometimes sign on to a particular case or file an amicus brief and take it to an appellate court. An amicus brief (*amicus curiae*, friend of the court) is generally filed by business or trade associations, unions, government, and nonprofit organizations in support of one of the litigants in a civil lawsuit. The federal court system is divided into 13 appellate circuits with multiple district federal courts in each circuit. Each of these circuits has a different balance of the judges regarding their judicial philosophical leanings. The Ninth Circuit Court of Appeals covering states on the West Coast tends to have a more liberal reputation, while the Fifth Circuit Court of Appeals covering Texas, Louisiana, and Alabama has a more conservative reputation. As a result, where a federal lawsuit is initially filed may well heavily influence its outcome, by laying the legal grounds. This

---

6 *Brown v. Board of Education of Topeka* (1954) was a landmark decision of the U.S. Supreme Court in which the Court ruled that U.S. state laws establishing racial segregation in public schools are unconstitutional, even if the segregated schools are otherwise equal in quality. It was handed down on May 17, 1954. The Court's unanimous decision stated that "separate educational facilities are inherently unequal" and therefore violate the Equal Protection Clause of the 14th Amendment of the U.S. Constitution.

is especially important if the USSC refuses to grant a *writ of certiorari* for a case and the appellate court's decision becomes final. Organizations wishing to make policy changes through the judicial process are strategic in terms of where they originate a lawsuit.

The USSC has original jurisdiction only on suits between states, cases involving foreign ambassadors, and a couple other special areas. Most of its cases are the result of its granting a *writ of certiorari*, a request by the USSC to send the case forward. Each year there are approximately 7,000 such requests. The Court accepts only about 100 to 150 of those requests. In those cases rejected by the USSC, the decision by the last appellate court hearing the case is upheld. Generally, the USSC will tend to only hear cases from the one of its U.S. circuit court of appeals or a state supreme court. Generally, a litigant needs to exhaust its appellate opportunities before seeking a *writ of certiorari* from the USSC. It takes four of the nine justices on the Court to grant a *writ of certiorari*. The USSC can refuse to hear a case for any reason and does not need to explain why. If two federal circuit appellate courts have made different rulings on similar cases, the USSC is more likely to take the case. However, even if members of the Court generally support a plaintiff's case, it may decide that it is not the right case to use for its decision since there are other issues in that case that muddy the legal question that the Court wishes to address. The Supreme Court prefers to take cases in which the issues are clear and not confounded by other factors.

Writs of certiorari come to the USSC and are put into a "cert pool" on a weekly basis. Those are divided among the justices who are participating in the cert pool. Each justice in the cert pool will then assign cases to one of their three of four law clerks. The clerk will read the petition and write a memorandum summarizing the case and make a recommendation as to whether the USSC should hear the case. These memorandums are circulated to the other justices and then discussed at the Justice Conference.

Once granted *certiorari*, the case is placed on the docket for oral argument. Each side can write a brief of no more than 50 pages. A date is then set for oral argument sometime between October and April. If the federal government is a party to the case, the Solicitor General of the United States argues the federal government's position.

The oral argument lasts for an hour, each side having a half hour to make its case. Each justice will have reviewed the case with their clerks. The lawyers for each side are frequently interrupted in their oral presentation and asked to respond to questions from individual justices. The questions asked by each justice are frequently used by court analysts to infer how that justice might vote on the case. The justices meet on Wednesday and Friday afternoons in the Justice Conference to discuss cases. No outside people are allowed in the room and the chief justice begins talking about the case with each justice taking their uninterrupted turn in order of their seniority on the USCC. After the discussion, the chief justice begins the vote with the associate justices voting in order of seniority.

The chief justice or the most senior justice voting in the majority assigns one of the justices to write the majority decision of the USSC. The most senior justice in dissent may write or assign another justice to write a dissenting opinion. Sometimes decisions are unanimous. Dissenting opinions are not mandatory. Justices can concur with the majority or minority decision and yet write a partial dissent. A justice may write a partial dissent due to a disagreement over some of the reasoning used in the majority's decision but agree with the decision itself. Decisions of the Court can run over 100 pages. The justice writing the majority opinion will work with their law clerks as well as other justices on various circulated drafts. The drafts of the majority opinion are designed to keep the majority vote intact and perhaps gain the vote of an additional justice who may be on the fence or be willing to join the majority but write a partial dissent. This process may take months. It is hard to predict what will be the impact of the 2022 leak and its subsequent investigation of Justice Samuel Alito's draft majority opinion of *Dobbs v. Jackson Women's Health Organization* (2022). See **Breakout Box 3.5**.

There is then a final vote on the case by the justices and then a scheduled pronouncement from the bench as to the decision of the Court. In rare cases, there may be an oral dissent from the bench to make the dissent even more emphatic and more public. Dissents are important in laying the legal foundation for potentially overturning or modifying the Court's future rulings. Opinions are typically released on Monday, Tuesday, or Wednesday mornings when the justices meet in the court room but hear no arguments. This schedule is maintained throughout the term until May and June, during which the Court sits only to announce its opinions. There are generally several rulings coming in the final days of the Court's term. The USSC generally recesses at the end of June and begins again in October.

Rulings by the USSC are binding on all federal and state courts. Appealing a case to the Supreme Court can take years, a great deal of money, and skilled lawyers specializing in federal and constitutional law. There is, in fact, no guarantee the case will even be heard by the USSC. To declare that you will take the case to the Supreme Court implies overcoming many difficult hurdles over which you have no control. Despite that, the USSC remains an important avenue for establishing public policy.

The USSC's landmark decision of *Roe v. Wade* (1973) established policy regarding the right of women to seek an abortion.[7] This decision was based on the USSC precedent regarding the right to privacy and substantive rights of liberty under the 14th Amendment.[8] Since then, multiple states have passed numerous laws limiting that right to seek an abortion based on the stage of pregnancy, requiring women to undergo specific medical procedures, or enforcing special regulations of facilities providing abortions, and so forth. This has resulted in a series of judicial rulings limiting the timing and geographic access to abortion services. In the 1992 decision of *Planned Parenthood of Southeastern Pennsylvania v. Casey* (1992)

---

7   *Roe v. Wade* was a landmark 7-2 decision written by Justice Blackman and was decided on January 22, 1973. The Court ruled that the Due Process Clause of the 14th Amendment contained the right to privacy that protects a pregnant woman's liberty to choose to have an abortion. The decision used a progressive trimester basis to balance the rights of the woman and the rights of the fetus. In the first trimester, the woman's rights were dominant with succeeding trimesters the state could pass specific restrictions on the right to an abortion.

8   Section 1 of the 14th Amendment reads as follows: "All persons born or naturalized in the United States, and subject to the jurisdiction thereof, are citizens of the United States and of the State wherein they reside. No State shall make or enforce any law which shall abridge the privileges or immunities of citizens of the United States; nor shall any State deprive any person of life, liberty, or property, without due process of law; nor deny to any person within its jurisdiction the equal protection of the laws" (Const. amend. XIV, § 1).

the USSC reinforced the precedent of *Roe v. Wade* (1973) and substituted viability of the fetus as the point when states could invoke restrictions. Some states have continued to enact laws more tightly restricting the right to an abortion. Federal courts have taken various positions on those restrictions. The culmination of these efforts occurred in 2021 with the Texas Heartbeat Act, Senate Bill 8. See **Breakout Box 5.2**. The unique feature of this legislation was that the state of Texas was not the enforcement mechanism and therefore not subject to judicial review. The law allowed anyone to file a civil lawsuit against an abortion provider or anyone who helped a woman to obtain an abortion after cardiac activity was detected (typically 6 weeks). If the suit was successful, the plaintiff would receive $10,000 plus the cost of legal fees.

Breakout Box 5.2

TEXAS HEARTBEAT ACT

The Texas Heartbeat Act, Senate Bill 8 (SB 8) legally bans abortions in Texas after detectable cardiac activity, or 6 weeks into a pregnancy. The law provides exceptions for medical emergencies but has no exceptions for rape or incest. Under the law, enforcement is not done by the state but by a provision in the law that allows anyone to file a private lawsuit against an abortion provider or anyone who aids and abets a woman who receives an abortion after cardiac activity is detected. The plaintiff does not need to live in Texas. A successful plaintiff can be awarded $10,000 plus legal fees. Some other states' attempts to limit abortion have been held in violation of *Roe v. Wade* and others have been allowed. In this case, the civil enforcement mechanism means Texas does not have to defend the constitutionality of the law in court because it is technically not involved in the law's enforcement.

On September 1, 2021 the USSC declined to hear an emergency appeal by abortion providers, patients, and clinics in Texas (*Whole Woman's Health v. Jackson*, 2021) to prevent the Texas law from going into effect. As a result, the law went into effect on September 1, 2021. The USSC decision in the case was an 8-1 opinion written by Justice Gorsuch on December 10, 2021. Justices Alito, Kavanaugh, and Barrett joined the opinion in full. Justice Thomas filed an opinion concurring in part and dissenting in part. Chief Justice Roberts filed an opinion concurring in the judgment in part and dissenting in part, in which Justices Breyer, Sotomayor, and Kagan joined. Justice Sotomayor also filed an opinion concurring in the judgment in part and dissenting in part which Justices Breyer and Kagan joined. By the decision, the USSC remanded the case to the lower Texas courts where the case will be argued and likely find its way back to the USSC at some future date.

This has important significance in terms of a legal strategy to allow enforcement of legislation by private civil lawsuits. Other states have begun to copy this strategy for abortion and still other states have threatened to use this legal strategy to cover other topics. In 2022 the

California legislature began debating a proposed law copying the Texas civil litigation and citizen bounty payments to limit the sale of assault weapons and ghost guns in the state.

References

Roe v. Wade, 410 U.S. 113 (1973). https://supreme.justia.com/cases/federal/us/410/113
Whole Woman's Health v. Jackson, 595 U.S. ___,141 S. Ct. 2494 (2021). https://www .supremecourt.gov/opinions/21pdf/21-463_new_8o6b.pdf

It is important for the USSC to be perceived as nonpartisan, reinforcing the principle that "justice is blind" (the unbiased application of the law based on facts and evidence) with decisions based upon the law and not on the political opinions of justices. However, justices are also human; they bring with them personal experiences that impact their legal and philosophical perspectives. Periodically the USSC has been criticized for its politically oriented rulings. For example, the Hughes Court (1932–1937) continued to overturn popular New Deal legislation. This led to a proposal by President Franklin Delano Roosevelt (which was later abandoned) to pass the Judicial Procedures Reform Bill of 1937 to authorize additional justices to the Supreme Court.[9]

During the 1960s and 1970s there were attempts to impeach Chief Justice Earl Warren and Associate Justice William O. Douglas for their liberal opinions on the USSC. Billboards around the United States called for the removal of the chief justice. On April 15, 1970, House minority leader Gerald Ford on behalf of President Richard Nixon called for the impeachment of Justice Douglas. The House Judiciary Committee held a 6-month investigation, but nothing came of it. Both Warren and Douglas served until their retirement.

The increasing partisan Senate treatment of both Republican and Democratic nominees to the USSC and many USSC decisions based on party lines from *Bush v. Gore* (2000) to *Dobbs v. Jackson Women's Health Organization* (2022) have revived the perception of a partisan USSC.[10] One of the decisions that demonstrated the political tensions on the USSC was *National Federation of Independent Business v. Sebelius* (2012). See **Breakout Box 5.3**. Congressional Republicans had attempted to delay repeal, defund, or PPACA over 70 times. The National Federation of Independent Business sued in a Florida district court challenging the individual mandate provision and the expansion of Medicaid with the penalty of a loss of Medicaid funds for states that did not comply. Twenty-six states and a few individuals joined the suit. The case made its way through the appellate courts and was given a *writ of certiorari* by the USSC. This was a judicial vehicle

---

9 Judicial Procedures Reform Bill of 1937 was introduced on behalf of President Franklin Roosevelt to authorize the addition of up to six judges for those on the Supreme Court over the age of 70. It is frequently called the "court packing plan." The Democratic Chair of the Senate Judiciary Committee held up passage of the bill, and later the Judiciary Committee issued a negative report on the proposal. It was never passed.

10 *Bush v. Gore* was an unsigned decision of the USSC on December 12, 2000 that stopped a recount of the disputed Florida vote count in 2000 presidential election. The decision gave George W. Bush a majority in the Electoral College.

for invalidating PPACA; in fact, the four justices in the minority declared they would have to invalidate the law in its entirety. However, Chief Justice Roberts writing the 5-4 majority opinion and using judicial restraint held the act was a constitutional use of the federal government's taxing authority but held that the loss of Medicaid funds was impermissibly coercive, and therefore the penalty was invalid. In upholding PPACA the case can be seen on one hand as the Court being nonpartisan in one of the most contentious partisan battles. Chief Justice Roberts has been cognizant of the need for the USSC to maintain its legitimacy among the populace. On the other hand, Justice Roberts was immediately criticized for not overturning PPACA.

In 2022, the USSC granted *certiorari* to *Dobbs v. Jackson Women's Health Organization* (2022). This resulted in the landmark ruling overturning *Roe v. Wade* and *Planned Parenthood of Southeastern Pennsylvania v. Casey*. See **Breakout Box 3.5**. This will be a focus of judicial policy making for years to come. It raises the question as to whether the USSC is just another political body. The popular election of state judges (some through party identification) has also raised questions as to the nonpolitical nature of the court system at the state level as well.

Breakout Box 5.3

NATIONAL FEDERATION OF INDEPENDENT BUSINESS, ET AL. V. KATHLEEN SEBELIUS, SECRETARY OF HEALTH AND HUMAN SERVICES, ET AL.

The Patient Protection and Affordable Care Act was passed by the 111th Congress and signed into law by President Barack Obama on March 23, 2010. The National Federation of Independent Business sued in a Florida district court challenging the individual mandate provision and the expansion of Medicaid with the penalty of a loss of Medicaid funds for states that did not comply. Twenty-six states and a few individuals joined the suit.

The case was initially heard in a Florida federal district court. It ruled that PPACA was unconstitutional and struck down the entire law. The case was appealed by the government to the Eleventh Circuit Court which agreed that the individual mandate was unconstitutional but that it was severable so that the rest of the act could remain intact. The case was then appealed to the USSC which granted *certiorari* on November 14, 2011. It consolidated the case with two similar cases. The case was unusual in that it was argued on three separate occasions, March 25, 26, and 27, 2012. The case was decided on June 28, 2012.

There were multiple concurring opinions and dissenting opinions. Chief Justice John Roberts, Jr., was the author of the 5-4 majority decision with Justices Ginsburg, Breyer, Sotomayor, and Kegan joining the majority decision. The majority decision ruled that the individual mandate was constitutional under the power of Congress to tax. The government had argued that it was justified by the Commerce Clause and the Necessary and Proper Clause. Roberts had contended in the majority decision that neither clause could be used to justify a penalty for a person failing to engage in an economic activity (not buying health insurance). The majority decision ruled that the penalty of losing Medicaid funds was impermissibly coercive nature and thus invalid. While agreeing with Roberts on the constitutionality of PPACA, Justices Ginsberg, Breyer, and Kagan wrote a concurrence/dissent opinion arguing that the use of the Commerce Clause and the Necessary and Proper Clause was also valid for authorization of the act. Justices Ginsberg and Sotomayor also wrote a concurring opinion with a partial dissent saying that the Medicaid expansion was valid even if states lost access to previous existing Medicaid funds.

Justice Kennedy wrote the dissent along with Justices Scalia, Thomas, and Alito, in which they stated that they would have struck down PPACA in its entirety. They criticized Chief Justice Roberts for calling the mandate a tax when it had been described by the law as a penalty. They maintained PPACA could not be justified under the Commerce Clause because it applied to individual inaction as well as action. They also found that conditioning Medicaid funding on expanding Medicaid was unconstitutional and again they would strike down the entire law. In addition, Justice Thomas wrote a separate dissent criticizing the expansion of the federal use of the Commerce Clause since *Wickard v. Filburn* (1942).

The decision did not invalidate any specific provision of PPACA, but it did limit how it could be implemented, especially regarding the Medicaid penalty. There were continued attempts by Republicans in Congress to repeal PPACA, but none succeeded.

References

National Federation of Independent Business v. Sebelius, 567 U.S. 519 (2012). https://www.supremecourt.gov/opinions/11pdf/11-393c3a2.pdf

Wickard v. Filburn, 317 U.S. 111 (1942). https://supreme.justia.com/cases/federal/us/317/111

STATE AND LOCAL GOVERNMENTS

If you think that the federal policy process is complicated, examining state policy processes is even more complicated because all states are different. Although most state structures may be recognizable from one state to the next, the political processes will vary in important ways to tilt the legislative process one way or another. As noted before, states have different numbers of legislators and staffing. In addition, some state legislatures are authorized to meet for a very limited number of days. There are generally provisions for the governor or the legislature to declare the need for a special session to deal with a particular issue. Some states pass biennium budgets rather than an annual budget. Some states require that all submitted bills must be reported out of legislative committees with a recommendation to pass or not, while others allow committees to bury legislative proposals. Ethics and lobbying regulations may vary considerably between states.

A state's flexibility to conduct major public health activities may be limited since its public health department may be largely dependent on federal grants rather than state funds. Even federal block grants come with certain federal restrictions as to their use. Federal grants supplying personnel to conduct epidemiologic research, sponsor state maternal and child health programs, or maintain a public health laboratory may underpin the state's public health efforts. States with very limited state funds for public health will thus have less flexibility as to what public health initiatives can be undertaken at the state level.

State borders are fixed. However, people flow from one state to another for work, recreation, medical care, and so forth. Although there are examples of states formally agreeing to collect comparable data and sharing it, this is not standard practice among states. Patients may seek medical care in bordering states. Does State A's data represent the total experience of its population by including those who obtain medical care from State B? During the COVID-19 pandemic, states varied in their willingness to provide COVID-19 vaccines for workers or students from out-of-state even though the vaccines were free from the federal government. Where was that person's vaccination recorded? If a person tests positive for COVID-19 while visiting another state or a student returns home from an out-of-state university, where did the person contract COVID-19 and where is it recorded?

National political activity tends to be covered by multiple news agencies with major news bureaus in Washington, DC, that carry news on legislation being proposed by the executive branch or members of Congress. Members of Congress use the news media and social network media to tell their constituents about what is happening at the federal level. In addition, national media carry commentary reflecting various points of views on issues of the day. However, state government activity tends to receive much less media coverage. Depending on the size of the media market, most local news outlets may not have any of its reporters based in the state capital. There may be only one major media outlet with its own bias covering state politics. The latter has become more common with the general decline in investigative reporters at local news outlets and the consolidation of news media. At the same time, the role of unedited social media has exploded, changing the nature of news and commentary being consumed by the public. Examining the policy process at the state and local levels requires digging into the details of the political culture, structure, and processes within each jurisdiction.

There is one similarity among all states that is different from that of the federal government. Unlike the federal government, states cannot have deficit operating budgets. The federal deficit (the difference between revenue and expenditures for a given year) and the federal debt (the number of accumulated deficits over multiple years of borrowing) have been a point of contention since the founding of the republic. Periodically, Congress must raise the debt ceiling so as not to default on existing debt. Debt can accumulate through increasing expenditures and not increasing income or by reducing income (tax cuts) and not reducing expenditures. The national debt has been accumulated by both Republican and Democratic administrations.

When governors run for national office, they frequently brag that they know how to balance a budget because they cannot legally have a deficit at the state level. However, that is only partially true. The state's operational budget must be balanced each year or rely upon the existence of contingency funds (rainy day funds from previous years' surpluses) to make up any operational budget shortfall. However, unlike the federal government, states also have a separate capital budget, which includes expenditures for buildings, roads, sewage and water treatment plants, and other infrastructure projects. States pass bonds (debt) to pay for most of their infrastructure projects. There is no comparable capital budget at the federal level, except for the highways through the federal Highway Trust Fund. Federal capital expenditures are included in the annual federal budget. Consequently, states do indeed issue a great deal of debt.

Congress would have to pass a law allowing states to declare bankruptcy. Instead, when multiple states are having difficulty balancing their budgets, such as during a recession or the coronavirus pandemic of 2020 to 2021, Congress usually passes supplemental funds to be given to the states. The federal government basically bails out the states from their projected deficits. For example, the American Rescue Plan Act of 2021 provided $350 billion in emergency funding to state, local, territorial, and Tribal governments. As a result, many states have experienced budget surpluses during the COVID-19 pandemic, despite declining economies and tax revenues. The federal government rescued all states whether their politicians supported the American Rescue Plan or opposed it. Local governments such as municipalities, counties, school districts, and tax districts have also received a share of this federal support. Unlike states, local governments can and have declared bankruptcy under Chapter 9 of the federal bankruptcy code.

SUMMARY

The American political system is a complex system. Novices frequently think that they can go to Washington or their state capital and quickly make major changes. The policy process tends to be a long game. See **Figure 5.1** as a visualization of the maze.

There is seldom a quick policy fix, and if it is sold as such, it is probably going to result in failure or have serious unintended consequences. The legislative process was designed to create a difficult path for any legislation. Every administration or politician must confront unforeseen events that might suddenly change the political atmosphere as to what is politically possible. Even after the passage of a particular law, it may take years for results to materialize and to reap the accolades or condemnation for its impact. Decades later, there may be an historical reevaluation of the impact of policies or a reassessment of it based on changing values. Despite all the obstacles, a single public health law can improve the health and well-being of thousands or millions of people whether it be at the national, state, or local level.

DISCUSSION QUESTIONS

- Staff play an influential role in policy development. To what extent should the role of staff be improved or minimized?

- Discuss the advantages and disadvantages of requiring all legislative bills to be reported out of committee for a vote by both chambers?

- Should there be a House and Senate committee focused on public health?

- How should the Senate rule on the filibuster be changed?

- What, if any, changes in the USSC would make it more responsive to public opinion?

KEY TERMS

Administrative Procedures Act
American Rescue Plan Act of 2021
amicus brief
appropriation committees
authorization committees
budget committees
Bush v. Gore (2000)
Civil Rights Act of 1964
cloture
conference committee
congressional calendars
Congressional Record
congressional staff
Dobbs v. Jackson Women's Health Organization (2022)
Executive Order 12898
executive orders
federal depository libraries
Federal Register
filibuster
guidelines
House Committee of the Whole

House Rules Committee
House Ways and Means Committee
National Federation of Independent Business v. Sebelius (2012)
Omnibus Budget Reconciliation Act
Planned Parenthood of Southeastern Pennsylvania v. Casey (1992)
pocket veto
Roe v. Wade (1973)
Rucho v. Common Cause (2019)
rules and regulations
signing statements
special committees
standing committees
unanimous consent
United States Code
USSC minority dissent
USSC majority opinion
veto
writ of certiorari
writ of mandamus

A robust set of instructor resources designed to supplement this text is located at http://connect.springerpub.com/content/book/978-0-8261-8543-3. Qualifying instructors may request access by emailing textbook@springerpub.com.

REFERENCES

Administrative Procedures Act, Pub. L. No. 79-404, 60 Stat. 237 (1946). https://www.justice.gov/sites/default/files/jmd/legacy/2014/05/01/act-pl79-404.pdf

Allen, S. J. (2014, October 14). *That Lyndon Johnson quote (part 2).* Capital Research Center. https://capitalresearch.org/article/that-lyndon-johnson-quote-part-2

American Rescue Plan Act, Pub. L. No. 117-2, 135 Stat. 4 (2021). https://www.govinfo.gov/content/pkg/PLAW-117publ2/pdf/PLAW-117publ2.pdf

Baker v. Carr, 369 U.S. 186 (1962). https://supreme.justia.com/cases/federal/us/369/186

Brown v. Board of Education of Topeka, 347 U.S. 483 (1954). https://supreme.justia.com/cases/federal/us/347/483

Bush v. Gore, 531 U.S. 98 (2000). https://supreme.justia.com/cases/federal/us/531/98

Civil Rights Act, Pub. L. No. 88-352, 78 Stat. 241 (1964). https://www.govinfo.gov/content/pkg/STATUTE-78/pdf/STATUTE-78-Pg241.pdf

Clinton v. City of New York, 524 U.S. 417 (1998). https://supreme.justia.com/cases/federal/us/524/417

Congressional Budget and Impoundment Control Act, Pub. L. No. 93-344, 88 Stat. 297 (1974). https://www.govinfo.gov/content/pkg/STATUTE-88/pdf/STATUTE-88-Pg297.pdf

Congressional Review Act, Pub. L. No. 104-121, 110 Stat. 847 (1996). https://www.govinfo.gov/content/pkg/PLAW-104publ121/pdf/PLAW-104publ121.pd

Dobbs v. Jackson Women's Health Organization, 597 U.S. ___ (2022). https://www.supremecourt.gov/opinions/21pdf/19-1392_6j37.pdf

Exec. Order No. 12866, 58 Fed. Reg. 51735 (September 30, 1993). https://www.archives.gov/files/federal-register/executive-orders/pdf/12866.pdf

Exec. Order No. 12898. 59 Fed. Reg. 7629 (February 16, 1994). https://www.archives.gov/files/federal-register/executive-orders/pdf/12898.pdf

Exec. Order No. 13985. 86 Fed. Reg. 7009 (January 20, 2021). https://www.federalregister.gov/documents/2021/01/25/2021-01753/advancing-racial-equity-and-support-for-underserved-communities-through-the-federal-government

Exec. Order No. 13990. 86 Fed. Reg. 7037 (January 20, 2021). https://www.federalregister.gov/documents/2021/01/25/2021-01765/protecting-public-health-and-the-environment-and-restoring-science-to-tackle-the-climate-crisis

Exec. Order No. 14008. 86 Fed. Reg. 7619 (January 27, 2021). https://www.federalregister.gov/documents/2021/02/01/2021-02177/tackling-the-climate-crisis-at-home-and-abroad

Inflation Reduction Act, Pub. L. No. 117-169, 136 Stat. 1818 (2022). https://www.congress.gov/bill/117th-congress/house-bill/5376/text

Library of Congress. (n.d.). *Compiling a federal legislative history: A beginner's guide: Presidential signing statements.* https://guides.loc.gov/legislative-history/presidential-communications/signing-statements

Loving v. Virginia, 388 U.S. 1 (1967). https://supreme.justia.com/cases/federal/us/388/1

Mascarenhas, M., Grattet, R., & Mege, K. (2021). Toxic waste and race in twenty-first century America: Neighborhood poverty and racial composition in the siting of hazardous waste facilities. *Environment and Society, 12,* 108–126. https://doi.org/10.3167/ares.2021.120107

National Conference of State Legislatures. (2022, January 13). State and federal environmental justice efforts. https://www.ncsl.org/research/environment-and-natural-resources/state-and-federal-efforts-to-advance-environmental-justice.aspx

National Federation of Independent Business v. Sebelius, 567 U.S. 519 (2012). https://www.supremecourt.gov/opinions/11pdf/11-393c3a2.pdf

Obergefell v. Hodges, 576 U.S. 644 (2015). https://www.supremecourt.gov/opinions/14pdf/14-556_3204.pdf

Patient Protection and Affordable Care Act, Pub. L. No. 111-148, 124 Stat. 119 (2010). https://www.congress.gov/111/plaws/publ148/PLAW-111publ148.pdf

Perls, H. (2020, October 12). *EPA undermines its own environmental justice programs.* Harvard Law School. https://eelp.law.harvard.edu/2020/11/epa-undermines-its-own-environmental-justice-programs/#:%7E:text=There%20is%20no%20federal%20law,their%20authorities%20under%20other%20statutes

Planned Parenthood of Southeastern Pennsylvania v. Casey, 505 U.S. 833 (1992). https://supreme.justia.com/cases/federal/us/505/833

Roe v. Wade, 410 U.S. 113 (1973). https://supreme.justia.com/cases/federal/us/410/113

Rucho v. Common Cause, 588 U.S. ___ (2019). https://www.supremecourt.gov/opinions/18pdf/18-422_9ol1.pdf

United Church of Christ Commission for Racial Justice. (1987). *Toxic wastes and race in the United States: A national report on the racial and socio-economic characteristics of communities with hazardous waste sites.* United States Nuclear Regulatory Commission. https://www.nrc.gov/docs/ML1310/ML13109A339.pdf

U.S. Constitution, amend. XIV, §1.

U.S. Environmental Protection Agency. (2022, August 5). *Environmental justice.* https://www.epa.gov/environmentaljustice

Vizcarra, H., & Perls, H. (2021, March 3). *Biden's week one: Mapping ambitious climate action.* Harvard Law School. https://eelp.law.harvard.edu/portfolios/environmental-governance/bidens-week-one-mapping-ambitious-climate-action

Whole Woman's Health v. Jackson, 595 U.S. ___ (2021). https://www.supremecourt.gov/opinions/21pdf/21-463_new_8o6b.pdf

CHAPTER 6

POLITICAL CULTURE

This chapter discusses the importance of the political culture in the policy-making process. We begin by describing what is part of a nation's political culture and then provide examples of the dominant American political culture. We focus particularly on the rise of partisanship in our political system in national, state, and local politics. The previous chapters have provided you with knowledge of the U.S. political structure, process, and culture. In the next chapter we shift focus to doing a health policy analysis.

LEARNING OBJECTIVES

Be able to:

- Describe the general importance of political culture within the policy-making process.
- Describe aspects of the dominant American political culture and differences among the American population.
- Describe the rise of partisanship in the American political culture.

Political culture is a more difficult aspect to cover because it both influences the creation of the political structure and process and is reinforced by those same political structures and processes. In addition, it is more amorphous and changing. Political culture includes the accepted norms of behavior that are expected within the political system. All governments depend on unwritten rules that are understood to create the boundaries of political actions. Changes in these assumed protocols or boundaries may strengthen democracy or weaken it.

Those on both the political right and the left have made political culture a more sensitive topic. Those on the right attack a "woke" political culture or "political correctness" and those on the left attack remnants of sexism, racism, and nativism that remain within our political culture. Some see multiculturalism as divisive and some view as it as a strength. The intent here is not to provide a complete discussion of our political culture. There are multiple resources for a more in-depth examination of the American political culture (Carr, 2007; Edelman, 1967;

Hofstadter & Lasch, 1974; Levitsky & Ziblatt, 2018; Welch, 2013; Wiarda, 2018).[1] Instead, the intent here is to make public health policy analysts aware of its importance and to demonstrate its importance to public health policy.

THE NATURE OF POLITICAL CULTURE

Political culture can be defined as the norms, traditions, roles, and values of a society's political history that are articulated or practiced as largely unexamined assumptions that are passed along to future generations. It includes moral judgments, religious beliefs, political and historical myths, customs and accepted practices, and beliefs as to what makes good social order and political system. It shapes what policies are important and how the political system actually works regardless of what is on paper. In one sense it reflects the remnants of previous political and value conflicts, but it is more than history because it is continually evolving. One of the outstanding things about political culture is that one tends to not think about it, especially if one knowingly or unknowingly benefits from it.

Political structures and processes are visible in day-to-day activities that are highly visible and reported in the news, but the political culture tends to remain in the background. However, one becomes acutely aware of it when visiting a different country or state. Suddenly, things that citizens take as normal regarding the government or political activity is marginally or even radically different. As mentioned previously, the notion that Americans tend to define *freedom* as "freedom from" rather than "freedom to" is just one of those unexamined aspects of our political culture. In other countries political leaders and political systems are perceived differently. Simple things such as the ubiquitous presence or absence of the national flag, unarmed police, jaywalking, political graffiti, what is considered news, and so forth may be different. How people view government institutions, the bureaucracy, the police, national holidays, or paying taxes varies widely. Citizens, members of the military, politicians, bureaucrats, newscasters, and so forth think and behave differently in other countries.

There is a dominant political culture that tends to be accepted by a major section of the population and then there are micropolitical cultures, which may deviate in certain respects from the dominant political culture. Not everyone agrees with the dominant political culture. This may sometimes be the result of historical evolution (e.g., French and English Canadian provinces) or the incorporation of different ethnic groups into the nation state (e.g., Switzerland). Colonialism can have a legacy on the political culture of a nation state (Chigudu, 2021). Some segments of the population within the nation or state may not be in sync with certain aspects of the dominant political culture. In the United States we are all aware of cities that are "blue islands" within "red states" and "red islands" within "blue states." Some population voices may be invisible, undervalued, or unrecognized. Those who do not feel reflected by the dominant political culture due to the lack of representation or political power may feel a sense of disconnect and may create their own micropolitical culture or attempt to alter the dominant political culture. There are large Native American reservations such as the Navajo Reservation within Arizona and

---

1   As an example of how scientific knowledge itself can be framed as a product of a dominant political culture, and a discussion of alternative framings, see Lupien et al. (2022) and Prescod-Weinstein (2022).

other states that have very different political cultures from the dominant state political culture. There may be political jurisdictions in which nepotism may be a part of the micropolitical culture, but it is an anathema in the dominant political culture. There are political jurisdictions traditionally dominated by religious, racial, or ethnic groups that influence the political culture.

Political scientist Deborah Schildkraut (2014) has written an analysis of American social identity and political culture. She states that social identity refers to "the part of a person's sense of self that derives from his or her membership in a particular group and the value or meaning that he or she attaches to such membership" (Schildkraut, 2014, p. 443). She further contends that American identity consists of two sets of norms. One set is intended to apply to natural rights that "all men" can follow, which can be traced back to the ideals in the Declaration of Independence. The other set of norms depends on one's race, religion, gender, and other attributes. Other scholars have revisited this theme in the context of the response to the COVID-19 pandemic. For example, Ananthaswamy (2020) discusses Schildkraut's views in relation to the perception of mask orders and social distancing guidelines as threats to personal freedom. Inherent conflicts between "freedom and order" and "freedom and equality" are discussed. For example, people wanted to be able to have the personal freedom to engage in their daily life activities, while also expecting the government to impose some level of order and security. Choosing personal freedom for some individuals might restrict the freedom of other people (e.g., those already suffering from comorbidities) to engage in their own activities, thereby exacerbating health disparities. Schildkraut notes that while other democracies "might be more likely to pick equality over freedom when those two conflict; in the U.S., we tend to pick freedom, although there are certainly exceptions … compared with other countries, we also have the complexity of federalism where we value devolving power to the states in some areas, but not others. And people like to celebrate their state identities. Part of our national character is the immense variation across the states, and all that feeds into our response to the pandemic" (Ananthaswamy, 2020, p. 2, quoting Schildkraut). These sets of norms can sometimes contradict each other, and the evolution of these identities shapes the nation's ability to confront pandemics, both historically and today (Webster et al., 2022).

Political systems do not leave the development of political culture to chance. Political culture is associated with nation-building, the intentionally designed things done by the political system to develop a national psyche as what it means to be an American as opposed to a Swede, or a Californian as opposed to a Mainer. Relatedly, Jones (2014) created a TEDx Emory Talk on allegories of race and racism and our ability to recognize them. All political systems shape their political culture through its public education system; influence or control of print and social media; control of the internet; institutionalization of wealth and capital; creation and celebrations of holidays; the celebration of selected heroes; and other attempts to build a sense of being part of a shared community. Why do we all know about and celebrate President Lincoln and not President Pierce? Who has a monument in Washington, DC, or in our state capitals and what do they symbolize? When are monuments taken down?

While political culture tends to change gradually, when examined over time, the changes can be so substantial that it may seem like a different country. The political culture of the Pilgrims in the Plimoth Plantation is vastly different from that of Plymouth, Massachusetts today. In a similar vein, the political culture during the writing of the U.S. Constitution (not just the provision counting slaves as three-fifths of a person) is very different from that of today. What was politically acceptable regarding policies impacting Native Americans, slaves, or women is not acceptable in today's political culture. One merely needs to witness how Reverend Martin Luther King, Jr., who was once investigated by the Federal Bureau of Investigation (FBI), jailed, demonized, and murdered, now has a national monument in Washington, DC, and a federal holiday named after him.

Revolutions tend to result in more than a regime change. Revolutions are also generally accompanied by major shifts in the political culture. The French Revolution of 1789, the Russian Revolution of 1917, the 1989 Velvet Revolution in Czechoslovakia, or the 2005 Orange Revolution in Ukraine resulted in major shifts in political cultures as well as regime changes. While a regime change remains an important element of any revolution, one can make the argument that the resulting shift in political culture may be equally or more significant. Political institutions without a supporting political culture are bound for failure.

A major historic event experienced by a country or state can result in substantial changes in political culture, for example, the presidential election of 1860, the Great Depression, the war in Vietnam, 9/11, landmark Supreme Court decisions, the presidential elections of 2016 and 2020, and the storming of the U.S. Capitol on January 6, 2021. These events have had a substantial impact on our political culture and will continue to do so for years. Similarly, future major national events will lead to additional changes. Political culture is a work in progress that may be reinforced, weakened, or destroyed.

The first description of the American political culture was done (not surprisingly) by an outsider, Alexis de Tocqueville, from France. His visit to America in 1831 resulted in the publication of the book *Democracy in America*. He described a very different political culture than that of European nations, one based on the "equality of conditions" (Tocqueville, 2002). He observed that a formal rigid social structure did not exist in the United States as it did in European countries. There were no hereditary titles. Accordingly, men (but not women, Black people, or Native Americans)[2] could be judged on their abilities rather than their inheritance. Meritocracy remains part of our political culture and has been expanded to include other groups. Meritocracy praises the self-made individual. Even immigrants can make it in America; it is the land of opportunity.

As mentioned previously, the original 13 colonies had a very different historical experience than those territories in the West that later became states. Those western states did not directly experience the Revolutionary War but were more impacted by their geography and frontier experience. The distrust of executive powers was deeply ingrained in the original 13 colonies and therefore New England remains having comparatively weak governors. As pointed out in Chapter 4, more democratic practices (initiatives, referendums, recalls, and the election of judges) tended to develop in the western states and not the original 13 colonies. Slavery was experienced by one part of the country as an essential underpinning of the economy and by another as a troubling moral conflict between the ideal of America and

---

2 The epidemic known as the Great Dying killed large numbers of Indigenous people in the 1600s, reflecting a frequently ignored aspect of public health history prior to the American Revolution (Marr & Cathey, 2010).

the reality of America. The experience of the Civil War and the civil rights movement of the 1960s continue to impact states' political cultures differently. Women became part of the political landscape with the enactment of the 19th Amendment. Native Americans became part of the political culture even later. Some perceive the federal government as a protector of individual rights and others perceive it as an intruder of individual rights. Black Lives Matter and the militia movement continue to influence our political culture.

There is not room here to cite all the influences that have shaped our shared and differing political cultures. Consequently, we will only touch upon a few of them. What is important for the thoughtful public health policy analyst is to understand the political culture within their geopolitical environment. Even towns within the same state may have subtle but important differences in their political cultures. A policy may fit well within one political culture and not within another.

EXAMPLES OF THE DOMINANT AMERICAN POLITICAL CULTURE

The concept of natural rights is embedded within our political understanding as to the limits of the political system. It is notable that the second sentence of the Declaration of Independence reads, "We hold these truths to be self-evident, that all men are created equal, that they are endowed by their Creator with certain *unalienable Rights, that among these are Life, Liberty and the pursuit of Happiness*" (Jefferson, 1776, para. 2, emphasis added). These unalienable rights cannot be taken away by government. Natural rights are fundamental to the concept of limited government.

Another overriding aspect of the U.S. political culture is the focus on individualism and libertarianism. The role of the political system is to solve social problems that the individual or small groups cannot solve on their own. Where that line exists between the two sets of social problems is a constant source of debate. Compared to other countries, the United States is much more focused on the importance of "freedom from." This is reflected in our politics in that we tend to think that individuals should be free to pursue their own self-interest and that they are the creators of their own destiny. Consequently, social support systems (childcare, pensions, national health insurance) in the United States are typically seen very differently from those in other nations. The difference rests on the cultural perception of the role of the state and individual responsibility.

American exceptionalism is another part of our dominant political culture. American exceptionalism is the belief that the United States is different from all other countries. Accordingly, it rightfully plays an outsized and positive role in the world compared to other countries. Some point to John Winthrop's portion of his 1630 sermon cited as "City Upon a Hill" (2020) as an early example of this perspective since within the sermon Boston was envisioned as a new type of community that would be a beacon of hope for the world to copy. The establishment of a republic in 1789 that inspired other countries to overthrow monarchies and establish republics is also part of this historical element of American exceptionalism. Our entrance into World Wars I and II, the Marshall Plan for rebuilding Europe, and the establishment of the International Monetary Fund of the United Nations, as well as the creation of multiple military alliances such the North Atlantic Treaty Organization (NATO) and Southeast Asia Treaty Organization (SEATO), are examples of this outsized perception of ourselves as the leader of the "free world." The resistance to the 2022 Russian invasion of Ukraine has reinforced the notion of American exceptionalism. Of course, American exceptionalism is not universally accepted by other nations or even by some in the United States (Archer, 2018). The inheritance from our Indigenous, colonial, and postcolonial periods is complicated, but in parts of the United States such as Native American reservations, it plays an important role in the political culture.

The belief that power corrupts, and that therefore power must be distributed rather than concentrated, also plays an important role in our dominant political culture. We saw how this value was used by the authors of the Constitution to design our federal political structure. This notion is also related to the perceived value of keeping decision-making as close to the people as possible. Consequently, state and local governments tend to be favored over the federal government within our dominant political culture.

Distrust in human nature and the political system is also part of the dominant political culture. In some political cultures, people have confidence that the political system will generally do what is socially beneficial. Americans, despite patriotically praising the United States, have an underlying distrust of both politicians and the political system. This view is probably made most explicit and famous by President Reagan's inaugural address (1981) that "government is not the solution to our problem; government is the problem" (para. 9). Government is not to be trusted; it is perceived as being incompetent, wasteful, and self-interested. No set of data can repudiate those perceptions and any example of a governmental mistake merely reinforces the belief. This distrust is reflected in various aspects of our political culture; for example, many public health COVID-19 tasks were delegated to private for-profit organizations.

Trust becomes important when enacting health policy. In colonial times when a disease could wipe out a community, closing a port, imposing a quarantine, and isolating infected people were taken as necessary public health actions to protect the community. Even if the science was not settled as to the cause or its means of transmission, actions impinging on the freedom of individuals for the safety of the community was a given. As demonstrated by the experience of COVID-19, our political culture has changed regarding the balance between individual freedom and public health. Masks, a relatively mild preventive measure compared to isolation on an island, are perceived by many as a major invasion of individual freedom. Even as the COVID-19 epidemic continues, policies have been enacted in some political jurisdictions to limit the state or local government's ability to declare a state of emergency and/or take actions that have been scientifically demonstrated to protect public health.

An analysis of the difference between the experience of COVID-19 in Australia and in the United States indicated that trust in the government and trust in science resulted in a dramatic difference in the speed and effectiveness of the Australian conservative government's policies on minimizing deaths from COVID and the speed of population vaccinations (Cave, 2022). Australians have a more favorable view of government and public health professionals and were more receptive to lockdowns, closing borders, and receiving vaccinations. As a result, 84.73% of all Australians were fully vaccinated as of data in mid-2022 compared to 66.96% of the United States (Coronavirus Resource Center, 2022b). Deaths from COVID were 30.66 per 100,000 population in Australia compared to 303.40 per 100,000 in the

United States, or almost 10 times higher in the United States (Coronavirus Resource Center, 2022a). The lack of trust can have lasting consequences. One explanation for the slow uptake of vaccinations among Black people in the United States was the long-standing distrust of medicine and public health due to the 1932 Tuskegee syphilis experiments on Black individuals (Gamble, 1997).

This lack of political trust has taken a partisan turn. Among Democrats, 89% trust the Food and Drug Administration (FDA) and 84% trust the Centers for Disease Control and Prevention (CDC). Among Republicans, 41% trust the CDC and 43% trust the FDA (Sparks et al., 2022, Figure 17). An analysis of a new data dashboard with Microsoft AI for Health released by Brown School of Public Health demonstrated that in the United States 318,000 COVID-19 deaths could have been prevented if every state reached 100% vaccination; if that level had been reached, about 50% of the COVID deaths of those 18 years old and older from January 1, 2021, to April 2022 would have been preventable (Simmons-Duffin & Nakajima, 2022). States varied considerably; red states had a larger percentage of preventable deaths than did blue states (Simmons-Duffin & Nakajima, 2022).

The peaceful transfer of power and the sanctity of elections has been another hallmark of our political culture. Despite major political differences between various factions, when one party loses an election, it concedes the loss and facilitates the transfer of political power to the winner. Former President Donald Trump's refusal to accept the legitimacy of the 2020 presidential election results and subsequent attempts to disrupt the certification of Electoral College votes of the 2020 election have been seen as destabilizing our dominant political culture.[3] In parallel with the acceptance of the peaceful transfer of power is the tradition that the U.S. military plays no role in certifying or removing a civilian government.

Capitalist competition has become another hallmark of our dominant political culture. The dominant culture believes that competition is good and leads to social betterment. This perspective reinforces our capitalistic economic system. We are more likely to praise private enterprise than government activities. It is somewhat ironic that we tend to trust private enterprise designed to yield monetary profits and over whom we have little control more than we do public entities designed to benefit the commonweal and are controlled by popular elections and legislative oversight. From a public health perspective this distrust has a negative impact on such things as public health surveys, vaccination campaigns, and so forth.

Another aspect of our political culture is that the United States is a melting pot. Except for Native Americans, we are all immigrants from some period in our nation's history and have blended together. An important normative assumption of the melting pot is that those coming here should be part of the blend. Adopting the English language and American way of life are expected within the melting pot. Some countries, including the United States during certain periods of history, make immigration and citizenship difficult. Canada, a country that also welcomes immigrants, has a different perception of the blend of immigrants. Instead of a melting pot, it celebrates its diversity by describing the mix of cultures as a mosaic rather than a melting pot.

There are other elements of the dominant and micropolitical cultures that could be discussed here. However, what is important is that the public health policy

---

3 U.S. House of Representatives Select Committee to Investigate the January 6th Attack on the United States Capitol.

analyst be sensitive to those elements that have an influence over the acceptance or resistance to proposed health policies and how best to adapt existing paradigms to different political cultures.

NONPARTISAN EFFORTS

Historically, bureaucrats were hired and fired based upon their political loyalty rather than their expertise. The local postmaster was a political appointee. City bosses ruled with an iron fist. The United States went through a progressive period (late 1800s–1916) in which there were social and political reforms to confront problems of urbanization, industrialization, and corruption. One of those efforts was to decrease the unbridled partisanship of the federal bureaucracy. One of the first and most important steps was the passage of the Pendleton Civil Service Reform Act of 1883. It mandated that most positions in the federal government be awarded based upon merit and not party affiliation. The Civil Service Reform Act has been amended several times to create a largely nonpartisan professional workforce at the federal level. This model was generally followed by state governments. As discussed in previous chapters, while top bureaucratic positions are politically appointed to reflect election results, the bulk of the executive branch's bureaucracy remains nonpartisan. Since the bulk of positions do not change from one administration to the next, there is a pool of federal workers with expertise and a collective memory of the success and failures of past policy efforts.

There have been other efforts to decrease partisanship as well. During the same period many state and local elections became nonpartisan. We previously discussed the strength and weakness of nonpartisan elections. In addition, during the 1960s and 1970s there were attempts to professionalize state legislators and turn away from "citizen legislators." The latter are part-time legislators who meet for a short period of time and who do not generally have staffs or even offices. Citizen legislatures favor people who can afford to leave a full-time position, for example, retirees and professionals paid by salary rather than hourly wages (e.g., law firms that encourage their law partners to be politically active to attract additional clients). The perceived need for increased professionalization came from the notion that legislation had become more complex and time consuming. There was a perceived need for legislators who met for most of the year and had professional staffs to assist in both policy research and constituent service.

PARTISANSHIP

One changing aspect of our political culture that needs to be discussed in some detail is the role of partisanship. Even though political parties did not exist in our early national political experience, political disagreements were very intense. During and after the American Revolution, British loyalists were persecuted, with many of them fleeing to Canada. After the establishment of the United States political opponents were frequently called enemies. In 1798 the Alien and Sedition Act was passed by the Fifth Congress, allowing the federal government to imprison or deport noncitizens considered to be dangerous and making it a crime for citizens to make false statements critical of the government. Political rivals such as Aaron

Burr and Alexander Hamilton dueled, with Hamilton dying the next day from his wounds in 1804. From 1830 to 1860 there were 125 incidents of physical violence on the floor of Congress (Levitsky & Ziblatt, 2018). The Civil War was, of course, the ultimate partisan battle.

As explained by Levitsky and Ziblatt (2018), extreme partisanship did not really decline until, the election of 1876 when Republican President-elect Rutherford B. Hayes promised to remove federal troops from the South, allowing the end of Reconstruction. Without federal support, the electoral process returned to regional one-party domination and an acceptance of racial inequality by the dominant political culture in the South. This accommodation was disrupted in the 1960s with the civil rights movement and most notably by the Civil Rights Act of 1964 providing federal protection of civil rights. This also resulted in a major ideological realignment of the two major political parties. After signing the Civil Rights Act of 1964, Democratic President Lyndon Johnson reportedly told his aide Bill Moyers, "We have lost the South for a generation" or something to that effect (Allen, 2014).

By the 1880s the political culture began to be more open to democratic reforms. This began an era when political culture reflected what Levitsky and Ziblatt refer to as "institutional forbearance," the recognition that even if one had legal power, self-restraint and tolerance were important to maintain the public good (Levitsky & Ziblatt, 2018). As a result, political parties no longer perceived each other as enemies set out for the destruction of the other. Members of the two opposing parties could see each other as a pool of potential converts and not as enemies. Compromise became acceptable and bipartisan support for legislative proposals was possible. The height of attempts of diminished legislative partisanship was in the 1950s. This is when political scientists tended to critique the two American parties as being Tweedledee and Tweedledum. As a result, the American Political Science Association (1950) published a paper calling for the political parties to differentiate more to make them more responsible to voter preferences.

As pointed out by Klein (2020), increased differentiation of political parties does not necessarily lead to extremism, but to an increased ability for the voter to sort out the differences between them. A test of this came in the 1964 presidential election. Phyllis Schlafly's self-published book, *A Choice Not an Echo* (1964), was written to advance the candidacy of Barry Goldwater and as a rebuke of the Republican Eastern Establishment. Moderate Republicans were booed at the 1964 Convention. However, that clear choice resulted in a landslide loss for Goldwater. Instead, Democrat Lyndon Baines Johnson became president with strong Democratic majorities in both houses of Congress. Similarly, when Democrats nominated a more ideological George McGovern for president in 1972, they too lost in a landslide.

While having different overall philosophies regarding taxes and social hot button issues, the members of the two political parties still saw opportunities for cooperation. Both parties were "big tent" parties welcoming different types of candidates, supporters, and voters. Political donors and lobbyists contributed to both parties since it was more about gaining access to decision makers than supporting a particular ideology. Congressional Representatives and Senators could argue on the floor of their respective houses and then go for drinks and/or dinner afterward. They could oppose each other on some issues and join together on others. Symbolic of this collegial relationship was the working relationship between the liberal lion Senator Edward Kennedy (D-MA) and the social and fiscal conservative Senator Orin Hatch (R-UT). While clearly representing their different parties and being from very different backgrounds, they could work together on legislation. It was relatively safe for Democrats and Republicans to vote to support their legislation if the two of them could reach an agreement.

When did all this change? There are many historical examples of the American shift to increased partisanship. Each political party can point to multiple incidents when the other party violated protocol or slighted the other party (e.g., the Democratic rejection of a President Reagan's Supreme Court nominee Robert Bork or the Republican impeachment of President Clinton) and the need for retaliation.

However, one seminal event for greater partisan politics in the U.S. Congress was Newt Gingrich and Dick Armey's *Contract with America* for the 1994 midterm congressional election. The *Contract with America* was introduced shortly before the election as a list of policies Republicans would enact in the House in its first 100 days if they gained control of the House of Representatives (Riley, 1995). Its focus was on traditional Republican policies such as shrinking the size of government, promoting lower taxes, initiating a line-item budget veto, and enacting term limits, tort reform, and welfare reform. However, the *Contract* avoided mentioning divisive social policy issues such as abortion. The 1994 congressional elections resulted in the Republicans gaining control of both the House and the Senate. What was different about the *Contract with America* was that it was a *contract* and as such it was seen has something that had to be executed. As the first Republican Speaker of the House of Representatives in 40 years, Newt Gingrich centralized control under the Speaker and increased rewards for party loyalty instead of seniority. The Republicans also instituted term limits for Republican chairs of committees to make room for more "Republican" Republicans. This resembled a parliamentary type of government whereby Republican members were expected to follow leadership rather than respect seniority or committee chair fiefdoms. By the end of the 100 days, the House had passed nine of the 10 items in the Contract.

As a result of the 1994 midterm elections, the Republicans had also picked up eight Senate seats to take control of that chamber as well. However, due to staggered Senate terms only 13 Republicans were involved in the 1994 election and they had not based their campaigns on the House's *Contract with America*. As a result, House-passed legislation bogged down in the Senate. However, the lesson learned was that party leadership, discipline, and partisanship was politically beneficial.

Partisanship of Congress has since increased exponentially. Politically motivated oversight hearings, the refusal of the Senate to consider a presidential appointment to the U.S. Supreme Court (USSC) due to the proximity of a presidential election while approving another president's appointment while voting for the next president was underway, two House impeachments of a U.S. president along partisan lines and equally partisan votes of acquittals by the U.S. Senate, name calling and breaks of protocol, fights over the Senate filibuster, and other events have all led to a major change in congressional political culture. One can add any number of incidents to the list. However, it was not unusual in the 116th Congress for issues to be decided strictly on party-line votes. Collegial relations across the aisle are more strained.

At the beginning of each new Congress, both parties develop rules for their party caucus (House Democrats, 2021; House Republicans, 2021). The caucus includes only members of that party, although declared Independents can be invited to join a party caucus. Republican Speakers of the House now abide by the Hastert Rule, which was instituted in the 1990s by then Speaker Dennis Hastert (R-IL). Under the Hastert Rule, a Republican Speaker of the House of Representatives can only bring a bill to the floor if a majority in the Republican caucus in the House favors that legislation. This disadvantages any House-proposed legislation that may have a large bipartisan majority but not a majority within the Republican caucus. Although the rule is informal and exceptions have been made, the rule tends to weaken possibilities for bipartisan legislation.

One of interesting aspects of the current increased partisanship is the concurrent weakening of the political parties (Klein, 2020). Political parties used to control a major part of financial support for their political candidates. However, due primarily to the landmark USSC decision of *Citizens United v. FEC* (2010), money is increasingly raised by Political Action Committees (PACs; Connected PACs, Association PACs, Ideology PACs, Super PACs), small donor online fundraising, self-funding, and other financial mechanisms that typically bypass control by the political party. For example, according to the Brennan Center for Justice, Super PAC spending for midterm elections increased from $62.6 million in 2010 to $822 million in 2018 (Vandewalker, 2020). In addition, party nominees are increasingly determined by primaries rather than party conventions. Congressional campaigns have become more national with well-financed ideological individuals, corporations, PACs and identity political organizations. As a result, those wishing to run for office can merely declare their candidacy under a political banner and raise their own money with little obligation to their political party.

Sitting members of Congress are now afraid of being "primaried" by more ideologically pure candidates within their own party. To be labeled a Republican in Name Only (RINO) is an open invitation to be primaried. Examples from both parties have become more common. For example, Representative Kurt Shrader (D-OR) was defeated in the Democratic primary in Oregon in 2022 by a more progressive candidate, Jamie McLeod-Skinner. Liz Cheney (R-WY), the third ranking House Republican, was stripped of her party leadership role and was primaried due to her vote in favor of impeaching former President Donald J. Trump and her participation on the U.S. House of Representatives Select Committee to Investigate the January 6th Attack on the United States Capitol.

Political parties have in the past tended to be more pragmatic "big tent parties" looking for candidates and voters that would broaden their base of appeal among the electorate rather than responding to an ideological wing of the party. However, as Klein (2020) notes, to raise your own money you must stand out and be loud. The latter is done by creating villains, controversies, focusing on identity politics and nationalizing your campaign. House and Senate races are seen through an ideological lens more than on local issues or differences in policy positions. Identity politics is described as candidates and voters taking on the identity of a particular gender, race, religion, sexual orientation, or environmentalist, such as Sagebrush Rebels, Oath Keepers, Pro-Life, and so forth. Political candidates try to excite and appeal to these identities. Campaigns become less of a difference over the particulars of policy than a campaign of good versus evil. Politics becomes personal and name calling becomes acceptable. Obtaining something is less important than winning it all. Older members of Congress regret the increased partisan nature of both chambers, and some have retired as a result.

Partisanship has tended to increase exponentially since 2009. One of the major problems with this hardening of partisanship is the threat to what is understood as democracy in the United States. In their study of multiple countries that have turned from democracy toward authoritarianism, Levitsky and Ziblatt (2018) note that there are four key common denominators: (1) a rejection or weak commitment to the democratic rules of the game such as denying the legitimacy of elections, (2) denial of the legitimacy of political opponents such as calling opponents criminals or unpatriotic, (3) the toleration or encouragement of violence such as not condemning political violence or encouraging private militias, and (4) readiness to curtail civil liberties of opponents such as restricting freedom of the press or attacking news as lies. While the United States has always had antidemocratic and authoritarian politicians, such individuals have tended to have been isolated. However, some things have changed. Social media has become a platform for widespread dissemination of ideology, conspiracies, and misinformation. Well-financed ideologically oriented think tanks have focused on all levels of the political system. A former president has been investigated for interfering with counting the Electoral College vote. Antidemocratic policies are being advocated by multiple national and state political figures (Levitsky & Ziblatt, 2018).

Derogatory name calling and personal attacks have become common. There has also been an increase in political violence in the United States with attacks on the U.S. Capitol and threats of violence against the legislators, judges, the FBI, election officials, public health personnel, and others. How this change in the political culture will impact those willing to participate in the political process is yet to unfold. How this violence will affect the decision-making process is also yet to be determined. The ultimate test is what this increased violence in our political culture will do to our constitutional democracy.

STATE AND LOCAL POLITICAL CULTURES

Within the United States, state political cultures are variations on a theme; while there are some overriding similarities, there are also stark differences among the states. There may be regional infusions of political culture such as "Midwestern nice" and "volunteerism." Some states may intentionally celebrate their cultural differences with an adjacent state. Arizona and California have very different political cultures and neither shies away from the contrast. Despite both being small population rural states, the political culture of Vermont (having a self-identified democratic socialist as one of its U.S. senators) is not the same as that of solidly red Idaho. States vary greatly in terms of their political cultures despite sharing certain aspects of the dominant U.S. political culture. The influence of Scandinavians on Minnesota political culture; the influx of waves of French Canadians, Irish, and Italian immigrants in New England during the industrial revolution; the influence of the Russian Jewish immigration in New York City; the influence of Mexican and Central and South American immigrants in the West and South; the influence of Asians in California;

and the influence of the Cuban refugees in South Florida are but examples of the importance and variation of political cultures within the United States.

The recent increase in federal partisanship has also become apparent at state and local levels. State, county, mayoral, judgeship, secretaries of state, and local school board elections have all become more partisan affairs. Partisan national ideological divisions sometimes play an outsized role in state and local affairs. Seeking common ground is frequently perceived as surrendering to the enemy. Partisanship in the United States is still evolving. State and local governments have not been immune from such violence especially regarding school board members and election officials. State and local governments are so different that one would need to analyze each one as to the degree in which partisan politics plays a role in policy making. The U.S. political system has experienced much of this in the past.

SUMMARY

As a public health policy analyst, you need to be cognizant as to what the political culture is like in your geopolitical area. This chapter described some elements of our dominant political culture. Which of those elements does your political system share, or which additional elements are powerful factors that you need to consider? Violating perceived political culture norms may severely impact the feasibility of your policy proposal no matter how rational or well developed it may be. To ignore the traditionally accepted prerogatives of a powerful legislative committee chair may seriously impact your chances of success. We consider this further in Chapter 15. It is unknown when or whether there will be a toning down of partisanship and a return to some form of "institutional forbearance" as part of our political culture. Although a political strategy to get your policy adopted may be legal, does it fit within the political culture? How can your policy be changed to fit into the existing political culture, or alternatively, how can the political culture be modified to make your policy more acceptable?

DISCUSSION QUESTIONS

- Describe what you believe to be the most significant aspect of the American political culture influencing public health policy.
- To what extent do you believe the increased partisanship in the political process is good or bad?
- To what extent is institutional forbearance a positive or negative element?
- How can popular trust be built back into the American political system?
- How does your state's political culture differ from that of the dominant American political culture?

KEY TERMS

Alexis de Tocqueville
Alien and Sedition Act of 1798
American exceptionalism
bipartisanship
Citizens United v. FEC (2010)
citizen legislators
Contract with America
dominant political culture

Hastert Rule
melting pot
partisanship
Pendleton Civil Service Reform Act
  of 1883
Political Action Committees (PACs)
political culture

A robust set of instructor resources designed to supplement this text is located at http://connect.springerpub.com/content/book/978-0-8261-8543-3. Qualifying instructors may request access by emailing textbook@springerpub.com.

REFERENCES

Allen, S. J. (2014). *"We have lost the South for a generation": What Lyndon Johnson said, or would have said if only he had said it.* Capital Research Center. https://capitalresearch.org/article/we-have-lost-the-south-for-a-generation-what-lyndon-johnson-said-or-would-have-said-if-only-he-had-said-it

American Political Science Association. (1950). Toward a more responsible two-party system: A report. *American Political Science Review, 44*(3, Pt. 2 Suppl.). https://www.jstor.org/stable/i333592

Ananthaswamy, A. (2020, December 17). How the belief in American exceptionalism has shaped the pandemic response. *Smithsonian Magazine.* https://www.smithsonianmag.com/history/how-uss-values-and-american-exceptionalism-have-shaped-our-pandemic-response-180976573

Archer, S. (2018). *Sharks upon the land: Colonialism, Indigenous health, and culture in Hawai'i, 1778–1855.* Cambridge University Press. https://doi.org/10.1017/9781316795934

Carr, C. L. (2007). *Polity: Political culture and the nature of politics.* Rowman & Littlefield Publishers.

Cave, D. (2022, May 15). How Australia saved thousands of lives while Covid killed a million Americans. *The New York Times.* https://www.nytimes.com/2022/05/15/world/australia/covid-deaths.html

Chigudu, S. (2021). An ironic guide to colonialism in global health. *The Lancet, 397*(10288), 1874–1875. https://doi.org/10.1016/s0140-6736(21)01102-8

Citizens United v. FEC, 558 U.S. 310 (2010). https://supreme.justia.com/cases/federal/us/558/310

Civil Rights Act, Pub. L. No. 88-352, 78 Stat. 241 (1964). https://www.govinfo.gov/content/pkg/STATUTE-78/pdf/STATUTE-78-Pg241.pdf

Coronavirus Resource Center. (2022a, May 16). *Mortality analyses.* Johns Hopkins Coronavirus Resource Center. https://coronavirus.jhu.edu/data/mortality

Coronavirus Research Center. (2022b). *Understanding vaccination progress.* Johns Hopkins Coronavirus Resource Center. https://coronavirus.jhu.edu/vaccines/international

Edelman, M. (1967). *The symbolic uses of politics.* University of Illinois Press.

Gamble, V. N. (1997). Under the shadow of Tuskegee: African Americans and health care. *American Journal of Public Health, 87*(11), 1773–1778. https://doi.org/10.2105/ajph.87.11.1773

Hofstadter, R., & Lasch, C. (1974). *The American political tradition and the men who made it.* Vintage Books.

House Democrats. (2021, January 14). *Rules of the demographic caucus: 117th Congress.* https://www.dems.gov/imo/media/doc/DEM_CAUCUS_RULES_117TH_April_2021.pdf

House Republicans. (2021, March 17). *Conference rules of the 117th Congress.* https://www.gop.gov/conference-rules-of-the-117th-congress

Jefferson, T. (1776). *Declaration of independence.* National Archives. https://www.archives.gov/founding-docs/declaration-transcript

Jones, C. P. (2014, July 10). *Allegories on race and racism* [Video]. YouTube. https://www.youtube.com/watch?v=GNhcY6fTyBM

Klein, E. (2020). *Why we're polarized.* Avid Reader Press.

Levitsky, S., & Ziblatt, D. (2018). *How democracies die.* Broadway Books.

Lupien, P., Rincón, A., Lalama, A., & Chiriboga, G. (2022). Framing Indigenous protest in the online public sphere: A comparative frame analysis. *New Media & Society.* https://doi.org/10.1177/14614448221074705

Marr, J. S., & Cathey, J. T. (2010). New hypothesis for cause of epidemic among Native Americans, New England, 1616–1619. *Emerging Infectious Diseases, 16*(2), 281–286. https://doi.org/10.3201/eid1602.090276

Prescod-Weinstein, C. (2022). *The disordered cosmos: A journey into dark matter, spacetime, and dreams deferred.* Bold Type Books.

Reagan, R. (1981, January 20). *Inaugural address 1981.* National Archives. https://www.reaganlibrary.gov/archives/speech/inaugural-address-1981

Riley, R. L. (1995). Party government and the contract with America. *Political Science & Politics, 28*(04), 703–707. https://doi.org/10.1017/s1049096500058893

Schildkraut, D. J. (2014). Boundaries of American identity: Evolving understandings of "Us." *Annual Review of Political Science, 17*(1), 441–460. https://doi.org/10.1146/annurev-polisci-080812-144642

Schlafly, P. (1964). *A choice not an echo.* Pere Marquette Press.

Simmons-Duffin, S., & Nakajima, K. (2022, May 13). *This is how many lives could have been saved with COVID vaccinations in each state.* NPR. https://www.npr.org/sections/health-shots/2022/05/13/1098071284/this-is-how-many-lives-could-have-been-saved-with-covid-vaccinations-in-each-sta

Sparks, G., Lopes, L., Montero, A., Hamel, L., & Brodie, M. (2022, May 4). KFF COVID-19 vaccine monitor: April 2022. KFF. https://www.kff.org/coronavirus-covid-19/poll-finding/kff-covid-19-vaccine-monitor-april-2022

Tocqueville, A. (2002). *Democracy in America* (H. C. Mansfield & D. Winthrop, Trans.). University of Chicago Press.

Vandewalker, I. (2020, January 14). *Since citizens united a decade of super PACs.* Brennan Center for Justice. https://www.brennancenter.org/our-work/analysis-opinion/citizens-united-decade-super-pacs

Webster, D. G., Aytur, S. A., Axelrod, M., Wilson, R. S., Hamm, J. A., Sayed, L., Pearson, A. L., Torres, P. H. C., Akporiaye, A., & Young, O. (2022). Learning from the past: Pandemics and the governance treadmill. *Sustainability, 14*(6), 3683. https://doi.org/10.3390/su14063683

Welch, S. (2013). *The theory of political culture.* Oxford University Press.

Wiarda, H. J. (2018). *Political culture, political science, and identity politics: An uneasy alliance.* Routledge.

Winthrop, J. (2020). *A model of Christian charity: A city upon a hill.* Cosimo Classics.

CHAPTER 7

BEGINNING YOUR PUBLIC HEALTH POLICY ANALYSIS

This chapter outlines the process for conducting your health policy analysis. Your assignment may vary depending on your organization or policy maker. You need to understand their expectations for a policy analysis. We present several formats used in public health. We provide multiple resources to examine both peer-reviewed and grey literature for doing your research. Finally, we provide advice regarding the structure of your analysis such as writing an executive summary, the importance of defining terms, and the potential for appendices. The next chapter is more specific in noting resources for conducting a health policy analysis.

LEARNING OBJECTIVES

Be able to:

- Assess the motivations for conducting a policy analysis.
- Describe some existing frameworks for conducting a policy analysis.
- Identify sources of evidence found in the literature.
- Describe grey literature and how it can be utilized.
- Discuss stakeholder assessments.
- Explain the specific steps of the policy analysis.

Before getting into the substance of the policy analysis, it is important to discuss some of the pieces of your policy analysis that are helpful in making it more useful to readers. Remember that depending on your assignment, you may begin at different stages of the policy process wheel. See **Figure 4.1**. You or your organization will determine which elements are necessary and which are optional. For example, your analysis might focus more on policy implementation rather than on policy adoption. You may be asked to focus on one policy or to compare alternative policies.

You may find yourself preparing this analysis for a nonprofit health advocacy group, a legislator, a state agency, a governor's office, a federal agency, a lobbying firm, or any of a myriad of other types of organizations doing policy analysis. We will use the generic term *policy maker* throughout the rest of this book to represent this broad array of decision makers and policy influencers. You may have worked in your organization for years or just begun. In either case, you will need to clearly understand the operating procedures of your organization as well as understand its personalities and culture. You may be conducting the analysis as part of a Health Impact Assessment (HIA; Bhatia, Farhang, & Lee, 2010; Cooke et al., 2010; Dannenberg et al., 2019), which we discuss later in this chapter. Your organization may have a standard format for policy analysis. If you work in public health, the Centers for Disease Control and Prevention (CDC) provides guidance on the POLARIS website about policy analysis (CDC, n.d.-d). Sometimes a policy maker may prefer a different format, such as a Policy Brief. See the Appendix for additional resources. It is important to make your policy analysis fit the expectations of your organization.

You will need to understand the motivations behind your organization's pursuit of such an analysis. At first, this may appear to be obvious. However, there may be other motivations involved such as gaining political capital with various stakeholders. We will use a politician as our primary example here, but the same applies for organizations. The concept of political capital is borrowed from economics. Capital is a resource that can be accumulated and then converted for something of value later. Politicians accumulate political capital by supporting or opposing key legislation, using their party or committee leadership positions, gaining editorial endorsements, raising campaign contributions, providing constituency services, praising or endorsing another politician, and so forth. Political capital provides politicians with potential influence to be used later. Politicians will save their political capital and then spend it judiciously to gain support for their own policy priorities, to get an assignment on an important legislative committee, to resist pressure from a major campaign contributor, or to gain some other personal priority. Gambling one's political capital on an initiative may yield a high payoff or lead to a significant loss. Toward the end of their political career, one may wish to use all their remaining political capital to pass legislation that has been personally important to them but has been too politically costly in the past to support. They may now be increasingly concerned about their legacy. One thing you should ask yourself is, how much political capital do you think your policy maker is willing to expend on this policy? It is important to understand the multiple motivations policy makers have in undertaking a potentially long-term investment of political capital.

A ROADMAP FOR WRITING A POLICY ANALYSIS REPORT

There is no single "one-size fits all" approach to writing a policy analysis. However, in this section we provide some examples and templates to help organize your thoughts. One template is an HIA, which is an assessment process to help communities, decision makers, and practitioners make informed choices about prospective (upcoming) policies that may affect public health (Bhatia, Branscomb, et al., 2010; Bhatia, Farhang, & Lee, 2010). HIA is a prospective analytic tool, so it is intended to be used before a policy is adopted or before implementation funds are allocated and when there is adequate time to inform the decision-making process. The choice of whether to use an HIA approach would depend on whether the initial step of the HIA process (screening) determines that an HIA is warranted and would be valuable in a particular decision-making context (The Pew Charitable Trusts, 2018).[1] The CDC also provides an archive of practical tools and resources for HIA (CDC, n.d.-a). Steps that are relevant to the HIA process are highlighted in italics in **Table 7.1**.

CONSIDERATION OF POLITICAL SCIENCE THEORY

We suggest that you access additional references about political science and policy science theory to help guide your approach. For example, we briefly discuss Kingdon's "multiple streams" approach (Kingdon, 1984) and Sabatier's advocacy coalition approach (Sabatier, 2007; Sabatier & Jenkins-Smith, 1993) in Chapters 10 and 12. They are among the most widely used theories in public health. Additional theoretical references relevant to public health policy (Amri & Drummond, 2021; Baumgartner & Jones, 1991; Clarke et al., 2016; Jones et al., 2017; Okeke et al., 2021; Paniagua, 2022; Watson, 2014; Weible et al., 2020) are cited at the end of this chapter and in the Appendix.

ASSESSING THE EVIDENCE
Peer-Reviewed Literature

You will need to begin to find innovative programs and evidence as to which programs have been demonstrated to be effective. Even though you might have multiple criteria for success (see Chapters 8 and 13), effectiveness is a major criterion that would be used to assess any policy. One would not wish to waste public resources by recommending programs or policies that did not work. Therefore, you should first determine whether any peer-reviewed literature or reports speak to the effectiveness or impact of policies similar to yours. What does the literature say about whether the policy you are analyzing is likely to result in favorable outcomes?

Peer-reviewed literature is one of the best sources of that information. There is a note of caution here since there is a publication bias in favor of studies that result in positive outcomes. Those studies that do not show a positive result (null studies) tend have a more difficult time being published even though the lack of a relationship is just as important as the existence of a relationship.

Peer-reviewed studies are also one of the easiest sources to access due to the multiple centralized electronic databases that are available. If you are not familiar with the public electronic databases, you should access a research university librarian to provide you with some initial assistance. They can ease your initial search and highlight major resources. Research university libraries generally have

---

1 The Health Impact Project, a collaboration of the Robert Wood Johnson Foundation and the Pew Charitable Trusts, provides practical HIA tools and resources that help communities, agencies, and other organizations take action to improve public health. The toolkit offers examples of Health Impact Assessments, guides, and other research to support policy makers' efforts to consider health when making cross-sector decisions.

TABLE 7.1 TEMPLATE FOR HEALTH POLICY ANALYSIS REPORTS

	SECTIONS TO INCLUDE IN A POLICY ANALYSIS REPORT HIA (CDC, N.D.)		
	GENERAL REPORT TEMPLATE	**HIA TEMPLATE**	**CROSSWALK: STEPS OF THE HIA PROCESS**
1	Table of contents		N/A
2	Executive summary		N/A
3	List of abbreviations/definitions		N/A
		ANALYSIS	
4	**Problem Definition and Statement of the Policy Issue** ■ Assessing the evidence; using peer-reviewed and grey literature (Chapter 7) ■ Background Section (Chapter 10) ■ Framing the Issue (Chapter 11) ■ Using data, analytics, and health science research methods to help make your case (Chapters 7, 8, and 12; Bir & Freeman, 2016) ■ Considering the health effects associated with the issue (Chapters 7, 8, 11, and 12)	**Problem Definition and Statement of the Policy Issue** ■ Assessing the evidence; using peer-reviewed and grey literature (Chapter 7) ■ Background Section (Chapter 10) ■ Framing the Issue (Chapter 11) ■ Using data, analytics, and health science research methods to help make your case (Chapters 7, 8, and 12) ■ Considering the *health and equity effects* associated with the issue (Chapters 7, 8, 11, and 12) ■ *Including direct and indirect effects associated with decisions made outside traditional biomedical arenas (e.g., agriculture, environment, infrastructure, labor, education)*	**HIA Screening Step:** Identify policy issues and decisions for which an HIA could potentially be useful. Determine whether an HIA would be feasible, given the time and resources available. How might the HIA add value to the decision process?

5	Values and Stakeholder Analysis (Chapter 12)	Values and Stakeholder Analysis (Chapter 12)	HIA Scoping Step:
	■ Which policy makers are sponsoring or authorizing the policy or proposed decision?	■ Which policy makers are sponsoring or authorizing the policy or proposed decision?	Determine which health impacts to focus on in the HIA, given available time and resources.
	■ Who is likely to support it, and who is likely to oppose it?	■ Who is likely to support it, and who is likely to oppose it?	Data availability and/or data collection should also be considered.
	■ Which coalitions and alliances are important? Could new collaborations be formed?	■ *Are persons from affected communities represented? How might you use the HIA process to increase community engagement?*	Establish ethical relationships with community members, representatives of community-based organizations, health department staff, social service agencies, policy makers, urban/rural planners, nonprofits, advocacy groups, and other stakeholders from relevant sectors.
	■ Which sets of values might you consider to help bring stakeholders together?	■ Which coalitions and alliances are important?	Establish a workplan for completing the HIA (goals, timeline, participant roles, stakeholder involvement, health impacts to be considered, research questions, methods of analysis, communication strategies, and reporting format).
	■ Use data to inform this section, as discussed in Chapters 8 and 9. Social network analysis (Chapter 12) can also be helpful for this section.	■ *Could the HIA process facilitate new collaborations, particularly across sectors?*	
	■ Qualitative research can add insights regarding stakeholder perspectives.	■ Which sets of values might you consider to help bring stakeholders together?	
	■ The CDC POLARIS Stakeholder Analysis Worksheets can help to support this section: www.cdc.gov/policy/analysis/process/docs/table1.pdf www.cdc.gov/policy/analysis/process/docs/table2.pdf Brugha and Varvasovszky (2000) provide additional insights on how to conduct a stakeholder analysis. Please see the Appendix for additional resources, including other examples of stakeholder worksheets and policy process tools.	■ Use data to inform this section, as discussed in Chapters 8 and 9. Social network analysis (Chapter 12) can also be helpful for this section.	
		■ *PAR and CBPR methods can be particularly helpful in supporting equity (Arcaya et al., 2018).*	
		■ Qualitative research methods can add insights regarding stakeholder perspectives.	

(continued)

TABLE 7.1 TEMPLATE FOR HEALTH POLICY ANALYSIS REPORTS *(continued)*

SECTIONS TO INCLUDE IN A POLICY ANALYSIS REPORT HIA (CDC, N.D.)

	GENERAL REPORT TEMPLATE	HIA TEMPLATE	CROSSWALK: STEPS OF THE HIA PROCESS
6	***Develop Criteria for Assessment (Chapters 8 and 13)*** ■ What criteria will you use to assess the impacts of the policy (and/or policy alternatives) for the issue? (Chapters 8 and 13) ■ For example, what might be the impacts in terms of effectiveness, equity, efficiency, and feasibility? What would the impacts be in terms of sustainability? ■ Which populations might be the "winners" and "losers"? ■ Use data and health science research methods to inform your assessment, as described in Chapters 8, 9, and 12. ■ Mapping tools, spatial analysis, econometrics, and qualitative methods can also be very helpful in this section.	***Develop Criteria for Assessment (Chapters 8 and 13)*** ■ What criteria will you use to assess the impacts of the policy (and/or policy alternatives) for the issue? (Chapters 8 and 13) ■ For example, what might be the impacts in terms of effectiveness, equity, efficiency, and feasibility? What would the impacts be in terms of sustainability? ■ Which populations might be the "winners" and "losers"? *■ How are vulnerable populations affected? How will health disparities be addressed?* ■ Use data and health science research methods to inform your assessment, as described in Chapters 8, 9, and 12. ■ Mapping tools, spatial analysis, econometrics, and qualitative methods can also be very helpful in this section. *■ PAR, CBPR, and EJ paradigms can support the HIA process (Arcaya et al., 2018).*	**HIA Assessment Step:** Delineate the pathways by which the policy alternatives could impact health, including vulnerable groups that may be affected. Data science tools (see Chapters 9 and 12) such as causal loop diagrams, system dynamic models, spatial analysis, social network analysis, and other qualitative, quantitative, and participatory action research methods can be used to support this step. Prior research, literature reviews, meta-analyses, and analytic reports relevant to your context can also be utilized in this section. If possible, engage experts in data science, library science, epidemiology, biostatistics, and/or economics to assist with more advanced analytic functions.

7	*Review the Policy Options (Chapter 14)*	*Review the Policy Options (Chapter 14)*	**HIA Assessment and Recommendations Steps:**
	■ What are the possible policy alternatives for the issue? ■ Summarize each policy option. ■ Clarify the trade-offs. ■ Who will be the "winners" and who may be the "losers"? ■ Review the pros and cons of each policy alternative. ■ What types of health, economic, social, and environmental impacts would the decisions have? Use the criteria you selected (Chapter 13). ■ Consider the fact that "doing nothing" (or maintaining the status quo) is actually a political choice with its own health implications that should be specified. ■ When possible, quantify the health impacts that may be associated with each policy option. ■ Use qualitative methods to add contextual information.	■ What are the possible policy alternatives for the issue? ■ Summarize each policy option. ■ Clarify the trade-offs. ■ Who will be the "winners" and who may be the "losers"? ■ Review the pros and cons of each policy alternative. ■ *How will different population subgroups be affected? How will vulnerable populations be affected? What will be the impact on health disparities?* ■ What types of health, economic, social, and environmental impacts would the decisions have? Use the criteria you selected (Chapter 13). ■ Consider the fact that "doing nothing" (or maintaining the status quo) is actually a political choice with its own health implications that should be specified. ■ When possible, quantify the health impacts that may be associated with each policy option. ■ Use qualitative methods to add contextual information.	If possible, quantify the health impacts that may be associated with each policy option, as well as the economic and equity impacts. Use qualitative methods to add contextual information. This will help to strengthen the assessment by clarifying the trade-offs for different population subgroups.

(continued)

TABLE 7.1 TEMPLATE FOR HEALTH POLICY ANALYSIS REPORTS (*continued*)

SECTIONS TO INCLUDE IN A POLICY ANALYSIS REPORT HIA (CDC, N.D.)

	GENERAL REPORT TEMPLATE	HIA TEMPLATE	CROSSWALK: STEPS OF THE HIA PROCESS
8	**Recommendations and Strategies** ■ Based on the criteria you identified and your analytic assessment, what recommendations would you make? (Chapter 15) ■ Do some alternatives appear to benefit health more than others (or mitigate negative health impacts than others)? ■ In what ways, and for whom? ■ Simulation analysis and systems science methods ((Chapter 9) can be particularly helpful in terms of exploring the potential impacts of different policy scenarios. Modeling, spatial analysis, and econometric analyses can also be helpful in this section.	**Recommendations and Strategies** ■ Based on the criteria you identified and your analytic assessment, what recommendations would you make? (Chapter 15) ■ Do some alternatives appear to positively affect health (or mitigate negative health effects) more than others? In what ways, and for whom? ■ *How is equity considered? Who participated in the process? Who was not represented? Which sectors were not at the table?* ■ Simulation analysis and systems science methods (Chapter 9) can be particularly helpful in terms of exploring the potential impacts of different policy scenarios. Modeling, spatial analysis, and econometric analyses can also be helpful.	**HIA Recommendations and Reporting Steps:** Summarize each policy option. Suggest practical actions to promote positive health effects and/or minimize negative health effects. Present HIA results to decision makers, affected communities, and other stakeholders using PHRASES or other culturally sensitive communication strategies. If possible, engage a communication science professional to assist with telling your story in a culturally sensitive manner.

9	Evaluation	Evaluation (to be conducted after the decision is made)	HIA Monitoring and Evaluation Steps:
	■ What outcomes can be measured? Which health indicators changed? (Review your criteria from Chapter 13, and use health science research methods as described in Chapters 9 and 12.) ■ Why might the decision have unfolded the way it did? What factors might help to explain the process? ■ Utilize health science research methods and analytic tools described in Chapter 9. Meta-analytic tools (Bir & Freeman, 2016) and case study methods (Yin, 1994) can also be helpful.	■ *What impact did the HIA have on the decision process?* ■ What outcomes can be measured? Which health indicators changed? (Review your criteria from Chapter 13, and use health science research methods as described in Chapters 9 and 12.) ■ *Can environmental justice indicators be measured?* ■ Why might the decision have unfolded the way it did? What factors might help to explain the process? ■ Utilize health science research methods and analytic tools described in Chapter 9. ■ *Consider ways to utilize PAR and tools such as community mapping and social network analysis to assess changes in collaborations and stakeholder relationships.*	Evaluate the HIA's impact on the decision and its effects on population health status. Who participated in the process, and who did not? Were any new collaborations or relationships formed? How was social capital affected? Assess the differential impacts on vulnerable populations and marginalized groups. If possible, engage experts in evaluation, community-based participatory research, epidemiology, Geographic Information Systems, biostatistics, and/or economics to assist with this section.
	References		
	Appendices (additional data, visuals, tables, maps, graphs/diagrams, Photovoice, media resources, etc.)		

CBPR, community-based participatory research; CDC, Centers for Disease Control and Prevention; EJ, environmental justice; HIA, Health Impact Assessment; PAR, participatory action research; PHRASES, Public Health Reaching Across Sectors.

Source: Centers for Disease Control and Prevention. (n.d.). Healthy places: *Health Impact Assessment resources.* U.S. Department of Health and Human Services. https://www.cdc.gov/healthyplaces/hiaresources.htm

free access to many of these databases as well as access to individual peer-reviewed journals, allowing you to read specific articles. Librarians can also provide valuable guidance as to how to search the literature in a professional, systematic, and replicable way by using search strings, MeSH (Medical Subject Headings), and relevant key words. They can help you find summaries of prior literature (collectively referred to as systematic reviews, scoping reviews, meta-analysis, and other types of reviews). Many local hospitals have their own libraries that contain clinical journals.

Because you are dealing with health, one of the most useful sources of peer-reviewed literature is the National Institutes of Health's National Library of Medicine's PubMed (https://pubmed.ncbi.nlm.nih.gov). This database catalogs most major peer-reviewed journals in the field of medicine, public health, and environmental health. While mainly covering U.S. peer-reviewed journals, this database also includes the more influential health journals in other countries. By entering a public health topic, you are likely to receive thousands of citations. You then need to narrow the topic to receive citations that are more targeted. You can then scan those citations for the articles that seem to be the most current or relevant to your policy initiative.

One of the things that you would want to look for within the PubMed citations is a systematic review article. These articles typically have *systematic review* in the title. They are particularly helpful because they summarize the findings of the published literature between given years for a particular topic. Some systematic reviews may be for minority populations; some may be for other countries; some may be more recent than others. You will want to scan this list for those systematic reviews that appear to be the most applicable to your policy topic and are the most recent. These systematic reviews will be helpful in highlighting the seminal works that you should read. Systematic reviews tend to identify areas where there is basic consensus within the literature and where there are differences. They may point to especially innovative policies or programs. They will discuss important data and methodological differences among the various studies. The bibliographies of these systematic reviews will cite those individual studies that are most applicable to your policy (see **Breakout Box 7.1**).

There are other databases for law (Westlaw, www.westlaw.com) and business (Business Source Premier, www.ebscohost.com/academic/business-source-premier). Both of these indices may also be useful for health policy analyses depending on your topic. Additional resources are provided in the Appendix.

A similar type of study that you should attempt to locate is a meta-analysis (Bir & Freeman, 2016). A meta-analysis combines data from multiple studies and then produces a summary statistical estimate of "pooled effect" or the overall effectiveness. A meta-analysis is useful in examining the statistical strength of individual studies as well as coming up with one number showing the effect size (generally a decimal from .00 to 1.00) of the variables under investigation. By combining multiple studies, a meta-analysis has the impact of expanding the size of the population represented by only one study (adding strength to the relationship) and potentially the inclusion of important subpopulations representing different ethnic groups, ages, and so forth. You need to examine the criteria used by the authors for including studies in their meta-analysis. The inclusion of poorly designed studies weakens any meta-analysis conclusion. Some of these

Breakout Box 7.1

USING SYSTEMATIC REVIEWS TO INFORM POLICY ANALYSIS

Although one might think that there is a lot of evidence comparing various childhood obesity programs and policies, in reality comparative effectiveness research is an emerging science, especially in community settings. An example of a systematic review of childhood obesity programs can be found in an article by Bleich et al. (2013). The authors systematically reviewed community-based childhood obesity prevention programs in the United States and other high-income countries.

To find relevant studies, the authors searched databases including Medline, Embase, PsychInfo, CINAHL, clinicaltrials.gov, and the Cochrane Library. Only studies published in English were included. To be eligible for inclusion, obesity interventions had to have been implemented in the community setting; have at least 1 year of follow-up after baseline; and compare results from an intervention group to a comparison group. This yielded nine community-based studies for inclusion: five randomized controlled trials and four nonrandomized controlled trials with comparison groups. One study was conducted only in the community setting, three were conducted in the community and school setting, and five were conducted in the community setting in combination with at least one other setting (such as the home). Outcome measures included changes in body mass index (BMI) and health behaviors.

After synthesizing the data, the authors graded the quantity, quality, and consistency of the best available evidence by adapting an evidence grading scheme recommended in the *Methods Guide for Conducting Comparative Effectiveness Reviews* (Chang, 2011). Results showed that desirable changes in BMI were found in four of the nine studies. Two studies reported statistically significant improvements in behavioral outcomes (e.g., physical activity and vegetable intake).

The authors concluded that the strength of evidence is "moderate" that a combined diet and physical activity intervention conducted in the community setting with a school component is more effective at preventing obesity or overweight compared to other types of interventions or no intervention. A "moderate" rating indicates that the authors had moderate confidence that the evidence reflects the true effect, and further research may change our confidence in the estimate of the impact over time. However, the authors emphasize that even if interventions have a modest effect on individual body weight, the cumulative population-wide impact has the potential to yield significant public health benefits. The authors also recommend more research using consistent methods in order to better understand the comparative effectiveness of childhood obesity prevention programs in community settings.

Thought Questions

Imagine that you are doing an analysis for a policy maker who is generally supportive of community-based childhood obesity programs and wants to continue dedicating funds to them. She is running against a conservative opponent who doesn't feel that tax dollars should be used to fund programs of uncertain impact. How would you help your policy maker to:

1. Understand the evidence presented by Bleich et al. (2013) including its strengths and limitations?

2. Frame a message that aligns with her supportive stance for community-based obesity prevention programs, while not misconstruing the current state of the science?

3. Recognize how her opponent may frame the evidence presented above as indicative that these programs don't work, and how she might counter such an argument?

References

Bleich, S. N., Segal, J., Wu, Y., Wilson, R., & Wang, Y. (2013). Systematic review of community-based childhood obesity prevention studies. *Pediatrics, 132*(1), e201–e210. https://doi.org/10.1542/peds.2013-0886

Chang, S. M. (2011). The Agency for Healthcare Research and Quality (AHRQ) Effective Health Care (EHC) Program methods guide for comparative effectiveness reviews: Keeping up-to-date in a rapidly evolving field. *Journal of Clinical Epidemiology, 64*(11), 1166–1167. https://doi.org/10.1016/j.jclinepi.2011.08.004

meta-analyses will be more applicable to your potential policy concern than others, so be selective. Because meta-analyses tend to be statistically complex, you might want to consult with someone who is comfortable in interpreting statistical analyses.

There are peer-reviewed journals covering both general and specialty areas within medicine and public health. It is impossible to list all the sources. Some health science journals are more theoretical, and some are more oriented toward practitioners. Unless you are already familiar with these journals, a librarian in a health-oriented library can help guide you in terms of finding key relevant journals.

Your task is to select the most relevant articles that reflect the variety and richness of the information on your topic that is available to you through peer-reviewed journals and/or reports from leading health organizations such as the CDC and the World Health Organization (WHO; www.who.int/tools/health-impact-assessments). Using the lens of the Health in All Policies (HiAP) described in Chapter 1 should lead you to other policy areas that may have lessons that can be applied to your policy concerns. This can help you to frame the policy issue from a multisectoral perspective, which may enable you to garner additional partners and collaborators who are likely to support your proposal.

Grey Literature

While peer-reviewed articles are an important source of policy information, they also have their weaknesses, especially for public health policy analysis.

Peer-reviewed literature is developed by academics to further the literature in their discipline. Their research agendas may not match the policy needs of the national, state, or local governments. Peer-reviewed journals also have their own interests and agendas and may not give precedence to articles that are policy or practice oriented. Due to the length of time needed for their analytical studies, peer-reviewed literature may not contain the most recent evidence.

Grey literature includes agency reports, monographs, white papers, policy issue briefs, or technical reports that are not published by a general commercial publisher. Grey literature tends to be written for specific audiences and have low print runs or may only be available in electronic format. It might be a policy issue brief written by state agency or a regional or national private organization. Indeed, your own public health policy analysis may become part of the grey literature. Grey literature may go through some form of internal review process by the organization publishing the material, but it is generally not reviewed by an impartial panel of external reviewers. A document written by a state agency about one of its programs may be useful, but it may not be critical of its own program unless it is laying the foundation for obtaining additional resources or policy authority.

One of the places to look for policies/programs described by grey literature is to look at publications by geopolitical units (national, state, or local governments). State governments are frequently viewed as being a source of policy experimentation. Associate Justice Brandeis of the U.S. Supreme Court is generally attributed with calling states "the laboratory of democracy" in the United States (*New State Ice Co. v. Liebmann*, 1932). The experience of a state or local public health program is less likely to be published in a peer-reviewed journal due to its narrow or local reader interest. If the authors demonstrate that a state program/policy has potential national significance, it has a better chance of being published in a peer-reviewed journal, especially one that is practitioner oriented.

Accessing grey literature can be difficult. There are some useful sources such as The New York Academy of Medicine (Current Grey Literature Report, 2016; www .greylit.org/reports/current). It publishes a list of recent state-published reports along with an electronic source to access the original report. One can search by author, title, publisher, or date of publication but not by topic. However, it is a very useful resource to keep abreast of what has been recently produced by state agencies throughout the country.

Because most grey literature appears on agency websites, you can use a commercial browser. However, such documents will not usually be the first page of a search engine's browser results unless you are very specific in terms of title and state. Consequently, the search for grey literature can be time consuming.

Access to grey literature creates a problem of credibility. Some research groups have a particular ideological bias. It is certainly wise to seek information reflecting different political ideologies, such as a conservative perspective from The Heritage Foundation (www.heritage.org) or a liberal perspective from The Center for American Progress (www.americanprogress.org) to learn of different political takes on the issue. Accessing ideologically different sources will allow you to gain insight to potential allies and opposition. However, recognizing and acknowledging potential bias is important in building the credibility of your own analysis. Many of these sources of grey literature may have policy research sounding names and a national board of advisors. They may employ PhD fellows to write reports and policy briefs for them. Examine the credentials of the people associated with these organizations. Some produce quality work, but you should be aware of the organization's political/policy agenda. While grey literature is an important source of information, be vigilant of political biases that may impede their methodological rigor. Since grey literature generally lacks peer review, by using it you have the increased burden of screening the good from the bad. Citing questionable sources as your evidence undermines the credibility of your analysis.

A state's website may not have a very user-friendly search engine. Consequently, finding a particular article can be frustrating. In addition, articles may be taken down and no longer be accessible. Readers may not be able to actually access the original source.

Some policy papers blur the distinction between peer-reviewed and grey literature. The Rand Corporation (www.rand.org) is one of the largest and most respected U.S. private research corporations that produce both grey literature and peer-reviewed publications. It produces very reputable research and even has its own policy research PhD program. Federal government agencies frequently contract with Rand to do sophisticated analyses in a wide variety of policy areas. It publishes some of its own studies and also submits articles to peer-reviewed journals. The Henry J. Kaiser Family Foundation also falls into this area as well. It would be difficult to write a comprehensive review of Medicare, Medicaid, or healthcare reform policy without using analytical material and data from the Henry J. Kaiser Family Foundation (www.kff.org).

Another important source for a variety of policy issues is the Brookings Institution (www.brookings.edu). It publishes policy articles and books in a wide variety of areas. It includes blogs as well as articles by many distinguished authors. It also has a section devoted to public health issues.

Another important type of organization to access are private foundations that sponsor research and demonstration projects around the country or in specific regions. Within healthcare, there are many such foundations; one that is particularly notable is the Robert Wood Johnson Foundation (www.rwjf.org). It is the largest health-focused foundation in the United States, and it is renowned for funding model demonstration programs around the country that implement innovative solutions at the state and local level. Robert Wood Johnson Foundation publishes *Issue Briefs* that highlight successful programs it has funded around the country. For example, on the topic of childhood obesity there is an issue brief describing successful childhood obesity programs (Robert Wood Johnson Foundation, 2016). Two CDC national collaborative networks, the Physical Activity Policy Research and Evaluation Network (PAPREN; https://papren.org) and the Nutrition and Obesity Policy Research and Evaluation Network (NOPREN; https://nopren .ucsf.edu/about-us) offer practical resources for finding obesity-related studies, including both peer-reviewed and grey literature. Healthy Places by Design (healthyplacesbydesign.org) is also a good source of practical, community-level policy and environmental change initiatives across the country. Many of these community initiatives have been rigorously evaluated.

If you decide to deal with state or local initiatives for your policy, you should be especially sensitive to what local foundations have funded as demonstration programs in your geographic area. Many states now have relatively large state-/local-based health foundations as a result of the sale of their nonprofit hospitals to for-profit corporations. These foundations have become important sources for funding local healthcare demonstration projects.

Another source of policy at the state level is the National Conference of State Legislatures (NCSL; www.ncsl.org). It is a bipartisan organization that conducts research and discusses policy issues. Its website is a great source for summaries of legislation introduced state by state on various topics with an electronic link to the bill in each state. The NCSL also conducts conferences for state legislative leaders to share information. It has a section on healthcare and provides a good source of information as to what is currently happening in individual states. The American Legislative Exchange Council (ALEC; 2022) has gained national attention for providing model legislative initiatives for states to copy. ALEC's political agenda favors limited government, free markets, and states' rights.

Policy institutes in academic institutions are also an important source of policy ideas and evaluations of existing programs. They can also be advocates for certain policy initiatives. Some have close ties with state governments and others remain independent of political forces. Such institutes may focus on a particular topic such as mental health, climate change, domestic violence. Others might focus on regional areas or rural/urban areas. Some of these centers receive federal funds to serve as national or regional centers for expertise in policy development. These centers generally produce both grey literature and peer-reviewed literature.

There are also federal sources of grey literature that should be considered. We have previously mentioned the Congressional Budget Office (CBO), which provides studies on policies that have a budgetary impact (www.cbo.gov). The CBO is a nonpartisan branch of the U.S. Congress that does research for members of Congress. The CBO is careful to protect its independence and be nonpartisan in its assessments. It also provides Congress with the official cost estimates for the costs or savings of any proposed legislation. Its estimates of the cost of legislative proposals can be critically important in congressional debates on proposed bills. Because its studies are nonpartisan, it has a great deal of credibility within and outside Congress.

Another federal agency that is important to consult is the Government Accountability Office (GAO; www.gao.gov). It too is a nonpartisan agency of the U.S. Congress that produces studies at the request of individual members of Congress. Being nonpartisan, the agency has credibility within and outside Congress. It produces high-quality work. However, while the agency is nonpartisan, the questions that they are asked to examine may be quite partisan. Members of Congress or their staff may be looking for evidence to support their political position. Therefore, the question being asked of the GAO may be politically slanted. Members of Congress are looking for a timely response. The amount of available data at the time may be limited or the time needed for a more comprehensive review involving a more sophisticated study design may not be available.

GAO and CBO officials will testify before congressional committees and their testimony will be contained in committee reports. Some of their reports may appear in the form of a letter of reply to a particular member of Congress. If your policy proposal involves impacting (expanding, contracting, or eliminating) an existing federal program, the CBO and GAO are critical sources of information. The documents produced by these two agencies are readily available to congressional staff and they will use them to support or oppose your policy initiative. It is best to know what has been produced since they will carry weight with members of Congress and their staffs.

Another important source for public health policy alternatives is The Community Guide (https://thecommunityguide.org). This guide is developed by the U.S. Preventive Services Task Force to make recommendations regarding the current body of evidence on different preventive health programs. It uses criteria to evaluate the level of evidence available for different preventive strategies. For example, it provides an assessment (High, Moderate, or Low) on the certainty of net benefit for a particular intervention strategy and then a letter grade (A, B, C, D, Insufficient Evidence) as to the magnitude of the impact of such a preventive strategy. Strategies graded A or B are generally recommended for adoption. Those with a grade of C are recommended if there are other considerations that support this strategy. A grade of Insufficient Evidence is given if there is not a consensus among a panel of experts as to the benefit of such a preventive strategy. The Task Force has gained increased national significance in the implementation of the Affordable Care Act. Only those preventive procedures rated A or B can be cited by the Secretary of Health and Human Services as a required preventive procedure for health insurance policies.

If one looks at The Community Guide (n.d.) for strategies for obesity prevention programs featuring "Increasing Water Access Combined with Physical Activity Interventions in Schools," the score given is "Insufficient Evidence." This complicates your policy analysis in that there is no consensus among public health experts as to whether these particular school-based obesity prevention programs are effective or not. To date there is a lack of consensus demonstrating that they are effective. If your policy proposal fits within a category that receives a high grade from *The Community Guide*, this would bolster your argument for its adoption.

It is also important to be aware of programs authorized by past legislation. Due to of the passage of the American Recovery and Reinvestment Act of 2009, the U.S. Department of Health and Human Services (DHHS) received $650 million for a Prevention and Wellness Initiative (DHHS, 2009). Part of this money was devoted to a competitive grant program for local communities to focus on programs leading to increased levels of physical activity, improved nutrition, decreased overweight/obesity prevalence, decreased tobacco use, and decreased exposure to secondhand smoke. Knowing what programs have been funded will provide you with examples throughout the country on different approaches that are being tried and evaluated.

One would also want to be familiar with efforts by the National Academy of Sciences to address the issue of obesity (www.nationalacademies.org/our-work/roundtable-on-obesity-solutions). Because obesity has become such a major health problem for years, national resources such as the Institute of Medicine (IOM) have developed frameworks to address the problem. In previous years, the IOM published a major work entitled *Bridging the Evidence Gap in Obesity Prevention: A Framework to Inform Decision Making* (Kumanyika et al., 2010). In addition, it has developed the L.E.A.D. framework, which is an approach to identify, evaluate, and compile evidence specific to obesity (Kumanyika et al., 2010). The L.E.A.D. framework calls for **L**ocating evidence using a transdisciplinary systems perspective to understand obesity as a complex population-based problem, **E**valuating evidence based on standards of quality of evidence, **A**ssembling evidence that is relevant, and informing Decisions by using the evidence in decision-making processes.

Evidence-Based Practice for Public Health (EBPH) provides an electronic search engine to find the best evidence to support effective interventions (University of Massachusetts Medical School, 2017). The Cochrane Public Health Group (https://ph.cochrane.org) was established in 2008 to undertake systematic review of public health interventions. HIA is also a valuable tool for analyzing the health impact of policies outside the traditional healthcare sector, reflecting the HiAP perspective (Fielding & Briss, 2006).

ENGAGING KEY STAKEHOLDERS

You should consider engaging with a select number of key stakeholders to better understand the values held by supporters and opponents of your policy, and to identify potential community partners with whom you can collaborate. These partners might include state and local policy makers, health department staff, representatives from community-based organizations, advocacy groups, nonprofits, academic researchers, and other important stakeholders. Contacting these stakeholders will provide you with a beginning knowledge of what public health experts regard as innovative or successful efforts. Depending on their tenure longevity, they will know about programs that have been tried in the past and failed. Given your level of skills, resources, and time frame, you may engage stakeholders through interviews, listening sessions, focus groups, and/or other qualitative research methods as discussed in Chapter 9. In some cases, you may need to get approval from your organization's Institutional Review Board (IRB) prior to collecting information from stakeholders.

Do not underestimate the expertise that is available within the bureaucracy of your own state government, including public health and related agencies. Because many of them have continuous contact with the federal government officials through national or regional offices, they are valuable resources on national policy and state policy. They will be knowledgeable about federal regulations and their potential impact on policy implementation. They attend national professional meetings where they learn from their counterparts in other states. You may be relatively new to the issue; they are not. You might hear, "We tried that 5 years ago, and it did not work" or "It just will not work here." There may be some truth to that, or it may be an excuse for turf protection. Either way, these perspectives are valuable, especially if these are the same people who will be responsible for implementing your policy after its adoption. They may be aware of some pitfalls that may undermine your policy's intent. These professionals are also sensitive to the politics of the geopolitical area. The best-designed program can be a failure because it does not account for the politics or value conflicts within a particular geopolitical system. Stakeholders are discussed further in Chapter 12.

Another group that is generally overlooked in policy analysis are those who are not organized into an interest group, but who might be the most impacted by the policy. This frequently means consumers and vulnerable populations. For example, if your policy included a proposed change in the Supplemental Nutrition Assistance Program (SNAP), important, organized stakeholders representing agricultural interests and grocery stores would have representatives who you could contact to obtain their perspectives. However, any change in a program for vulnerable populations may have dire consequences. Too often policy is designed at the 10,000-foot level and not at the level where the impact is felt the most. You should attempt to gain input from any population that is directly impacted by the policy or program. Lower income persons using SNAP are generally not organized and, therefore, tend to lack their own political advocacy group. Public health departments will hopefully be sensitive to their perspectives. There may be surveys of recipients available, but it is unlikely that these will give you the information as to how your specific proposal will create intended and unintended consequences. Because public health policy is literally impacting people's lives, it is important to understand a recipient's perspective. This is your opportunity to make other voices heard. There are specific methods and entire courses on working with stakeholders, and community engagement; training is important particularly when engaging with vulnerable populations.

SOME SPECIFICS FOR WRITING YOUR REPORT

Here, we describe potential sections of your report that will support your analysis by making it more user friendly. The core analytic sections of your report are discussed in subsequent chapters.

Table of Contents

A table of contents provides a basic outline of your policy analysis. As such it can be initially used as a map for how the document is to be read. It may seem like an obvious portion of any document, but it is frequently omitted even though it can be done fairly quickly. Page numbers generally accompany where sections and subsections begin, allowing the reader to go directly to the section of interest, either initially or later. If the document is lengthy, one may wish to add subheadings to the table of contents to provide more exact locations for significant sections of the report. If the document is short, perhaps there is no need for a table of contents; section headings may be sufficient. The key here is to place oneself in the role of the reader so as to make the document as user friendly as possible.

Executive Summary

This section has to be written at the end of your analysis. However, it normally appears as one of the front sections of your finished policy analysis. Policy makers generally have a short time window to read any one document. Some people mistake an executive summary for an introduction. The latter tells the reader what is to be expected in the document and perhaps some background material to introduce the subject. In contrast, an executive summary condenses the document into a few pages, covering all the essential elements needed to understand its conclusions.

There is no magic number of pages for an executive summary. Some policy makers may have no artificial page limit, others prefer five pages, and some prefer one page. The shorter the executive summary, the more difficult it is to write and the more you have to assume about the reader's knowledge. Since you have a personal investment in the document, you probably believe that every paragraph is essential to the logic of the document. This might be the time for you to ask someone else to edit your executive summary. Having another person critique the executive summary can give you insight as to what might be missing or what might be overkill.

The executive summary has to be sensitive to the policy makers for whom it is written. Everyone comes to a policy issue with a different level of expertise. Some policy makers may have years of experience with an issue while others may find this a new area or an area of only partial interest. So, the executive summary will vary depending on the expertise of the prospective user(s) of the analysis. If the analysis is intended for the general public, the executive summary will probably have to be longer. The length is a judgment call based upon your knowledge of the intended audience.

Some policy makers prefer an executive summary that is to be used as logic map for the conclusion. From this perspective, it is read both before and after reading the analysis. It provides the reader with a roadmap as well as a summary of what is in the analysis. This type of executive summary can be less detailed because it assumes that the policy makers will actually read the entire policy analysis for its details.

Other policy makers use the executive summary as the only section that they will read. This places an additional burden on the author of the executive summary because the summary must be sufficiently comprehensive to prevent misinterpretation of the content yet fit within a page limitation. While the conclusion will be there, there may also be subtle but essential cautions or exceptions that might be overlooked by an exuberant policy maker. Some policy makers may read the executive summary and then only one of the core sections of the report (e.g., Recommendations and Strategies) for additional detail. Some may read it just prior to going into a committee meeting or a press conference. Understanding the audience and the proclivities of your policy maker is critical in writing a useful executive summary.

Due to the need for brevity, excessive words must be eliminated while the meaning remains sharp and unambiguous. Some may prefer to have bullets. However, the bullets need to be self-explanatory. Remember that the person reading the executive summary may not have read the report or may not have all the background that you possess. What may be clear to you as a bullet may not be clear to someone who has not read the details of your analysis.

Some readers are more visual in their ability to comprehend and retain information. Consequently, a graph or chart may be a meaningful way to communicate information in a small amount of space. However, this creates an additional burden since you must make sure that the graph or table is unambiguous and visually clean. A complicated figure within the executive summary is potentially harmful since it could be easily misinterpreted. The more you know about the people reading the report, the more likely the executive summary will be on target.

Definitions/Abbreviations

You may want to have an appendix in your final document that contains critical abbreviations and definitions for your policy. While you will finalize this list at the end of your analysis, it is best to keep a working copy as you go through the policy analysis.

The first section of any legislative bill is a list of definitions. There is an important reason for this. Once enacted, the bill becomes law, and the legislative intent must be unambiguous. It may sometimes seem obvious that people have a common understanding of a term. However, that is seldom the case, and the judicial system is filled with cases where people have different interpretations of what is meant by a single word or phrase.

For example, most people have a general understanding of what is meant by a hospital. The definition of a *hospital* for any proposed policy is actually quite complicated. There are various types of hospitals such as acute care hospitals, secondary and tertiary hospitals, rural hospitals, critical access hospitals, teaching hospitals, mental health hospitals, rehabilitation hospitals, military hospitals, veterans' hospitals, prison infirmaries, college infirmaries, and so forth. Some hospitals specialize in one disease (cancer) or one type of patients (children's hospitals). Some hospitals train physicians and other healthcare providers (e.g., teaching hospitals). Some hospitals are for-profit investor owned and some are nonprofit community-owned hospitals. Some hospitals are officially classified as small (e.g., 50 or fewer beds). Some hospitals have special policy problems, such as urban hospitals (serving a more indigent population) or rural hospitals (the need for telehealth). Among rural hospitals, some are legally classified as critical access hospitals and others are not. Does your policy proposal apply to all of these hospitals in the same way? Should some hospitals be exempt due to location, size, mission, and so forth? Therefore, you carefully define what is meant by a hospital in your policy analysis.

You should use standard, legal, or commonly accepted definitions whenever possible. If your policy substantially increases public funding for specific hospitals, other hospitals may wish to be included within the definition, thus increasing the cost of your policy. Alternatively, if your policy is more regulatory in nature, many hospitals may seek to be excluded from your policy proposal or lobby for the bill's defeat. Lobbyists representing different organizations will intensely focus on any definitions that are used in either the proposed bill or the regulations developed by a regulatory agency. What are the intended and unintended effects or alternative definitions? Legislators or stakeholders may support your legislation or at least refrain from opposing your policy with a simple change your definition.

Definitions are frequently needed for professionally used terms. There is a standard and accepted definition of obesity that has been developed by the CDC. It defines *obesity* using a formula comparing height to weight (mass): body mass index (BMI) = weight/(height)^2. For adults, being underweight is <18.5; normal is 18.5 to 24.9; overweight is 25.0 to 29.9; and obesity is 30.0+ (CDC, n.d.-e). This is the standard definition of obesity, and it is important to use that definition unless part of your policy proposal is to revise the standard definition. While people in public health understand the preciseness of that term, policy makers may not. It is also important to know that this CDC obesity formula does not apply to children since BMI is considered less reliable for children due to their growth spurts. There is a different definition of childhood obesity based on the age of the child and the 95th percentile on a CDC growth chart (CDC, n.d.-b). Some researchers prefer to use measures of waist circumference to measure abdominal adiposity, which is associated with risk for diabetes and cardiovascular disease (Harvard T. H. Chan School of Public Health, 2016). No matter which definition you use, you must be clear as to which one you are adopting for your analysis. You may have to explain why you are using that definition and not another.

Equally important for child obesity is the definition of a *child*. Is a child based upon a particular age range or is it defined as being enrolled in a primary or secondary educational system? Studies will be done using a particular definition; are different studies using comparable definitions? If you are comparing one state to another, do the two states use the same definition of a child as well as obesity?

Since obesity deals with both energy intake and output, it is important to also know what *physical activity* entails in terms of intensity, duration, and frequency. For example, how often (three times per week) does one have to swim and for how long (20 minutes or 50 laps) to qualify as exercise? The *Compendium for Physical Activities* provides formulas for estimating the metabolic equivalents (METs) for common physical activities (Ainsworth et al., 2000). Do all the sources you used in your analysis use METs as a uniform measure of exertion? Are you considering only leisure time (recreational) physical activity, or physical activity related to occupation as well?

All these concepts and terms need to be defined as precisely as possible so that your policy proposal is clear and to avoid needless opposition to your proposal based on a misunderstanding. Being as precise as possible is important to avoid potential political struggles down the road that could have been avoided in the first place if you had only been clear and precise in your definitions.

There are also definitions for concepts that might not be well known, but that are commonly used in the debate over your policy issue. The literature on obesity focuses on the importance of the *built environment* (streets, sidewalks, zoning, parks, bike paths, etc.) that either facilitate or create barriers for physical exercise. While this term is understood within the public health and research communities, it is less common within political circles. Clear definitions help to avoid having your policy maker tripped up by using the wrong term during a debate or news conference, not knowing the implications of a word or phrase being used. The more technical the policy area, the more important clear definitions become.

Public health surveys and surveillance systems, while useful for your analysis, are often filled with acronyms and abbreviations. For example, the National Health and Nutrition Examination Survey (NHANES) is one of the major data sources used for obesity research (CDC, n.d.-c). It is typically referred to by its initials NHANES and not its full title. In addition to knowing what the initials stand for, it is may also be important that your policy makers know essential facts about that data set. The fact that NHANES is a national data sample, that it is a continuous survey covering the noninstitutionalized population of the United States, that it contains clinical indicators of disease as well as individual self-reports, and that it is released every 2 years may or may not be important descriptors your policy maker might want to know if it is critical in your analysis. It is important that people reading your analysis know what NHANES represents. The important point here is that policy makers should have easy access to a list of critical terms and definitions.

In addition to specific obesity terms, it might be important to easily define general statistical terms that are commonly used in your analysis. You do not need to provide your policy makers with a tutorial on statistical interpretation; you merely need to make sure that your intended readers understand the implications and limitations of the analysis presented. Many policy makers may have never taken a course in statistics or may have taken one so long ago that it is not part of their normal thought process. Make sure your readers can make maximum use of the data and statistical analysis provided without distorting its implications. The CDC publishes introductory guides on epidemiology and biostatistics, which can help with these topics (Dicker et al., 2006).

References

You will need to include a bibliography with a list of references or works cited using a standard, professional citation style, such as that of the American Psychological Association (APA; Purdue Online Writing Lab, 2022). You should build this reference list as you go and use the full citation so that you can easily relocate it if needed. Your organization or policy maker may have their own stylistic preferences.

Other Appendices

In addition to the elements previously discussed, you might wish to make other documents or explanations available to the readers, but find that they would distract from the flow of your policy analysis. You might want to provide additional graphics, tables, and maps into an appendix. You may wish to provide a detailed description of a model program you found in another geopolitical area. You can refer to it in the text and then provide more detail in the appendix for those wanting more information. You might want to provide more detailed information on a critical study or a fuller explanation of a particular methodology. Some readers will use these appendices and others will not. If something is critical to understanding the policy analysis, it probably belongs in the body of your document.

SUMMARY

This chapter deals with some of the basics that you will need to consider as you begin planning your policy analysis before writing. Your policy analysis will most likely depend greatly on the assignment from your policy maker. Consequently, there is no one size fits all format. Alternative formats are available. Whether you are conducting an HIA or another type of public health policy analysis, carefully consider which components and what format would be most useful to your intended readers. We discuss the strengths and weaknesses of peer-reviewed and grey literature and where you can find assistance accessing them. We note the importance of accessing potential stakeholders. Finally, we discuss the components such as the executive summary, references, definitions, and so forth that you may wish to use.

All of these components require judgment calls based on the intended audience of your analysis and how it will be used. From the beginning you need to think about your audience and how best to facilitate their use of the report and to build confidence in the credibility of its findings. The next two chapters focus on data and methodology.

DISCUSSION QUESTIONS

- Examine how organizational missions of stakeholders might impact how they both approach a policy analysis and also how it may be used in practice.

- Explore how grey literature can be utilized in the policy analysis process and what the limitations of some sources are relative to peer-reviewed studies. What might be some approaches the analyst could take to improve these statements and uses of evidence?

- What are the challenges of creating an impactful yet clear executive summary?

- Discuss the idea of transparency of methods when doing a policy analysis.

- How could personal or professional values impact the framing of an analysis at the writing stage?

KEY TERMS

American Legislative Exchange Council (ALEC)
The Community Guide
Congressional Budget Office (CBO)
Evidence-Based Practice for Public Health (EBPH)
executive summary
Government Accountability Office (GAO)
grey literature
Health Impact Assessment

Institutional Review Board
L.E.A.D. framework
MeSH
National Conference of State Legislatures (NCSL)
peer-reviewed literature
POLARIS
political capital
PubMed
systematic reviews

 SPRINGER PUBLISHING **CONNECT™**

A robust set of instructor resources designed to supplement this text is located at http://connect.springerpub.com/content/book/978-0-8261-8543-3. Qualifying instructors may request access by emailing textbook@springerpub.com.

REFERENCES

Ainsworth, B. E., Haskell, W. L., Whitt, M. C., Irwin, M. L., Swartz, A. M., Strath, S. J., O'Brien, W. L., Bassett, D. R., Schmitz, K. H., Emplaincourt, P. O., Jacobs, D. R., & Leon, A. S. (2000). Compendium of physical activities: An update of activity codes and MET intensities. *Medicine and Science in Sports & Exercise*, 32(Suppl. 9), S498–S504. https://doi.org/10.1097/00005768-200009001-00009

American Legislative Exchange Council. (2022). *Model policies*. https://alec.org/model-policy

Amri, M. M., & Drummond, D. (2021). Punctuating the equilibrium: An application of policy theory to COVID-19. *Policy Design and Practice*, 4(1), 33–43. https://doi.org/10.1080/25741292.2020.1841397

Arcaya, M. C., Schnake-Mahl, A., Binet, A., Simpson, S., Church, M. S., Gavin, V., Coleman, B., Levine, S., Nielsen, A., Carroll, L., Ursprung, S., Wood, B., Reeves, H., Keppard, B., Sportiche,

N., Partirdge, J., Figueora, J., Frakt, A., Alfonzo, M., … , Youmans, T. (2018). Community change and resident needs: Designing a participatory action research study in metropolitan Boston. *Health & Place*, 52, 221–230. https://doi.org/10.1016/j.healthplace.2018.05.014

Baumgartner, F. R., & Jones, B. D. (1991). Agenda dynamics and policy subsystems. *The Journal of Politics*, 53(4), 1044–1074. https://doi.org/10.2307/2131866

Bhatia, R., Branscomb, J., Farhang, L., Lee, M., Orenstein, M., & Richardson, M. (2010, November). *Minimum elements and practice standards for Health Impact Assessment, version 2*. The Pew Charitable Trusts. https://www.pewtrusts.org/-/media/assets/external-sites/health-impact -project/hiaworkinggroup_hiapracticestandards_2009.pdf

Bhatia, R., Farhang, L., & Lee, M. (2010, November 1). *Minimum elements and practice standards for Health Impact Assessment*. GHPC Materials. https://scholarworks.gsu.edu/ghpc_materials/11

Bir, A., & Freeman, N. (2016, June). *Meta-evaluation: Using meta-analysis and data visualization to inform policy*. RTI International. https://www.rti.org/sites/default/files/rti_innovation_brief_meta -evaluation.pdf

Bleich, S. N., Segal, J., Wu, Y., Wilson, R., & Wang, Y. (2013). Systematic review of community-based childhood obesity prevention studies. *Pediatrics*, 132(1), e201–e210. https://doi.org/10.1542/ peds.2013-0886

Brugha, R., & Varvasovszky, Z. (2000). Stakeholder analysis: A review. *Health Policy and Planning*, 15(3), 239–246. https://doi.org/10.1093/heapol/15.3.239

Centers for Disease Control and Prevention. (n.d.-a). *Healthy places: Health Impact Assessment resources*. U.S. Department of Health and Human Services. https://www.cdc.gov/ healthyplaces/hiaresources.htm

Centers for Disease Control and Prevention. (n.d.-b). *Healthy weight, nutrition, and physical activity: Body mass index (BMI)*. U.S. Department of Health and Human Services. https://www.cdc.gov/ healthyweight/assessing/bmi/index.html

Centers for Disease Control and Prevention. (n.d.-c). *National Center for Health Statistics: NHANES: National Health and Nutrition Examination Survey*. U.S. Department of Health and Human Services. http://www.cdc.gov/nchs/nhanes.htm

Centers for Disease Control and Prevention. (n.d.-d). *Office of the Associate Director for Policy and Strategy: POLARIS policy analysis*. U.S. Department of Health and Human Services. https:// www.cdc.gov/policy/polaris/policyprocess/policy_analysis.html

Centers for Disease Control and Prevention. (n.d.-e). *Overweight & obesity: Defining adult overweight and obesity*. U.S. Department of Health and Human Services. http://www.cdc.gov/obesity/ adult/defining.html

Chang, S. M. (2011). The Agency for Healthcare Research and Quality (AHRQ) Effective Health Care (EHC) Program methods guide for comparative effectiveness reviews: Keeping up-to-date in a rapidly evolving field. *Journal of Clinical Epidemiology*, 64(11), 1166–1167. https:// doi.org/10.1016/j.jclinepi.2011.08.004

Clarke, B., Swinburn, B., & Sacks, G. (2016). The application of theories of the policy process to obesity prevention: A systematic review and meta-synthesis. *BMC Public Health*, 16(1), Article 1084. https://doi.org/10.1186/s12889-016-3639-z

Cooke, A., Friedli, L., Coggins, T., Edmonds, N., O'Hara, K., Snowden, L., Stansfield, J., Steuer, N., & Scott-Samuel, A. (2010). *The mental well-being impact assessment toolkit*. HIAConnect. http://hiaconnect.edu.au/wp-content/uploads/2012/05/MentalWellbeingImpactAssessment Toolkit20101.pdf

Current grey literature report. (2016, November). The New York Academy of Medicine. http://www .greylit.org/reports/current

Dannenberg, A. L., Rogerson, B., & Rudolph, L. (2019). Optimizing the health benefits of climate change policies using Health Impact Assessment. *Journal of Public Health Policy*, 41(2), 139–154. https://doi.org/10.1057/s41271-019-00189-y

Dicker, R., Coronado, F., Koo, D., & Parrish, R. G. (2006). *Principles of epidemiology in public health practice* (3rd ed.). U.S. Department of Health and Human Services. https://www.cdc.gov/ csels/dsepd/ss1978/index.html

Fielding, J. E., & Briss, P. A. (2006). Promoting evidence-based public health policy: Can we have better evidence and more action? *Health Affairs*, 25(4), 969–978. https://doi.org/10.1377/ hlthaff.25.4.969

Harvard T. H. Chan School of Public Health. (2016, April 13). *Waist size matters*. Obesity Prevention Source. https://www.hsph.harvard.edu/obesity-prevention-source/obesity-definition/ abdominal-obesity

Jones, C. M., Clavier, C., & Potvin, L. (2017). Adapting public policy theory for public health research: A framework to understand the development of national policies on global health. *Social Science & Medicine*, 177, 69–77. https://doi.org/10.1016/j.socscimed.2017.01.048

Kingdon, J. W. (1984). Agendas, alternatives, and public policies. Little, Brown, & Company.

Kumanyika, S. K., Parker, L., & Sims, L. J. (Eds.). (2010). *Bridging the evidence gap in obesity prevention: A framework to inform decision making.* National Academies Press. https://doi .org/10.17226/12847

New State Ice Co. v. Liebmann, 285 U.S. 262 (1932). https://supreme.justia.com/cases/federal/ us/285/262

Okeke, C., Manzano, A., Obi, U., Etiaba, E., Onwujekwe, O., Mirzoev, T., & Uzochukwu, B. (2021). Exploring mechanisms that explain how coalition groups are formed and how they work to sustain political priority for maternal and child health in Nigeria using the advocacy coalition framework. *Health Research Policy and Systems, 19*(1), Article 26. https://doi.org/10.1186/ s12961-020-00660-3

Paniagua, P. (2022). Elinor Ostrom and public health. *Economy and Society, 51*(2), 211–234. https://doi.org/10.1080/03085147.2022.2028973

Purdue Online Writing Lab. (2022). *APA formatting and style guide* (7th ed.). Purdue University. https://owl.purdue.edu/owl/research_and_citation/apa_style/apa_formatting_and_style _guide/general_format.html

Robert Wood Johnson Foundation. (2016, June 21). *Declining childhood obesity rates.* RWJF. https:// www.rwjf.org/en/library/research/2016/06/declining-childhood-obesity-rates.html

Sabatier, P. A. (2007). *Theories of the policy process* (2nd ed.). Westview Press.

Sabatier, P. A., & Jenkins-Smith, H. C. (1993). *Policy change and learning: An advocacy coalition approach (theoretical lenses on public policy).* Westview Press.

The Community Guide. (n.d.). *Obesity prevention and control: Increasing water access combined with physical activity interventions in schools.* https://www.thecommunityguide.org/findings/ obesity-prevention-control-increasing-water-access-combined-physical-activity-interventions -schools.html

The Pew Charitable Trusts. (2018, April 29). *HIAs and other resources to advance health-informed decisions: A toolkit to promote healthier communities through cross-sector collaboration.* Author. https://www.pewtrusts.org/en/research-and-analysis/data-visualizations/2015/hia-map?sor tBy=relevance&sortOrder=asc&page=1

University of Massachusetts Medical School. (2017). *Evidence-based practice for public health.* Lamar Soutter Library. https://library.umassmed.edu/ebpph/index.cfm

U.S. Department of Health and Human Services. (2009). *American Recovery and Reinvestment Act summary of the Prevention and Wellness Initiative—Community component.* https://www.cdc.gov/ chronicdisease/recovery/PDF/PW_Community_fact_sheet_final.pdf

Watson, T. (2014). Political science theory for public health practice. *American Journal of Health Education, 45*(6), 319–321. https://doi.org/10.1080/19325037.2014.949368

Weible, C. M., Nohrstedt, D., Cairney, P., Carter, D. P., Crow, D. A., Durnová, A. P., Heikkila, T., Ingold, K., McConnell, A., & Stone, D. (2020). COVID-19 and the policy sciences: Initial reactions and perspectives. *Policy Sciences, 53*(2), 225–241. https://doi.org/10.1007/s11077 -020-09381-4

Yin, R. K. (1994). *Case study research: Design and methods* (2nd ed.). SAGE Publications.

CHAPTER 8

HEALTH POLICY ANALYSIS FOUNDATIONS

The purpose of this chapter is to provide an overview of important concepts that you will need in doing your health policy analysis. We begin by examining the nature of health and the significance of the Health in All Policies (HiAP) for health policy analysis. The chapter includes a discussion of evidence-based health policy using criteria such as effectiveness, efficiency, equity, and feasibility. We then provide several integrative frameworks for health policy. Finally, we provide resources for organizations that have been involved in nationally based health policy analysis. You may wish to refer back to this chapter and earlier chapters, such as the policy wheel in Figure 4.1, as you work through the remainder of the textbook. The next chapter focuses on specific tools for quantitative and qualitative analysis.

LEARNING OBJECTIVES

Be able to:

- Understand the role of health services research on the framing of the health policy analysis.

- Describe the breadth of what constitutes health as reflected in HiAP and the Adelaide Statement.

- Determine the appropriate impact measure(s) for the health policy analysis, specifically:

  - Effectiveness as an outcome measure

  - Efficiency as an outcome measure

  - Equity as an outcome measure

- Examine some existing integrative frameworks for conducting health policy analysis.

- Identify sources of health policy analysis research.

HEALTH POLICY AND HEALTH SERVICES RESEARCH

Health policy is part of the larger field of health services research, an area devoted to the discovery of new information for the improvement of individual and population health. You may wish to review the conceptual model of the determinants of health in **Figure 1.1**. Due to the nature of health, both health services research and health policy analysis are interdisciplinary by nature, using the knowledge of both the biological sciences and the social sciences. The evolving fields of implementation science, decision science, data science, sustainability science, and Indigenous and feminist epistemologies also address health policy analysis (Bacchi, 1999; Brownson et al., 2006; Carroll et al., 2021, 2022; Clark, 2007; Clark & Dickson, 2003; Kingdon, 2003; Madahian et al., 2012; Sabatier & Jenkins-Smith, 1993; Stokols, 1992; Stokols et al., 1996).

Health is a complicated concept. The most famous definition of health comes from the World Health Organization (WHO): "[h]ealth is a state of complete physical, mental and social well-being and not merely the absence of disease or infirmity" (1946, preamble). This definition points to the comprehensive nature of health; there is both a physical health and mental aspect of health as well as a sense of well-being. The definition tends to be more aspirational with a focus on what it takes to achieve human potential rather than a description of reality. Individuals and societies transition from one state of health to another over time. Given the WHO definition, *health* may be a very temporary state.

Health is not a given. Societies create conditions that promote both disease and health. Refer back to **Figure 1.1** and **Breakout Box 1.1**. As demonstrated by Evans and Stoddart and other similar social-ecological and systems science models, societies produce health or disease through the interaction of multiple variables (e.g., policy, the natural and created environments [the built environment]; Evenson & Aytur, 2012), building medical care systems, as well as individual behavior (Evans & Stoddart, 2003; Huang et al., 2009; McLeroy et al., 1988; Stokols et al., 1996). Manipulating any one of these variables (e.g., education or the transportation systems) creates greater disease or health for individuals and for society. By implication, societies can influence their own health through their public policies (Brownson et al., 2009). The creation and distribution of wealth, the educational system, natural and built environments including but not limited to the creation of safe work environments, and access to the medical care system all play critical roles in determining the health status of a given population or a particular individual. All these inputs to health are shaped by the actions of both individuals and society through the policy process; the health of a society is not predestined and public policies play a major role in determining health.

Our understanding of how these different inputs affect health has changed over time. The evolution of the public health lexicon to include planetary determinants of health reflects this. For example, efforts to increase physical activity and improve nutrition in the general population were historically aimed at changing individual-level health behaviors. Individuals were told to exercise more and eat more healthy meals. The focus was to get the individuals motivated to change their behavior and to adopt healthy eating patterns. Thaler and Sunstein (2008) refer to this as "the nudge" or "libertarian paternalism." However, such approaches have been found to be minimally effective, costly, and difficult to sustain (Lyn et al., 2013).

As a result, public health professionals began to address this problem using a more comprehensive approach referred to as policy, systems, and environmental change. These initiatives are built upon the notion that individual decisions for healthy behavior can be facilitated or frustrated by political decision-making. This approach includes (a) policy interventions that seek to change laws, ordinances, regulations, or legislation (e.g., a city council zoning ordinance prohibiting fast food chains within a certain distance of a school); (b) system-level interventions that promote changes that impact organizations, institutions, or communities (e.g., a school deciding to buy a certain percentage of its cafeteria food from local sources, and training the food service staff to cook and serve vegetarian meals on certain days); (c) environmental interventions that involve changes to the physical environment (e.g., a school constructing bike lanes and bike storage facilities to encourage active transportation to school), often resulting from policy decisions such as zoning and transportation expenditures (Lyn et al., 2013); and (d) planetary health interventions that include incentives for electric vehicles (Peters et al., 2020), telehealth interventions (Aytur et al., in press), and sustainable "green" innovations in the healthcare delivery sector (Shaw et al., 2021). As illustrated by these examples, our increased understanding of the synergy of multiple factors of health, using a syndemic lens (Caron & Adegboye, 2021; Caron & Aytur, 2022; Singer et al., 2017), has complicated the policy process because one simple intervention is probably not sufficient.

HEALTH POLICY ANALYSIS

As a result of this more comprehensive and systematic understanding of the inputs to health, the breadth of *health policy* has increased dramatically. The Centers for Disease Control and Prevention (CDC) defines policy analysis as "the process of identifying potential policy options that could address your problem and then comparing those options to choose the most effective, efficient, and feasible one" (CDC, n.d.-b, para. 1).

Due to the multiple inputs to health status, the 2010 Adelaide Statement describes the need to approach health policy as HiAP (Krech et al., 2010; WHO & Government of South Australia, 2010). The Adelaide Statement emphasizes the need to examine all policies for their potential impact on population health and health equity. This is a significant broadening of the scope of the health sector within public policy making. The Adelaide Statement describes innovative models emerging from around the world. Of critical importance to the success of this approach will be an aggregation of evidence as to the impact of this approach in different geographic and political environments.

Health policy analysis is a type of applied research. While one might think that our healthcare system is evidence-based and dependent on what research demonstrates to be valuable, that is not always the case. In fact, it is not usually the case. Many health programs and proposals that have been demonstrated to have scientific validity never get broadly implemented, and even more commonly, many existing programs and practices in medicine have never been formally proved to be effective. The Institute of Medicine (IOM) has estimated that about 4% of health services have strong evidence to back them and that more than half have no or weak evidence to support them (Field & Lohr, 1992). Researchers have identified several aspects of policy analysis that need particular attention (Brownson et al., 2009; Krieger, Chen, et al., 2021; Krieger, Waterman, et al., 2021; Schmid et al., 2006). These include (a) documenting *how* an impact is achieved in a particular context; (b) understanding barriers to successful implementation; (c) delineating multiple outcomes that could be important (including unintended consequences and differential impacts on different vulnerable populations); and (d) developing tools to help prioritize policy choices, including specific criteria to evaluate policy impacts.

The importance of conducting sound health policy analysis is highlighted when one considers the problem of a chronic disease such as obesity. While there is much we know about the cause and consequences of obesity, how the political and health systems should respond to that knowledge becomes a focus of health policy analysis. For example, since older and minority populations are at heightened risk of diabetes, how should Medicare and Medicaid policies be developed to minimize the impact of diabetes on individuals, specific groups, and society (Fradkin, 2012)? Obesity has become an epidemic in the United States and many other developed countries, but logical, scientifically based, and culturally tailored programs to fight obesity tend to flounder for lack of political action.

There has been a rise in the importance of evidence-based medicine and evidence-based public health (Anderson et al., 2005; Brownson et al., 2009; Green, 2006; Kumanyika et al., 2012; Swinburn et al., 2005), underscoring the need for systematic evaluation of what works in medicine and public health. While this is encouraging, evidence-based healthcare is something that is easier said than done. Evidence-based health systems and policy remain the goal, no matter how difficult the path may be. With the explosion in social media's spread of disinformation, there has been a rise in the spread of unproven and even dangerous therapies. The COVID-19 pandemic has given rise to a distrust of medical professionals, therapies, and public health strategies such as vaccinations, isolation, and mask wearing (Krieger, Chen, et al., 2021; Krieger, Testa, et al., 2021; Krieger, Waterman, et al., 2021). The populist movement against science and professionalism raises generic problems that public health initiatives need to overcome.

EVIDENCE-BASED HEALTH POLICY

There is a great deal of literature focusing on medicine and the medical care system. Begley et al. (2004) created a useful paradigm of health policy analysis by dividing the literature into three areas of concern: effectiveness, efficiency, and equity. Other divisions of the literature could be feasibility, practicality, ideology, and sustainability, but we will focus on effectiveness, efficiency, and equity and feasibility in this chapter. Other public health factors are revisited in later chapters. This chapter provides a brief overview of these concepts.

Effectiveness

The effectiveness literature focuses on demonstrating what works to improve the health of the individual or the population. Certainly, public policies should encourage treatments that work and discourage those that waste resources or those treatments that do not improve the health of the population and/or potentially cause harm. During the COVID-19 pandemic, multiple unproven drugs and therapies were proposed on social media platforms. The licensure of health professionals, accreditation of healthcare organizations, and approval of pharmaceuticals are predicated on protecting the public from ineffective and harmful practices. Since the days of codeine-laced cure-alls, effectiveness and prevention from harm have been key components of public health policies.

Effectiveness needs to be discussed from two different perspectives: population effectiveness and medical effectiveness. Medical effectiveness tends to deal with individual patients and the social impact of a specific intervention. These interventions are typically evaluated by conducting clinical trials that take a similar group of people and then randomly assign them to either the prescribed treatment or a placebo procedure to test the effectiveness of the treatment.

Population effectiveness rests upon Geoffrey Rose's population strategy that has become the theoretical basis for public intervention to prevent disease (Rose, 1992). Rose maintained that prevention should not just focus on high-risk individuals, but on the entire population. Thus, reducing salt consumption benefits not only those with hypertension, but also those who are prehypertensive. By reducing the average intake of salt within the population, the entire population benefits. While this reduction of the average salt intake may not make a perceptible difference to some individuals, it is effective for the population as a whole.

In addition to the biological aspects of effectiveness, there are also the health system and social system aspects of effectiveness. For example, while certain pharmaceuticals have been demonstrated to be effective for diseases on the individual level, the lack of clinical facilities, refrigeration, social support systems, or cultural norms may prevent those same pharmaceuticals from being effective for the population in a developing country.

The focus on evidence-based medicine is not new. It gained a great deal of momentum with the pioneer work done by Wennberg and Gittelsohn (1973). Their research focused on the variation in the practice of medicine from one geographic area to another in the United States and what could potentially explain such variations. The Dartmouth Atlas documents the geographic variation in the practice of medicine within the United States (Dartmouth Atlas Project, 2022).

There is also great variation in health status across the United States. Studies conducted by the Joint Center for Political and Economic Studies have shown that life expectancy in some parts of the United States can vary by as much as 30 years when comparing one zip code to another (Virginia Commonwealth University, 2009). What tends to explain this variation? What are the consequences of this variation? Given that variation in medical care exists, what is the right level of medical care? Geographic variation has multiple potential explanations (Chen et al., 2021; Krieger, 2013; Krieger, Waterman, et al., 2021). How much variation is warranted and how much is unwarranted? How can reimbursement systems be restructured to create the right incentives for increased efficiency and effectiveness in medical care and public health? (Bernstein et al., 2011; Webster et al., 2022).

In some areas, such as pharmaceuticals, the federal government's Food and Drug Administration (FDA) is authorized to approve or disapprove medical interventions. Formal approval by the FDA does not end the process of evaluation of effectiveness because payers (Medicare/Medicaid and private insurance companies) make their own decisions regarding whether they will categorize the treatment as experimental and, therefore, not list it among their covered services. The 2021 FDA's approval of Biogen Inc.'s Aduhelm for Alzheimer disease was also met with a decision by the U.S. Centers for Medicaid and Medicare Services (CMS) that it would only approve Medicare payment for Aduhelm for patients enrolled in approved clinical trials. Consequently, approval does not equate with access.

The FDA is restricted in terms of its authority; while it has authority to approve appliances (e.g., implants) and pharmaceuticals, it is not authorized to approve or disapprove medical procedures. There has been medical controversy over the effectiveness of vertebroplasty, a surgical procedure used for people with severe back problems (Wulff et al., 2011). As a medical procedure, the FDA was not involved with its approval. Vertebroplasty became accepted in medical practice prior to any clinical trials demonstrating its effectiveness, and yet this procedure is widely performed and paid for by major insurance providers and Medicare in the United States.

The analysis of comparative effectiveness of medical procedures has the potential for a more precise recommendation for the most effective treatment for different sub-populations and the beginning of "personalized medicine." Frequently, the criteria for effectiveness do not consider the lived experience and perspective of the patient. This is particularly important in terms of considering the sequelae of a particular procedure. For example, prostate surgery may remove cancerous tissue, but due to the slow growing nature of prostate cancer in general, the patient might die of another disease before they would have died from prostate cancer. However, by undergoing the surgical procedure for prostate cancer the patient may have a diminished quality of life due to incontinence and impotence following the procedure. The effectiveness of such treatment from the patient's perspective is far from clear. The effectiveness of treatment is more complicated than merely the removal of cancerous tissue.

One of the classic studies of effectiveness was done by McGlynn et al. (2003) on the quality of care in the United States. It concluded that patients in the United States received a little more than half of what was recognized as quality care. The study sent a shock wave through the medical community, and it remains a seminal piece of evidence of the effectiveness of the practice of medicine.

Determining what is effective is not as clear as one might initially think. This is compounded by rapidly changing technology. What may appear to be effective today might be outmoded in the future. New technologies such as robotic surgery may initially be less effective but improve over time with additional professional experience and technological advances. If effectiveness is a major part of your policy proposal, you should access texts in epidemiology, biostatistics, and health services research.

Efficiency

A second major aspect of health policy analysis revolves around the issue of efficiency, the ratio of outputs to inputs. As indicated by Victor Fuchs in his groundbreaking book from 1974, "No country is as healthy as it could be; no country does as much for the sick as it is technically capable of doing. ... The grim fact is that no nation is wealthy enough to avoid all avoidable deaths" (p. 17). This recognizes the fact that societies have a limited number of resources and that spending in one area may reduce the ability for it to spend in another. One would want a healthcare system to maximize the health of the population but also to conserve society's resources for other sectors such as education or national defense. Typically, this is measured by the percentage of the gross national product spent on healthcare. By this measure the United States is an anomaly among other industrialized countries. The United States always leads the Organisation for Economic Co-operation and Development (OECD) countries in terms of the percentage of gross national product. OECD data for 2020 places the United States at 18.8% while Canada is 12.9%, the United Kingdom at 12.0%, France at 12.2%, and Sweden at 11.5% (OECD, 2022).

When a society realizes its resources are limited, one would hope that those medical services that do the least good are the ones to be reduced or eliminated in favor of those that that are more cost effective. A literature review of studies from 2012 to 2019 on waste in the healthcare system used the IOM delineated areas of potential waste (failure of care delivery, failure of care coordination, overtreatment or low-value care, pricing failure, fraud and abuse, and administrative complexity). The total estimated annual waste per year was between $760 billion and $935 billion. The largest areas were in pricing failure and administrative complexity (Shrank et al., 2019). The magnitude and the cause of the inefficiency of the U.S. medical system might be in dispute, but there is a consensus that there is a great deal of waste within the existing system. The amount of waste and inappropriate care was indeed popularized and became a factor in the political discussions for healthcare reform with Gawande's (2009) comparison of the differences in healthcare costs in two Texas communities.

Of course, one of the major areas of efficiency is the area of disease prevention and health promotion versus medical treatment. Public health advocates generally cite that the efficiency of the health system can be enhanced by preventing disease and disability in the first place. Studies using cost benefit and cost-effective analysis have demonstrated that prevention activities can save money by forgoing medical expenditures (Graham et al., 1998; Grosse et al., 2007; Mays & Smith, 2011). This aligns with the well-known proverb that an ounce of prevention is worth a pound of cure. Vaccines are a typical example of this policy focus on prevention. For example, a 2019 systematic review of the literature from 1980 to 2016 indicated that vaccines targeted for adults (e.g., influenza, hepatitis, pneumococcal) were all cost effective (Leidner et al., 2019). However, one must be careful to not state that all prevention programs are cost effective. If a disease is rare and the consequences of getting that disease are not too harmful, providing a vaccine to the entire population or even a large proportion of that population may be far more costly for society than providing medical care treatment for the few individuals who acquire the disease. Generally, however, disease prevention and promotion are less costly than treatment, especially when considering the potential adverse experiences of people with the treatment and disease sequelae. While many people are experiencing mild symptoms from the recent variants of COVID-19, those acquiring the symptoms of long COVID need to be considered (Nittas et al., 2022).

Allocative and Production Efficiency

Production efficiency is the more generally understood term of the two types of efficiency. It involves maximizing the ratio of outputs to inputs for producing a given item. For example, one can improve the production efficiency of a medical practice by utilizing physician assistants or nurse practitioners. The latter health professionals are typically paid less than physicians and can perform many frequently performed tasks at a lower cost. The use of scheduling protocols can improve the flow of patients and, thereby, increase the number of people screened per day for imaging services, thus spreading the fixed costs of the service over more units of service (patients). Specialization, division of labor, and substitution of capital for labor are general strategies that are frequently used for increasing the production efficiency of particular units.

In contrast, allocative efficiency deals with maximizing outputs in society given limited resources; it focuses on the efficiency of one sector versus another. Making hospitals more productively efficient does not solve the inefficiency of treating people after they become sick. Shifting resources from medical care to public health could increase the allocative efficiency of the healthcare system by producing a healthy population, thus eliminating the need for hospital costs, even for efficient hospitals. Shifting resources from medical care to providing livable incomes for the poor, increased education, or improving the built environment in an inner city might improve the health status of the population at a much lower cost than increasing hospital care. Spending money on prevention or providing more general education to the population may produce much greater health at a lower cost to society. Whether the United States spends too much of its limited resources on medical care is an open allocative efficiency question.

Economic analysis is an entirely different area of policy analysis. If efficiency is a major focus of your policy proposal, you need to become familiar with the details of the various types of efficiency studies in greater detail than we can do here.

Equity

A third major area of concern for health policy analysis is that of equity; generally, this means promoting fairness within the public health system. This includes eliminating disparities in access to health-promoting resources for subpopulations (e.g., gender, sexual orientation, race, ethnicity, income, education, geography). It addresses how health policies can promote the elimination of unfair differences in health status. Why are certain minority populations differentially impacted by diabetes (Betancourt et al., 2012)? Black individuals have a very different life expectancy than do White individuals (Krieger, Chen, et al, 2021; Smedley et al., 2003). Former U.S. Surgeon General Dr. David Satcher calculated that 83,570 African Americans died in 2002 who would not have died if Black and White mortality rates were equal. This means that there were 229 "excess deaths" per day, or the equivalent of an airplane loaded with Black passengers crashing every single day of the year (California Newsreel, 2008). What policies or programs can be enacted to reduce such disparities? *Healthy People 2030* states that one of its seven Foundational Principles is "[a]chieving health and well-being requires eliminating health disparities, achieving health equity, and attaining health literacy" (Office of Disease Prevention and Health Promotion, n.d., para. 8).

Equity is divided into two aspects. One aspect is *procedural equity*, to assure that the processes in place are fair and do not discriminate. For example, current procedures exist to guarantee that those who receive organ transplants are not those with the most money or connections, but those who are in higher need and have higher chance of survival. The second aspect of equity is *substantive equity*, to reduce the disparities between survival rates that cannot be explained by biological conditions, for example, infant mortality rates for Black children. What policies or programs can be implemented to help reduce the disparity in outcomes among various populations for infant mortality? If equity becomes a major aspect of your policy proposal, you should access major texts in epidemiology and public health and medical ethics. The growing body of research examining the nuances of "justice" versus "equity" can also offer important insights (Braveman et al., 2011). The environmental justice lens (Bullard & Johnson, 2000) and the Health Impact Assessment (HIA) process described in Chapter 7 can help to integrate equity considerations into your policy analysis (Dannenberg, 2016; Dannenberg et al., 2008).

Feasibility

Another important area of concern is feasibility, or the practical operational factors associated with a policy's adoption and implementation. This is a very important aspect to consider in your policy analysis, and it depends on having access to contextual place-based information or local knowledge about the environment in which you are working. Working with stakeholders and partners who have this knowledge will greatly enable you to assess the feasibility of your policy proposal at this particular moment in time (CDC, n.d.-a, 2013). Your background research (Chapter 10) and stakeholder analysis (Chapter 12) will help you to assess feasibility. Accessing economic data and/or working with an economist to evaluate the costs and benefits associated with the proposed policy can also help to assess feasibility. Sometimes a policy change may not be feasible in a particular year, but it may become feasible over time.

INTEGRATIVE FRAMEWORKS

There are several integrative frameworks that enable health program planners, policy analysts, and evaluators to balance criteria when they analyze health programs and policies (Gielen et al., 2008; Glasgow et al., 2019; Green, 1974; Green & Kreuter, 2004; Kumanyika et al., 2012; University of Kansas Center for Community Health and Development, 2013). These include PRECEDE-PROCEED, RE-AIM, and L.E.A.D. (Locate evidence, Evaluate evidence, Assemble evidence, inform Decisions). The first two are discussed in the following sections; L.E.A.D. is discussed in more detail in Chapter 7.

PRECEDE-PROCEED

PRECEDE-PROCEED is an evaluation framework that was developed in 1974 by Dr. Lawrence Green (Green, 1974; Green & Kreuter, 2004). It describes a process that starts with desired outcomes and then works backward to identify the best combination of strategies for achieving those outcomes (Gielen et al., 2008). The framework assumes that the program participants (or consumers) will play an active role in defining their own problems, establishing their goals, and developing their solutions. Health behavior is conceptualized as being influenced by both individual and environmental factors, and the framework is broken into two distinct parts. The first, *PRECEDE* (**P**redisposing, **R**einforcing and **E**nabling

Constructs in Educational Diagnosis and Evaluation), provides an educational diagnosis. For example, predisposing factors include knowledge, attitudes, beliefs, personal preferences, existing skills, and self-efficacy toward the desired behavior change. Reinforcing factors include conditions that reward or reinforce the behavior change, such as social support, economic rewards, and social norms. Enabling factors include skills, availability and accessibility of resources, and other services that facilitate behavior change.

The second part of this framework, *PROCEED* (**P**olicy, **R**egulatory, and **O**rganizational **C**onstructs in **E**ducational and **E**nvironmental **D**evelopment), provides an ecological diagnosis. This framework has been widely used in public health and behavioral medicine (Freire & Runyan, 2006).

RE-AIM

Another framework that has gained popularity is RE-AIM (Reach, Effectiveness, Adoption, Implementation, Maintenance; Glasgow et al., 1999, 2019; King et al., 2010). RE-AIM provides a set of criteria for planning and evaluating interventions that are intended to be broadly implemented, including policy interventions. To facilitate translation of research to practice and policy, RE-AIM emphasizes balancing internal and external validity. It also describes specific ways of measuring the potential public health impact of a program or policy.

The RE-AIM framework can be useful in comparing different public health policies, determining whether certain subpopulations benefit more than others (equity) and identifying areas for integration of policies with other health promotion strategies (Jilcott et al., 2007; King et al., 2010). Application of the RE-AIM framework requires data or knowledge about the target population and the potential settings and organizations (e.g., clinics, worksites, schools) that can implement a policy change (Smith & Harden, 2021). Jilcott et al. (2007) describe how to apply RE-AIM to health policies, including policies that impact health in other sectors (such as urban planning policies that shape the built environment). Glasgow et al. (1999) offers examples based on actual community strategies employed in Colorado during the past 3 years (Nourish Colorado, 2022) as well as a 20-year review of RE-AIM evaluations (Glasgow et al., 2019).

Questions to consider for RE-AIM:

1. Whose health behaviors and health are to be improved?
2. Which stakeholders need to be included in the planning process, and which agencies are responsible for approving or adopting the policy change?
3. Which agencies are responsible for implementing the change?
4. Which agencies are responsible for maintaining the change?
5. What funding needs to be secured to implement and maintain the change?

The *Reach* portion of RE-AIM includes the absolute number, percentage, and representativeness of those affected by a policy or environmental change. For example, to apply RE-AIM to an obesity issue, imagine that a city council decides to build a new bike lane to increase active transportation. Which populations are likely to be affected the most? Does the bike lane connect a low-income neighborhood to a park or school, or does it connect a wealthy neighborhood to a commuter rail station?

Effectiveness in the RE-AIM framework involves using research methods to study who uses the bike lane. This may involve collecting data before and after the bike lane is built. Alternatively, one can sometimes make an educated guess by referring to published studies from similar communities that have constructed bike lanes. As mentioned previously, effectiveness may also involve measuring changes in risk factors (e.g., obesity) and/or disease rates in the target population, although this would involve a longer period of study. This can be achieved by collecting primary data, using secondary data from a surveillance system such as the Behavioral Risk Factor Surveillance System (BRFSS), or referring to published literature for estimates.

Adoption in the RE-AIM framework considers which political entity has the authority to decide to build the bike lane, and the process they use (e.g., the city council and the Department of Transportation would be responsible for making decisions about the bike lane and which funds could be used).

Implementation in the RE-AIM framework considers how the policy is actually carried out. For example, are enough funds to build the bike lane actually allocated? Is the project completed? Who enforces use of the bike lane (e.g., are police officers or crossing guards deployed to manage dangerous intersections)?

Maintenance has two considerations, one at the setting level and one at the individual user level. For example, who will make sure that the bike lane remains free from trash and debris? Will additional city funds be allocated to maintain it? At the user level, one can measure ridership at different points in time to determine whether people keep using the bike lane, or if use drops off after a period of time.

NATIONAL EFFORTS OF HEALTH POLICY ANALYSIS

Health policy questions have been with us for a very long time. Perhaps one of the earliest efforts in the United States to methodically address these issues based on evidence was the study done by the Committee on the Cost of Medical Care (1932) that produced a multivolume study of the U.S. healthcare system and made recommendations for its improvement. It is not surprising given the current debates on major health policy issues that the recommendations from the 1920s were not unanimous and that there was a spirited minority report.

Many of the recommendations of that committee would be familiar to current debates on healthcare policy. One of the consistent recommendations has been the collection of data to identify the precise nature of the problem. Within health policy, this is generally called *type one evidence* or descriptive epidemiology. It provides information to document the existence of a problem. An example of type one evidence would be the incidence rate of a specific disease that demonstrates either its increase or decrease over time. The collection of obesity data has done much to stimulate health policy action in the United States. It demonstrates the existence of an increasing population health problem. Type one evidence does not attempt to explain the cause of the problem or conclude that a particular solution is viable. That is the job of type two evidence, or analytic epidemiology. The collection of demographic, epidemiologic, and medical type one data has been an ongoing activity of federal, state, and local public health departments. In 1956 the National Health Security Act led to the establishment of the National Center for Health

Statistics (NCHS). Health data collection remains an important aspect of knowing where we are in terms of improving the health of the population. An important part of the public lens is recognizing that the conceptualization of evidence itself is socially produced and affected by power dynamics. Whose story is being told by the data? Whose knowledge is valued? Who is counted and by whom? We encourage readers to refer to the growing body of literature on minority populations and Indigenous epistemologies and other ways of knowing that are central to planetary health (Lewis et al., 2020; Prescod-Weinstein, 2020).

We have already discussed the importance of the Government Accountability Office (GAO) and the Congressional Budget Office (CBO) for policy analysis. There are other organizations that need to be mentioned as well.

Agency for Healthcare Research and Quality

Through the 1980s and 1990s there was a concerted effort to improve the analysis of the healthcare system through the establishment of the Agency for Health Care Policy and Research (AHCPR) that later became the Agency for Healthcare Research and Quality (AHRQ; www.ahrq.gov). Here the focus was not just on the collection of data, but the analysis of data to demonstrate that one approach may be more effective, efficient, or equitable than another. This is generally referred to as *type two evidence*. It requires a higher level of data analysis by considering confounding factors and potential spurious relationships. Many sponsored research projects are conducted and supported by the AHRQ as well as the National Institutes of Health (NIH), the CDC, and even the National Science Foundation (NSF) to demonstrate the efficiency, effectiveness, or equity of medical and public health practices. These studies are generally carried out by research universities or consulting companies as well as by private foundations (e.g., the Kaiser Family Foundation or the Robert Wood Johnson Foundation). In addition, most levels of public and private funding require formal evaluations of their sponsored projects. The lessons learned from these projects help to inform policy makers of the successes and failures of funded efforts to solve health problems. The products of these studies frequently end up in the peer-reviewed literature as well as grey literature.

The National Academy of Medicine (Institute of Medicine)

The Institute of Medicine (IOM; www.iom.edu) was founded in 1970 and is one of the five National Academy of Sciences. In 2015, the National Academy of Sciences voted to change the name of the Institute of Medicine to the National Academy of Medicine (NAM). The name change reflected efforts to better integrate the work of the National Academies of Sciences, Engineering, and Medicine.

The NAM is a private, independent entity that attempts to provide best evidence reports and information to the public and to decision makers. It has been an important source of information for shaping health policy discussions. Much of its work is the result of congressional mandates. Two of its most seminal works were *To Err Is Human* (Donaldson et al., 2000) and *Crossing the Quality Chasm* (IOM, 2001), which have been the foundation for much of the quality improvement work in the health sector. The publication *Bridging the Evidence Gap in Obesity Prevention: A Framework to Inform Decision Making* (Kumanyika et al., 2010) was a seminal work on the population health problem of obesity.

Patient-Centered Outcomes Research Institute

One of the contributions of the Patient Protection and Accountable Care Act of 2010 (PPACA) was the establishment of the Patient-Centered Outcomes Research Institute (PCORI; www.pcori.org). Its mission is to provide people with evidence-based information on the comparative effectiveness of various treatments. It is an independent quasi-public body. Its mandate is to improve the quality and relevance of evidence available to help patients, caregivers, clinicians, employers, insurers, and policy makers make better-informed health decisions (Garber, 2011). PCORI works with healthcare stakeholders to identify critical research questions and answer them through comparative clinical effectiveness research, or clinical effectiveness research (CER). It involves patients' perspectives in examining the outcomes of medical practices as well as innovative approaches to healthcare delivery.

Data science methods have begun to promote a movement toward personalized medicine, although a number of challenges still exist relative to the data, its computational complexity, and demonstrating improved outcomes relative to the standard of care (Fröhlich et al., 2018). We discuss these points in Chapter 9.

In 2021, the PCORI Board of Governors approved research funding totaling $49.5 million to support nine new comparative CER studies that aim to improve care for adults and children across a range of health conditions. Some of the funds focus on telehealth and mobile health strategies (mHealth), which are at the center of many clinical and public health policy discussions. For example, one study will compare the effects of an mHealth cognitive behavioral therapy (CBT) intervention to an intervention that provides financial rewards based on evidence of smoking abstinence, as well as to traditional cessation approaches.

PCORI is not a governmental agency, and it is limited in its ability to use cost-effective analysis or use its findings to recommend policy. One of PCORI's 2021 research awards was to Massachusetts Health Quality Partners to examine sickle cell disease (SCD) pain management outside clinical settings (Rabson, 2022). The results of these studies will potentially have major implications for the future allocation of scarce resources and improve the lives of patients.

Centers for Disease Control and Prevention

The CDC's Office of the Associate Director for Policy and Strategy (OADPS) supports policy analysts in building and translating evidence to determine "what works" in public health practice (CDC, 2021b). It also supports the CDC POLARIS website for policy analysis, which provides useful resources, downloadable tools, and worksheets to help guide your work (CDC, 2021a). Policy analysts can use the POLARIS tools to identify inputs such as data needed to assess political will, develop the policy, and identify stakeholders. They can then identify activities and outputs that are relevant to formulating policy such as engaging stakeholders, raising awareness, and drafting policy solutions (process evaluation). Intended outcomes are also identified, but these may change as the process evolves. Using emergent logic models (logic models that evolve over time), policy interventions can be examined in relation to the iterative policy process.

The Centers for Disease Control and Prevention Policy Research, Analysis, and Development Office

The CDC Policy Research, Analysis, and Development Office (CDC, n.d.-c) spearheads and coordinates policy work including establishing policy priorities at multiple levels (federal, state, local, global, and with the private sector); conducting policy analysis; developing and implementing strategies (e.g., regulatory, legal, economic) to deliver on policy priorities; and coordinating agency work with the healthcare system and relevant organizations to advance CDC's policy agenda (Leeman et al., 2011, 2012).

In addition, the CDC collects data, conducts and sponsors scientific research, administers national health efforts, promotes healthy and safe behaviors, and provides support to state, Tribal, and local health initiatives (www.cdc.gov). For example, obesity prevalence maps can be found on the CDC website (www.cdc.gov/obesity/data/prevalence-maps.html). The Nutrition and Obesity Policy Research and Evaluation Network (NOPREN) was funded by the CDC to conduct transdisciplinary nutrition- and obesity-related policy research and evaluation in certain states. NOPREN helps to promote understanding of the effectiveness of policies related to preventing childhood obesity through improved access to affordable, healthy foods and beverages in a variety of settings including communities, workplaces, healthcare facilities, childcare institutions, and schools (Ascher et al., 2012). Several of the state-level policy research examples showcased in this book were funded in part through the CDC's NOPREN initiative. Similarly, the Physical Activity Policy Research and Evaluation Network (PAPREN) is a CDC-funded network that brings diverse partners together to cocreate environments that maximize physical activity (https://papren.org). PAPREN advances the evidence base and puts research into practice through collaboration across multiple sectors with a shared vision of achieving healthy, active communities.

Other Policy Research Institutes

There are literally hundreds of health policy research institutes around the country. There are too many to list them all and many specialties in healthcare have their own major research institutes. Some of these are embedded in universities (public and private) and some of those are supported through federal and state grants or private funding. Some health institutes focus on rural healthcare (e.g., the six federally designated rural health research centers funded by HRSA's Office of Rural Health Policy (www.hrsa.gov/ruralhealth/policy/rhrcdirectory/index.html), and others focus on particular aspects of health such as disabilities (e.g., Association of University Centers on Disabilities, www.aucd.org). Some are focused on state health policy initiatives (e.g., National Academy for State Health Policy, www.nashp.org). The Rand Corporation (www.rand.org) has long been a center for major healthcare studies and reports. Rand continues to publish important health policy research, some of it published in peer-reviewed journals and others by Rand itself. The Henry J. Kaiser Family Foundation (www.kff.org) has been a source of important policy studies on Medicare, Medicaid, the uninsured, and healthcare reform. Most studies involving Medicare or Medicaid generally cite some information or analysis done by the Kaiser Family Foundation. Policy institutes also reflect the full political spectrum. The Heritage Foundation (www.heritage.org) and the CATO Institute (www.cato.org) have long been identified as a source of conservative and free market healthcare proposals. The Brookings Institution (www.brookings.edu) and the Center for American Progress (www.americanprogress.org) are sources for liberal policy research.

Human Impact Partners (HIP; www.humanimpact.org) is one of the few organizations in the United States that conducts policy analyses with an explicit focus on uncovering and addressing policies and practices that make communities less healthy and create health inequities. It emphasizes policies outside the medical arena (e.g., housing, education, transportation, urban planning). HIP aims to build collective power with social justice movements. One important process for considering such policies is HIA (Dannenberg et al., 2008; Rogerson et al., 2020). HIA is a practical tool that uses data, research, and stakeholder input to prospectively determine a policy's potential impact on the health of a population. HIAs also provide recommendations to address these impacts.

The above examples demonstrate the richness of governmental and nongovernmental research centers. There are many others that are relevant for particular areas of health policy analysis. For example, if you were focusing on a particular disease, there are national and state organizations that would be important resources. However, a limitation in heath policy analysis, and in health services research more generally, is that one often cannot get data at the appropriate geographic or temporal scale to perform a complete analysis. This is because data infrastructure and surveillance systems are fragmented and uneven in their coverage, due in part to significant underinvestment in public health in the United States (Maani & Galea, 2020), but also notions and rules for the privacy and security of health information. We explore these data issues further in Chapter 9.

SUMMARY

Health policy analysis is an area that requires knowledge and skills from a variety of disciplines and perspectives. In this chapter we discussed the importance of evidence-based health policy and the promise and problems associated with operationalizing it. We reviewed some major national organizations in the United States that provide resources for conducting policy analysis. While recognizing the importance of evidence-based health policy, it is also important to recognize the importance of ideology and differing sets of values in policy analysis.

In the next chapter we explore some sources of publicly available health data, major data collection systems, and the process of analyzing health policy using health services research methods, social science, and newer data science methods.

DISCUSSION QUESTIONS

■ Discuss what variables might be needed when taking an efficiency focus in a health policy analysis.

■ Discuss how taking an equity focus might contradict taking an efficiency focus in a health policy analysis.

■ How does using a broad framework like HiAP, both complicate and support a health policy analysis?

■ Examine one of the existing health policy frameworks and/or efforts. What variables are considered and what scope do they take?

■ Discuss the difference between analyzing a population and analyzing a health condition.

KEY TERMS

Adelaide Statement
Agency for Healthcare Research and
    Quality (AHRQ)
allocative efficiency
Centers for Disease Control and
    Prevention (CDC)
effectiveness
feasibility
National Academy of Medicine
    (NAM)

Patient-Centered Outcomes
    Research Institute (PCORI)
RE-AIM
PRECEDE-PROCEED
production efficiency
procedural equity
substantive equity
type one and type two evidence

SPRINGER PUBLISHING
CONNECT™

A robust set of instructor resources designed to supplement this text is located at http://connect.springerpub.com/content/book/978-0-8261-8543-3. Qualifying instructors may request access by emailing textbook@springerpub.com.

REFERENCES

Anderson, L. M., Brownson, R. C., Fullilove, M. T., Teutsch, S. M., Novick, L. F., Fielding, J., & Land, G. H. (2005). Evidence-based public health policy and practice: Promises and limits. *American Journal of Preventive Medicine, 28*(5), 226–230. https://doi.org/10.1016/j.amepre.2005.02.014

Ascher, W., Blanck, H., & Cradock, A. (Eds.). (2012). Evaluating policies and processes for promoting healthy eating: Findings from the Nutrition and Obesity Policy Research and Evaluation Network (NOPREN). *American Journal of Preventive Medicine, 43*(3 Suppl. 2), S85–S152. https://www.ajpmonline.org/issue/S0749-3797(12)X0005-9

Aytur, S. A., Smith, S, Humphreys, B., Corvini, M., Madison, M., & Thompson, T. (in press). Planetary health considerations in the context an occupational therapy telehealth intervention for families of children and youth with special health care needs. *Journal of Climate Change and Health*.

Bacchi, C. L. (1999). *Women, policy and politics: The construction of policy problems*. SAGE Publications.

Begley, C. E., Lairson, D. R., Balkrishnan, R., & Aday, L. A. (2004). *Evaluating the healthcare system: Effectiveness, efficiency, and equity* (3rd ed.). Health Administration Press.

Bernstein, J., Reschovsky, J. D., & White, C. (2011, April). *Geographic variation in health care: Changing policy directions*. National Institute for Health Care Reform, Policy Analysis No. 4. https://www.nihcr.org/analysis/geographic-variation/

Betancourt, J. R., Duong, J. V., & Bondaryk, M. R. (2012). Strategies to reduce diabetes disparities: An update. *Current Diabetes Reports, 12*(6), 762–768. https://doi.org/10.1007/s11892-012-0324-1

Braveman, P. A., Kumanyika, S., Fielding, J., LaVeist, T., Borrell, L. N., Manderscheid, R., & Troutman, A. (2011). Health disparities and health equity: The issue is justice. *American Journal of Public Health, 101*(S1), S149–S155. https://doi.org/10.2105/ajph.2010.300062

Brownson, R. C., Chriqui, J. F., & Stamatakis, K. A. (2009). Understanding evidence-based public health policy. *American Journal of Public Health, 99*(9), 1576–1583. https://doi.org/10.2105/ajph.2008.156224

Brownson, R. C., Royer, C., Ewing, R., & McBride, T. D. (2006). Researchers and policymakers: Travelers in parallel universes. *American Journal of Preventive Medicine, 30*(2), 164–172. https://doi.org/10.1016/j.amepre.2005.10.004

Bullard, R. D., & Johnson, G. S. (2000). Environmentalism and public policy: Environmental justice: Grassroots activism and its impact on public policy decision making. *Journal of Social Issues, 56*(3), 555–578. https://doi.org/10.1111/0022-4537.00184

California Newsreel (Producer). (2008). *Unnatural causes: Is inequality making us sick?* [TV Series]. PBS. https://unnaturalcauses.org

Caron, R. M., & Adegboye, A. R. A. (2021). COVID-19: A syndemic requiring an integrated approach for marginalized populations. *Frontiers in Public Health, 9*, Article 675280. https://doi.org/10.3389/fpubh.2021.675280

Caron, R. M., & Aytur, S. A. (2022). Assuring healthy populations during the COVID-19 pandemic: Recognizing women's contributions in addressing syndemic interactions. *Frontiers in Public Health, 10*, Article 856932. https://doi.org/10.3389/fpubh.2022.856932

Carroll, S. R., Herczog, E., Hudson, M., Russell, K., & Stall, S. (2021). Operationalizing the CARE and FAIR principles for Indigenous data futures. *Scientific Data, 8*, Article 108. https://doi.org/10.1038/s41597-021-00892-0

Carroll, S. R., Suina, M., Jäger, M. B., Black, J., Cornell, S., Gonzales, A. A., Jorgensen, M., Palmanteer-Holder, N. L., de la Rosa, J. S., & Teufel-Shone, N. I. (2022). Reclaiming Indigenous health in the US: Moving beyond the social determinants of health. *International Journal of Environmental Research and Public Health, 19*(12), Article 7495. https://doi.org/10.3390/ijerph19127495

Centers for Disease Control and Prevention. (n.d.-a). *A sustainability planning guide for healthy communities*. https://www.cdc.gov/nccdphp/dch/programs/healthycommunitiesprogram/pdf/sustainability_guide.pdf

Centers for Disease Control and Prevention. (n.d.-b). *Office of the Associate Director for Policy and Strategy: Policy analysis*. U.S. Department of Health and Human Services. https://www.cdc.gov/policy/polaris/policyprocess/policy_analysis.html

Centers for Disease Control and Prevention. (n.d.-c). *Office of the Associate Director for Policy and Strategy: Policy and strategy at CDC*. U.S. Department of Health and Human Services. https://www.cdc.gov/policy/index.html

Centers for Disease Control and Prevention. (2013). *A practitioner's guide for advancing health equity: Community strategies for preventing chronic disease*. U.S. Department of Health and Human Services. https://www.cdc.gov/nccdphp/dnpao/health-equity/health-equity-guide/pdf/HealthEquityGuide.pdf

Chen, J. T., Testa, C., Hanage, W. P., & Krieger, N. (2021). *Picturing prevention: Visualizing how vaccination profoundly protects your loved ones, you, and your community from hospitalization and death due to COVID-19 using real-life data from 12 US states (Jan–July 2021)*. Harvard Center for Population and Development Studies Working Paper, 21(4), 1–19. https://cdn1.sph.harvard.edu/wp-content/uploads/sites/1266/2021/08/21_C19_vaxxvisual_pop-center-working-paper_chen-et-al_submitted_0808_with-cover-and-abstract_final.pdf

Clark, W. C. (2007). Sustainability science: A room of its own. *Proceedings of the National Academy of Sciences, 104*(6), 1737–1738. https://doi.org/10.1073/pnas.0611291104

Clark, W. C., & Dickson, N. M. (2003). Sustainability science: The emerging research program. *Proceedings of the National Academy of Sciences, 100*(14), 8059–8061. https://doi.org/10.1073/pnas.1231333100

Committee on the Cost of Medical Care. (1932). *Medical care for the American people. The final report of the committee on the costs of medical care*. University of Chicago Press.

Dannenberg, A. L. (2016). Effectiveness of Health Impact Assessments: A synthesis of data from five impact evaluation reports. *Preventing Chronic Disease, 13*, E84. https://doi.org/10.5888/pcd13.150559

Dannenberg, A. L., Bhatia, R., Cole, B. L., Heaton, S. K., Feldman, J. D., & Rutt, C. D. (2008). Use of Health Impact Assessment in the U.S.: 27 case studies, 1999–2007. *American Journal of Preventive Medicine, 34*(3), 241–256. https://doi.org/10.1016/j.amepre.2007.11.015

Dartmouth Atlas Project. (2022, February 11). *Dartmouth atlas of health care.* https://www.dartmouthatlas.org

Donaldson, M. S., Corrigan, J. M., & Kohn, L. T. (Eds.). (2000). *To err is human: Building a safer health system* (Illustrated ed.). National Academies Press.

Evans, R. G., & Stoddart, G. L. (2003). Consuming research, producing policy? *American Journal of Public Health, 93*(3), 371–379. https://doi.org/10.2105/ajph.93.3.371

Evenson, K., & Aytur, S. (2012). Policy for physical activity promotion. In B. E. Ainsworth & C. A. Macera (Eds.), *Physical activity and public health practice* (pp. 321–344). CRC Press. https://doi.org/10.1201/b11718

Field, M. J., & Lohr, K. N. (Eds.). (1992). *Guidelines for clinical practice: From development to use.* National Academies Press. https://doi.org/10.17226/1863

Fradkin, J. E. (2012). Confronting the urgent challenge of diabetes: An overview. *Health Affairs, 31*(1), 12–19. https://doi.org/10.1377/hlthaff.2011.1150

Freire, K., & Runyan, C. W. (2006). Planning models: PRECEDE-PROCEED and Haddon matrix. In A. C. Gielen, D. A. Sleet, & R. J. DiClemente (Eds.), *Injury and violence prevention: Behavioral science theories, methods, and applications* (pp. 127–158). Jossey-Bass.

Fröhlich, H., Balling, R., Beerenwinkel, N., Kohlbacher, O., Kumar, S., Lengauer, T., Maathuis, M. H., Moreau, Y., Murphy, S. A., Przytycka, T. M., Rebhan, M., Röst, H., Schuppert, A., Schwab, M., Spang, R., Stekhoven, D., Sun, J., Weber, A., Ziemek, D., & Zupan, B. (2018). From hype to reality: Data science enabling personalized medicine. *BMC Medicine, 16*(1), Article 150. https://doi.org/10.1186/s12916-018-1122-7

Fuchs, V. R. (1974). *Who shall live? Health, economics and social choice.* Basic Books.

Garber, A. M. (2011). How the patient-centered outcomes research institute can best influence real-world health care decision making. *Health Affairs, 30*(12), 2243–2251. https://doi.org/10.1377/hlthaff.2010.0255

Gawande, A. (2009, May 25). The cost conundrum. *The New Yorker.* https://www.newyorker.com/magazine/2009/06/01/the-cost-conundrum

Gielen, A., McDonald, E., Gary, T., & Bone, L. (2008). Using the PRECEDE/PROCEED model to apply health behavior theories. In K. Glanz, B. K. Rimer, & K. Viswanath (Eds.), *Health behavior and health education: Theory, research and practice* (4th ed., pp. 407–433). Jossey-Bass.

Glasgow, R. E., Harden, S. M., Gaglio, B., Rabin, B., Smith, M. L., Porter, G. C., Ory, M. G., & Estabrooks, P. A. (2019). RE-AIM planning and evaluation framework: Adapting to new science and practice with a 20-year review. *Frontiers in Public Health, 9*(7), Article 64. https://doi.org/10.3389/fpubh.2019.00064

Glasgow, R. E., Vogt, T. M., & Boles, S. M. (1999). Evaluating the public health impact of health promotion interventions: The RE-AIM framework. *American Journal of Public Health, 89*(9), 1322–1327. https://doi.org/10.2105/ajph.89.9.1322

Graham, J. D., Corso, P. S., Morris, J. M., Segui-Gomez, M., & Weinstein, M. C. (1998). Evaluating the cost-effectiveness of clinical and public health measures. *Annual Review of Public Health, 19*(1), 125–152. https://doi.org/10.1146/annurev.publhealth.19.1.125

Green, L. W. (1974). Toward cost-benefit evaluations of health education: Some concepts, methods, and examples. *Health Education Monographs, 2*(Suppl. 1), 34–64. https://doi.org/10.1177/10901981740020s106

Green, L. W. (2006). Public health asks of systems science: To advance our evidence-based practice, can you help us get more practice-based evidence? *American Journal of Public Health, 96*(3), 406–409. https://doi.org/10.2105/ajph.2005.066035

Green, L., & Kreuter, M. (2004). *Health program planning: An educational and ecological approach* (4th ed.). McGraw-Hill.

Grosse, S. D., Teutsch, S. M., & Haddix, A. C. (2007). Lessons from cost-effectiveness research for United States public health policy. *Annual Review of Public Health, 28*(1), 365–391. https://doi.org/10.1146/annurev.publhealth.28.021406.144046

Huang, T. T., Drewnosksi, A., Kumanyika, S., & Glass, T. A. (2009). A systems-oriented multilevel framework for addressing obesity in the 21st century. *Preventing Chronic Disease, 6*(3), A82. https://www.ncbi.nlm.nih.gov/pmc/articles/PMC2722412

Institute of Medicine. (2001). *Crossing the quality chasm: A new health system for the 21st century.* National Academies Press. https://doi.org/10.17226/10027

Jilcott, S., Ammerman, A., Sommers, J., & Glasgow, R. E. (2007). Applying the RE-AIM framework to assess the public health impact of policy change. *Annals of Behavioral Medicine, 34*(2), 105–114. https://doi.org/10.1007/bf02872666

King, D. K., Glasgow, R. E., & Leeman-Castillo, B. (2010). Reaiming RE-AIM: Using the model to plan, implement, and evaluate the effects of environmental change approaches to enhancing population health. *American Journal of Public Health, 100*(11), 2076–2084. https://doi.org/10.2105/ajph.2009.190959

Kingdon, J. W. (2003). *Agendas, alternatives, and public policies.* Addison-Wesley Educational Publishers.

Krech, R., Valentine, N. B., Reinders, L. T., & Albrecht, D. (2010). Implications of the Adelaide statement on Health in All Policies. *Bulletin of the World Health Organization, 88*(10), 720. https://doi.org/10.2471/blt.10.082461

Krieger, N. (2013). Got theory? On the 21st c. CE rise of explicit use of epidemiologic theories of disease distribution: A review and ecosocial analysis. *Current Epidemiology Reports, 1*(1), 45–56. https://doi.org/10.1007/s40471-013-0001-1

Krieger, N., Chen, J. T., Testa, C., Waterman, P. D., & Hanage, W. P. (2021). *Political lean: A crucial variable for monitoring COVID-19 in the United States.* Harvard Center for Population and Development Studies Working Paper, 21(5), 1–14. https://cdn1.sph.harvard.edu/wp-content/uploads/sites/2623/2021/10/21_krieger-et-al_C19_political-lean-plus_HCPDS-working-paper_Vol-21_No-5_reduced-file-size.pdf

Krieger, N., Testa, C., Waterman, P. D., & Chen, J. T. (2021). *Go big on relief!—Repairing the commingled miseries of COVID-19 and US housing and food insecurity.* Harvard Center for Population and Development Studies Working Paper, 21(2), 1–9. https://cdn1.sph.harvard.edu/wp-content/uploads/sites/1266/2021/02/21_krieger-et-al_C19HH-pulse_HCPDS_Vol-21_No-2_Final.pdf

Krieger, N., Waterman, P. D., Chen, J. T., Testa, C., Santillana, M., & Hanage, W. P. (2021). *Plague of US missing COVID-19 data for race/ethnicity: Debacle continues with vaccination data.* Harvard Population Center for Development Studies Working Paper, 21(1), 1–5. https://cdn1.sph.harvard.edu/wp-content/uploads/sites/1266/2021/02/21_Krieger_Waterman-et-al_missing-data-on-race-continues-w_-vaccine_HCPDS-Vol-21_No-1_FINAL_AB.pdf

Kumanyika, S., Brownson, R., & Cheadle, A. (2012). The L.E.A.D. framework: Using tools from evidence-based public health to address evidence needs for obesity prevention. *Preventing Chronic Disease, 9,* E125. https://doi.org/10.5888/pcd9.120157

Kumanyika, S. K., Parker, L., & Sim, L. J. (Eds.). (2010). *Bridging the evidence gap in obesity prevention: A framework to inform decision making.* National Academies Press. https://doi.org/10.17226/12847

Leeman, J., Sommers, J., Leung, M. M., & Ammerman, A. (2011). Disseminating evidence from research and practice. *Journal of Public Health Management and Practice, 17*(2), 133–140. https://doi.org/10.1097/phh.0b013e3181e39eaa

Leeman, J., Sommers, J., Vu, M., Jernigan, J., Payne, G., Thompson, D., Heiser, C., Farris, R., & Ammerman, A. (2012). An evaluation framework for obesity prevention policy interventions. *Preventing Chronic Disease, 9,* E120. https://doi.org/10.5888/pcd9.110322

Leidner, A. J., Murthy, N., Chesson, H. W., Biggerstaff, M., Stoecker, C., Harris, A. M., Acosta, A., Dooling, K., & Bridges, C. B. (2019). Cost-effectiveness of adult vaccinations: A systematic review. *Vaccine, 37*(2), 226–234. https://doi.org/10.1016/j.vaccine.2018.11.056

Lewis, D., Williams, L., & Jones, R. (2020). A radical revision of the public health response to environmental crisis in a warming world: Contributions of Indigenous knowledges and Indigenous feminist perspectives. *Canadian Journal of Public Health, 111*(6), 897–900. https://doi.org/10.17269/s41997-020-00388-1

Lyn, R., Aytur, S., Davis, T. A., Eyler, A. A., Evenson, K. R., Chriqui, J. F., Cradock, A. L., Goins, K. V., Litt, J., & Brownson, R. C. (2013). Policy, systems, and environmental approaches for obesity prevention. *Journal of Public Health Management and Practice, 19*(Suppl. 1), S23–S33. https://doi.org/10.1097/phh.0b013e3182841709

Maani, N., & Galea, S. (2020). COVID-19 and underinvestment in the public health infrastructure of the United States. *The Milbank Quarterly, 98*(2), 250–259. https://doi.org/10.1111/1468-0009.12463

Madahian, B., Klesges, R. C., Klesges, L., & Homayouni, R. (2012). System dynamics modeling of childhood obesity. *BMC Bioinformatics, 13*(Suppl. 12), A13. https://doi.org/10.1186/1471-2105-13-s12-a13

Mays, G. P., & Smith, S. A. (2011). Evidence links increases in public health spending to declines in preventable deaths. *Health Affairs, 30*(8), 1585–1593. https://doi.org/10.1377/hlthaff.2011.0196

McGlynn, E., Asch, S., Adams, J., Keesey, J., Hicks, J., DeCristofaro, A., & Kerr, E. (2003). Quality of health care delivered to adults in the United States. *New England Journal of Medicine, 349*(19), 1866–1868. https://doi.org/10.1056/nejm200311063491916

McLeroy, K. R., Bibeau, D., Steckler, A., & Glanz, K. (1988). An ecological perspective on health promotion programs. *Health Education Quarterly*, 15(4), 351–377. https://doi .org/10.1177/109019818801500401

Nittas, V., Gao, M., West, E. A., Ballouz, T., Menges, D., Wulf Hanson, S., & Puhan, M. A. (2022). Long COVID through a public health lens: An umbrella review. *Public Health Reviews*, 43, Article 1604501. https://doi.org/10.3389/phrs.2022.1604501

Nourish Colorado. (2022, August 17). *Building resilient food systems.* https://nourishcolorado.org

Office of Disease Prevention and Health Promotion. (n.d.). *Healthy people 2030 framework.* Healthy People 2030, Office of Disease Prevention and Health Promotion, Office of the Assistant Secretary for Health, Office of the Secretary, and U.S. Department of Health and Human Services. https://health.gov/healthypeople/about/healthy-people-2030-framework

Organisation for Economic Co-operations and Development. (2022). *Health expenditure as a percentage of gross domestic product (GDP) in selected countries in 2020.* Statista Research Department. https://www.statista.com/statistics/268826/health-expenditure-as-gdp -percentage-in-oecd-countries

Peters, D. R., Schnell, J. L., Kinney, P. L., Naik, V., & Horton, D. E. (2020). Public health and climate benefits and trade-offs of U.S. vehicle electrification. *GeoHealth*, 4(10), Article e2020GH000275. https://doi.org/10.1029/2020gh000275

Prescod-Weinstein, C. (2020). Making Black women scientists under white empiricism: The racialization of epistemology in physics. *Signs: Journal of Women in Culture and Society*, 45(2), 421–447. https://doi.org/10.1086/704991

Rabson, B. G. (2022, March 4). *Engaging stakeholders to set new directions for sickle cell disease pain self- management research.* Patient-Centered Outcomes Research Institute. https://www.pcori.org/ research-results/2021/engaging-stakeholders-set-new-directions-sickle-cell-disease-pain-self -management-research

Rogerson, B., Lindberg, R., Baum, F., Dora, C., Haigh, F., Simoncelli, A. M., Parry Williams, L., Peralta, G., Pollack Porter, K. M., & Solar, O. (2020). Recent advances in Health Impact Assessment and Health in All Policies implementation: Lessons from an international convening in Barcelona. *International Journal of Environmental Research and Public Health*, 17(21), Article 7714. https://doi.org/10.3390/ijerph17217714

Rose, G. (1992). *The strategy of preventive medicine.* Oxford University Press.

Sabatier, P. A., & Jenkins-Smith, H. C. (1993). *Policy change and learning: An advocacy coalition approach (theoretical lenses on public policy).* Westview Press.

Schmid, T. L., Pratt, M., & Witmer, L. (2006). A framework for physical activity policy research. *Journal of Physical Activity and Health*, 3(s1), S20–S29. https://doi.org/10.1123/jpah.3.s1.s20

Shaw, E., Walpole, S., McLean, M., Alvarez-Nieto, C., Barna, S., Bazin, K., Behrens, G., Chase, H., Duane, B., el Omrani, O., Elf, M., Faerron Guzmán, C. A., Falceto De Barros, E., Gibbs, T. J., Groome, J., Hackett, F., Harden, J., Hothersall, E. J., Hourihane, M., ... Woollard, R. (2021). AMEE consensus statement: Planetary health and education for sustainable healthcare. *Medical Teacher*, 43(3), 272–286. https://doi.org/10.1080/0142159x.2020.1860207

Shrank, W. H., Rogstad, T. L., & Parekh, N. (2019). Waste in the US health care system: Estimated costs and potential for savings. *JAMA*, 322(15), 1501–1509. https://doi.org/10.1001/ jama.2019.13978

Singer, M., Bulled, N., Ostrach, B., & Mendenhall, E. (2017). Syndemics and the biosocial conception of health. *The Lancet*, 389(10072), 941–950. https://doi.org/10.1016/s0140-6736(17)30003-x

Smedley, B. D., Stith, A. Y., & Nelson, A. R. (Eds.). (2003). *Unequal treatment: Confronting racial and ethnic disparities in health care.* National Academies Press. https://doi.org/10.17226/12875

Smith, M., Saunders, R., Stuckhardt, L., & McGinnis, M. J. (Eds.). (2013). *Best care at lower cost: The path to continuously learning health care in America.* National Academies Press. https://doi .org/10.17226/13444

Smith, M. L., & Harden, S. M. (2021). Full comprehension of theories, models, and frameworks improves application: A focus on RE-AIM. *Frontiers in Public Health*, 9, Article 599975. https:// doi.org/10.3389/fpubh.2021.599975

Stokols, D. (1992). Establishing and maintaining healthy environments: Toward a social ecology of health promotion. *American Psychologist*, 47(1), 6–22. https://doi.org/10.1037/0003-066x.47.1.6

Stokols, D., Allen, J., & Bellingham, R. L. (1996). The social ecology of health promotion: Implications for research and practice. *American Journal of Health Promotion*, 10(4), 247–251. https://doi.org/10.4278/0890-1171-10.4.247

Swinburn, B., Gill, T., & Kumanyika, S. (2005). Obesity prevention: A proposed framework for translating evidence into action. *Obesity Reviews*, 6(1), 23–33. https://doi.org/10.1111/j.1467 -789x.2005.00184.x

Thaler, R. H., & Sunstein, C. R. (2008). *Nudge: Improving decisions about health, wealth, and happiness.* Yale University Press.

University of Kansas Center for Community Health and Development. (2013). *Chapter 2: Other models for promoting community health and development—Section 2: PRECEDE/PROCEED.* The Community Tool Box. https://ctb.ku.edu/en/table-contents/overview/other-models -promoting-community-health-and-development/preceder-proceder/main

Virginia Commonwealth University. (2009, October 1). *Place matters.* Center on Society and Health. https://societyhealth.vcu.edu/work/the-projects/place-matters.html?nav=200

Webster, D. G., Aytur, S. A., Axelrod, M., Wilson, R. S., Hamm, J. A., Sayed, L., Pearson, A. L., Torres, P. H. C., Akporiaye, A., & Young, O. (2022). Learning from the past: Pandemics and the governance treadmill. *Sustainability, 14*(6), Article 3683. https://doi.org/10.3390/su14063683

Wennberg, J., & Gittelsohn, A. (1973). Small area variations in health care delivery. *Science, 182*(4117), 1102–1108. https://doi.org/10.1126/science.182.4117.1102

World Health Organization. (1946, July 22). *Constitution.* Author. https://www.who.int/about/ governance/constitution

World Health Organization & Government of South Australia. (2010). *Adelaide statement on Health in All Policies: Moving towards a shared governance for health and well-being.* World Health Organization. https://apps.who.int/iris/handle/10665/44365

Wulff, K. C., Miller, F. G., & Pearson, S. D. (2011). Can coverage be rescinded when negative trial results threaten a popular procedure? The ongoing saga of vertebroplasty. *Health Affairs, 30*(12), 2269–2276. https://doi.org/10.1377/hlthaff.2011.0159

CHAPTER 9

HEALTH DATA AND ANALYTICAL METHODS

Health policy analysis is obviously only as good as the data that feeds it. As we have discussed, health is a complex construct that is affected by multiple factors across a number of levels of the social-ecological model: individual, interpersonal, organizational, economic, environmental, political, and many others. As such, it is often impossible to develop perfectly representative analytical models to describe health phenomena or predict health outcomes with a high degree of certainty. It is for this reason that the thoughtful analyst must be comprehensive and transparent when collecting and evaluating health data and research evidence.

LEARNING OBJECTIVES

To be able to:

- Identify and explore existing sources of public data.
- Discern between the different types of analytical studies.
- Understand various analytical functions and their uses.
- Explore data science tools and how they apply to policy analysis.
- Identify gaps in data and impacts for analysis.

Despite the call for evidence-based medicine and public health, evidence is frequently difficult to attain. Data are not always readily available, especially in the United States, where there is priority for privacy and proprietary ownership of health data. States generally have specific rules regarding the aggregation of data and the reporting of analysis to protect individuals from being identified. Specific health policies (e.g., Health Insurance Portability and Accountability Act [HIPAA], 1996) have tried to address these privacy rules for healthcare. Others related to how data can be stored and shared between patients, among providers, and within health records are continuously evolving, such as with the 21st Century Cures Act (2016). You should become familiar with the data collection policies of your state to understand the limitations of its use for analytical purposes.

Much health data in the United States is collected by private corporations (insurance companies, hospitals, clinics, physicians, etc.). Consequently, such data are proprietary and generally unavailable to the public or to researchers without specific authorization by the owners of the data. In addition, because collection of data tends not to be centrally governed in the United States, data are collected in different ways by different organizations and across different states, making comparisons between health data from different organizations often difficult. Organizations may use different identifiers of individuals, which makes tracking who people see, what services they get, or even where they live hard to connect. Variables are often defined in different ways, using different measurements with different cut-off points. An example is what might constitute someone who is prediabetic. Some organizations may create calculated or rules-driven fields that have a flag designating [not diabetic/prediabetic/diabetic] based on a summary of weight, medications used, and a measure of hemoglobin A1c. The cut-off points for HbA1c value, the weight value, and the medications can all vary by the rules that the organization has put in place.

Combining data from different organizations can become very difficult even if those private organizations give access to the data. Conversations among policy makers, practitioners, and private industry have centered on better data for decision-making and improving medical care. There has been much work done to transition to electronic medical records. Progress in interoperating those records, however, has been slow, largely due to the issue of patient confidentiality and privacy. Linking data across multiple sites of patient care becomes problematic when the data systems are privately developed and not interoperable or cannot talk to one another, use different values, or are on different proprietary software systems. Another complication is that proprietary data are generally not comparable to population-based census data, so it can be difficult to link these data sets to important demographic and socioeconomic information.

Interoperability is the function of connecting systems and sources of data between providers, insurers, and patients via electronic health systems. For the past nearly 20 years, promoting interoperability has been one of the primary roles of the U.S. Office of the National Controller (ONC) for health information technology within the U.S. Department of Health and Human Services (DHHS; www.hhs.gov). Given the length of time the effort has been underway, it is evident that there are a number of complex connections needed to create a seamless, yet respectful, private and secure set of systems. The ONC sets the information standards for a number of health-related issues such as patient and provider authentication, electronic prescribing, quality measurement, data transmission to public health agencies, and many others.

PUBLIC DATA

The federal government, through DHHS, also collects, hosts, and distributes much of the health data that are publicly available. This is frequently done through cooperative agreements with state governments. For example, hospital discharge data are collected through the Uniform Hospital Discharge Data System (UHDDS), although control and analysis of the data may vary from state to state. Other standardized data sets include the Uniform Ambulatory Care Data Set (UACDS), the Minimum Data Set (MDS 2.0) for Long Term Care and Resident Assessment Protocols, the Outcome Assessment Information Set (OASIS), the Data Elements for Emergency Department Systems (DEEDS), and the Essential Medical Data Set (EMDS).

Some of the more popularly used health data sources are:

- National Health Interview Survey (NHIS; www.cdc.gov/nchs/nhis.htm)
- National Health and Nutrition Examination Surveys (NHANES; www.cdc .gov/nchs/nhanes.htm)
- National Ambulatory Medical Care Survey (NAMCS; www.cdc.gov/nchs/ ahcd.htm)
- National Hospital Discharge Survey (NHDS; www.cdc.gov/nchs/nhds.htm)
- National Survey of Ambulatory Surgery (NSAS; www.cdc.gov/nchs/nsas .htm)
- National Home and Hospice Care Survey (www.cdc.gov/nchs/nhhcs.htm)
- National Nursing Home Survey (NNHS; www.cdc.gov/nchs/nnhs.htm)
- National Survey of Residential Care Facilities (NSRCF; www.cdc.gov/nchs/ nsrcf.htm)
- Centers for Disease Control and Prevention (CDC) Behavioral Risk Factor Surveillance System (BRFSS; www.cdc.gov/brfss)
- CDC Youth Risk Behavior Surveillance System (YRBSS; CDC, 2020)
- PLACES Data (www.cdc.gov/places/index.html)
- CDC/Agency for Toxic Substances and Disease Registry (ATSDR) Social Vulnerability Index (SVI; www.atsdr.cdc.gov/placeandhealth/svi/index.html)
- County Health Rankings & Roadmaps (www.countyhealthrankings.org)

The DHHS has other agencies involved in data collection. For example, the Agency for Healthcare Research and Quality (AHRQ) collects data under the Health Care Cost and Utilization Project (HCUP; AHRQ, 2022). The Surveillance Epidemiology and End Results (SEER; seer.cancer.gov) for cancer has been an important source of information on the experience of cancer patients. There are also national and state disease registries that collect information on specific diseases or in times of the COVID-19 pandemic (e.g., Johns Hopkins Coronavirus Resource Center at https://coronavirus.jhu.edu/about/how-to-use-our-data).

Some of the information collected by governments includes the entire population (Census and Vital Records, U.S. Census Bureau, www.census.gov) and Medicare (www.medicare.gov) and Medicaid (www.medicaid.gov) data sets, but most national data collection systems rely on samples of the population and not the total population. As a result, analyses using sample populations use extrapolations to the general population. This raises questions of external validity (the ability of the data to reflect the larger population).

For example, while Medicare data are complete and collected nationally, whether the experience of this subpopulation can be applied to the entire population composed of people ages 18 to 64 is questionable. An example of this is the literature on the geographic variation in medical practice. The only complete national data set that can address how extensive medical variation exists is Medicare data. One of the variables that influences medical expenditures is the health status of the population. Whether a Medicare recipient had insurance prior to being enrolled in Medicare could have a major impact on Medicare expenditures. Those individuals coming from areas with low employer health insurance may experience higher Medicare expenditures once they become eligible for Medicare due to their previous lack of health insurance. Consequently, additional Medicare expenditures in particular areas may have less to do with the "practice of medicine" than with the older population having been previously uninsured. Each data set has its own inherent strengths and weaknesses. When using a data set for policy analysis or relying on an article that uses a particular data set, make sure that you examine that data set's limitations. Many of the data sources described in this chapter also have online data aggregation and summation tools that can be utilized via the federal website. There may also be graphical interfaces and mapping functions available. It is important when using these to know how the estimates are being constructed (what are the numerator and denominator for any estimates or rates?) and what the inclusion and/or reporting parameters are for the data and its output, which is discussed more fully in the following paragraphs.

The primary way to become familiar with the strengths and weaknesses of any data set is to go the original source of the data set and examine the methodology used in data collection and the definition of its data elements. Another way to learn about the strength and weaknesses of data sets is to examine multiple studies using that data set. Through the peer review process, those studies will generally indicate some of the limitations of the data set within the methodology section of that study.

Data on various diseases differs greatly. Some diseases are "reportable" and, therefore, must be reported by medical providers to a central data source (typically a state Department of Public Health which then forwards it to the CDC). However, most diseases are not reportable and so our knowledge of the number and distribution of cases of those diseases generally rests on estimates from smaller population samples. In addition, many of these nonreportable diseases may be self-reported and, therefore, lack a professional formal diagnosis for verification. As a result, we have relatively precise numbers of people diagnosed with syphilis each year (a reportable disease) but much less precise numbers of those people with arthritis. Arthritis is a very debilitating and expensive disease, but its prevalence in the United States or in any state rests on estimates from population samples. Does a national sample of the prevalence of arthritis apply to a state with a large older adult population? Does that large older adult population (healthy older adults) reflect the average older adult population? Likewise, much of the United States data on the "obesity epidemic" is based on estimates derived from samples of the population. If the disease you are covering rests on estimates, you need to question how reliable your data might be. Does the data reflect only those who have been hospitalized for a particular diagnosis or does it include those living with the diagnosis in the community as well? Are the rates based on incidence rates (the number of new cases) or prevalence rates (the number of existing cases)?

A corollary question that needs to be asked regarding data collection is what level of precision is needed for your policy analysis? As indicated previously, the proportion of obese people in a particular state or the country rests on estimates. Who has made these estimates and how reliable is their methodology?

Does the organization providing the estimate have an incentive to exaggerate or underestimate the number? Given the sophistication of the estimates and the uniform nature of these estimates, what would be the practical policy impact of having a more precise number of obese people in the United States versus the current estimate? Does it really matter if the estimate is off plus or minus 1% or 3%? Given limited resources, is money better spent obtaining the exact number of obese people or funding services to treat the problem? The SEER for cancer has been an important source of detailed information on the cancer patients that has been useful in studying the etiology and treatment of cancer. However, the geographic areas included in SEER represent only 28% of the U.S. population (National Cancer Institute, 2022). What would be the cost of getting 80% or 100% of cancer patients? How much additional knowledge would we gain by having more data? Would the additional information be worth the cost? Would we learn more about rural populations or disadvantaged populations if we invested more in collecting data about these groups, which may be underrepresented in current data sets? These are important health policy questions.

Another source of data that is currently being used and discussed for health policy development is what are known as all payer claims data. Many states have either developed or are in the process of developing all payer claims databases (APCDs). These databases require all insurance companies selling policies in a state to provide the same proprietary data in an agreed-upon format to a central state data collection system. This has allowed those states implementing APCDs time to gain specific information on the utilization of health services by the commercially insured population within their states in addition to those insured in their Medicaid insurance systems. This data can be highly useful for understanding disease prevalence in populations, conducting surveillance of populations, and analyzing what care is or is not being received, where, and when for the insured population. However, these data systems are also limited. For example, claims are typically not processed for the uninsured population. In addition, unless the data system is set up to collect patient utilization in adjoining states, the data may not reflect insurance claims for people receiving medical services in other states. Also, most insurance data do not include socioeconomic or demographic information on patients, both of which are known to be major factors related to health disparities.

Changes in the healthcare system also influence the availability of data. For example, most states used to have relatively complete profiles of the utilization of health services by their Medicaid recipients through their own data collection. That information has been useful in designing Medicaid benefits as well as determining reimbursement levels. As more state Medicaid systems came to rely on private managed care entities to deliver services, Medicaid data became less accessible to researchers due to the fact that such data are now proprietary. Some states have been able to obtain some of this data by making agreements with their managed care companies to supply data to the state. The data provided may be in fixed formats rather than allowing the states to analyze data differently. These agreements need to be carefully constructed and open to renegotiation to make sure that the state has access to the data that it needs over time. Despite these agreements, receiving static statistical reports from a provider is not the equivalent of the state previously having the raw data to aggregate and analyze as needed.

In addition to disease and insurance data sets, there are public health surveillance systems administered by the CDC to estimate health behavior patterns and trends. For example, the *Behavioral Risk Factor Surveillance System* (BRFSS; CDC, n.d.-b) and the *Youth Risk Behavior Surveillance System* (YRBSS; CDC, n.d.-a) are important sources of information on behaviors and risk factors known to be associated with disease. The BRFSS is a cross-sectional telephone survey that state health departments conduct monthly over landline telephones and cellular telephones with a standardized questionnaire and technical and methodologic assistance from the CDC. The BRFSS is used to collect prevalence data among adult U.S. residents regarding their risk behaviors and preventive health practices that can affect their health status. Data are forwarded to the CDC to be aggregated for each state, returned with standard tabulations, and published annually by each state. The BRFSS uses sophisticated survey sampling techniques and weighting procedures to generate estimates representative of the U.S. population, including the District of Columbia and participating U.S. territories (www.cdc.gov/brfss/data_documentation/index.htm).

Because such data are collected at the state level, states and large metropolitan areas can be compared to each other on important behavioral characteristics such as smoking, the use of alcohol, or obesity. However, for a particular state it may be more important to look at variations within the state (e.g., urban vs. rural or one county vs. another county). Some states are now increasing the sample size for their BRFSS survey to be able to compare subpopulations or various counties within that state. However, this increases the cost of such surveys. Given tight state budgets, the additional costs may not be politically possible even though the health policy implications can be profound. You may want to examine whether your state's BRFSS reports provide you with the information that you need for your policy analysis.

The YRBSS monitors six categories of health-related behaviors and risk factors that contribute to the leading causes of death and disability among youth and adults in the United States. These include sexual behaviors related to unintended pregnancy and sexually transmitted diseases, behaviors that contribute to unintentional injuries and violence, alcohol and other drug use, tobacco use and substance use, dietary behaviors, and physical activity behaviors. The YRBSS also measures the prevalence of obesity, asthma, and other health-related behaviors as well as adverse childhood experiences. The YRBSS includes several components, including (1) a national school-based survey conducted by the CDC and (2) state, territorial, Tribal, and local surveys conducted by state, territorial, and local education and health agencies and Tribal governments.

Some states and larger local communities have developed Geographic Information Systems (GIS) and have begun using data visualization tools that allow health data to be displayed and analyzed spatially and longitudinally. Specific neighborhoods can be highlighted as having a high incidence of mortality, morbidity, or automobile collisions. Using these systems can be very effective in demonstrating where policy intervention might be most effective. However, such systems and capacities are very inconsistent across the United States. Foundations such as the Robert Wood Johnson Foundation (RWJF) have led efforts to make "place-based" health data more accessible. Some examples include:

- Environmental Protection Agency (EPA) Environmental Justice Screening (www.epa.gov/ejscreen)
- PLACES Data (www.cdc.gov/places/index.html)
- County Health Rankings & Roadmaps (www.countyhealthrankings.org and www.countyhealthrankings.org/explore-health-rankings/use-data/go -beyond-the-snapshot/find-more-data)
- America's Health Rankings (www.americashealthrankings.org)
- CDC/ATSDR Social Vulnerability Index (SVI; www.atsdr.cdc.gov/placeand health/svi/index.html)
- PolicyMap (www.policymap.com)

While it might appear that there is a great deal of data available, there are problems with any data source. The data that are available frequently does not match the problem being analyzed or the appropriate geographic scale for policy analysis. For example, age categories may not match or the definition of a disease using the *International Classification of Diseases* (*ICD*) codes may vary (CDC, n.d.-d). *ICD-10-CM* was released in 2014. Were studies used for your analysis based on *ICD-9-CM* or *ICD-10-CM* codes? Does it make a difference?

Use of data becomes even more complicated if you need to use more than one data set. Due to monetary constraints, many of these data systems are not collected every year. For example, one of the most important data sources is the U.S. Census because it is used as the denominator for disease/mortality rates. The Census also collects important socioeconomic data every 10 years. This 10-year gap is particularly important for communities that are growing or losing population rapidly or that have significant health problems in minority populations. The lack of timely Census information inhibits large-scale studies on the impact of socioeconomic variables (e.g., education, employment, income) on disease. Statistical estimates may be provided for interim periods for some of the Census data elements collected, but interim estimates are not provided for all.

An additional problem is that for those data systems that are collected on a regular basis there is always the temptation to change or add a question or modify a particular measure in order to better reflect current understandings or policy needs. For example, one might want to change the definition of "physical activity." Should it refer only to leisure-time physical activity, or should it include transportation and occupational activity as well? Any such changes must be done very conservatively because it can lead to the inability to compare results to previous years, thus losing the ability to do any trend analysis. One has to weigh the loss of longitudinal data against the use of a better definition or change of a survey question.

Standard data systems may not use the exact measure or variable that you need for your analysis. For example, a survey may collect "individual income" when "family income" or "household income" is really what is needed. The definition of a "family" versus a "household" can be very important. This becomes even more critical when one needs to link two or more data systems, each using its own definition for "family" or "household."

When one is confronted with imperfect data, one must either use a variable that is not quite right, but perhaps close enough, or go to the expense of collecting a new set of data (referred to as *primary data collection*). The new set of data might be better suited for the study, but the time and expense of collecting this new data set will probably be high. In addition, data collected for a particular study or policy may be challenged as being biased toward finding what was intended. There will be a natural suspicion as to the reliability and validity of the data that you collected for a specific purpose as opposed to a commonly used data set for which strengths and weaknesses are understood. Using a recognized national or state standard data set, with population-weighted estimates, also allows others to verify your findings. However, there are times when you may indeed want or need to collect very specific data for your policy initiative, especially if this is a relatively new area of policy analysis.

ANALYTICAL STUDIES

One needs to understand the strengths and weaknesses of types of health studies as well as data sets. Several frameworks have been created to weigh the level of evidence for healthcare studies. For example, Steinberg and Luce (2005) discuss the weight of individual methodologies. The following list is a modified version of their order of the strength of individual studies, from the most rigorous to the least.[1] However, all have a role in contributing to the understanding of a health policy issue.

There are various depictions of this list as a hierarchical "evidence pyramid" that provides a way to visualize the rigor and quality of evidence along with the amount of evidence available. For example, systematic reviews and other forms of evidence synthesis are often depicted at the top of the pyramid, followed by randomized controlled trials and cohort studies, with case control studies, cross-sectional studies, and reports toward the bottom. The pyramid generally represents a hierarchy of study designs ranked in order of internal validity (risk of bias).

- Systematic reviews and meta-analyses
- Randomized clinical trials
- Quasi-randomized (group randomized) trials
- Nonrandomized clinical trials
- Prospective or retrospective cohort studies
- Time-series studies
- Case control studies
- Cross-sectional studies
- Case series and registries
- Case reports

Murad et al. (2016) proposed a revised version of the evidence pyramid that acknowledges the importance of considering the methodological merits of different study designs in a more nuanced manner. For example, some scholars challenge the placement of systematic reviews and meta-analyses at the top of the pyramid because of their inherent heterogeneity (e.g., clinical, methodological, statistical),

---

1 The literature on novel designs such as pragmatic clinical trials is constantly evolving. We encourage readers to refer to additional sources on this topic, such as Weinfurt et al. (2017) and Oche et al. (2021).

often without full transparency about the analytical strategy being used, which could result in uncertainty and error. Thus, Murad et al. (2016) propose revising the pyramid by separating the types of study designs with wavy lines (rather than fixed lines) to delineate their fluidity and conceptualizing systematic reviews as a lens through which other groups of studies can be viewed, rather than inherently the most rigorous type of design.

The gold standard for medical studies has traditionally been the randomized clinical trial, especially a double-blinded clinical trial in which both patients and providers are blind in terms of those receiving treatment and those who are not. However, individual studies, even clinical trials, should not be taken in isolation. Weighing the level of evidence of a study is based on multiple factors. What are the hypothesized biological or social relationships that make the relationship between the intervention and outcome feasible? Is there a chain of reasoning that makes a causal relationship plausible? While clinical trials may be the preferred analytical method, time, expense, or ethical considerations may require other types of studies.

A single study is rarely conclusive. One should consider how many studies of the healthcare issue have been done and to what extent they reach a comparable answer. If there are few studies, the weight of a single clinical trial may be less convincing. To what extent do studies use different definitions, populations, or protocols for intervention? On the other hand, if different types of studies (cohort and clinical trials) come to the similar conclusion, there may be increased evidence. Is there a consistency of findings among the individual studies over time that use different populations? If studies confirm previous findings, there is a greater level of confidence in the results. Due to all these types of questions systematic literature reviews and meta-analyses literature reviews become important in weighing the level of evidence in favor or against a particular health policy proposal/program. Additionally, emerging analytical techniques from the fields of engineering and systems science are now being applied to policy analysis, particularly to enable us to visualize the simulated or projected outcomes of different policy alternatives (Madahian et al., 2012).

While clinical trials are considered the gold standard of evidence, care of accepting the results needs to be taken here as well. Clinical trials involve the provision of a treatment to one group and the lack of the same treatment to another. Both groups of patients are generally randomly assigned as to who receives treatment and investigators are careful to note any differences in the populations that might explain different outcomes other than the existence of treatment or not. Due to the random assignment of treatment, other confounding factors will, on average, be equally distributed between the two groups. If both the providers and the patients are unaware of who is receiving the intervention, it is a double-blind study and has increased credibility by removing potential provider bias.

Despite the historical reliance on clinical trials, there are multiple problems with them for the development of policy. Clinical trials are expensive and lengthy, and the sponsors of the clinical trials may have a substantial stake in the outcome. Therefore, there may be a built-in potential bias of the clinical trial in terms of seeking a favorable outcome. Another difficulty with clinical trials is the difference between efficacy (the demonstration of what works in a research setting) as opposed to effectiveness (the demonstration of what works in the real world;

Steinberg & Luce, 2005). This is especially important in the policy world where different demographic and social factors in the real world become important factors.

Clinical trials rely upon volunteers of both patients and providers to follow rigorous protocols. It may be difficult to get volunteer patients to participate in a clinical trial if there is a 50/50 chance that they will not receive the intervention, especially if this intervention "promises" a chance at survival. In addition, not all patient volunteers are accepted into clinical trials. Patients may have to have a certain level of the disease being studied and/or a lack of other diseases to be accepted into the study. These clinical trial participants become "ideal patients" who might benefit from the intervention. In addition, providers need to be recruited as well. These tend to be specialists dealing with the disorder in question with a greater level of expertise than the typical physician who may be treating patients in the real world. The selected providers are frequently compensated for recruiting participants and for their own participation in the trial. Clinical trials can also involve a relatively small number of participants due to the difficulty and expense of getting participants.

As a result, clinical trials tend to involve ideal patients and practitioners rather than routine patients and providers in general medical practice (Zuidgeest et al., 2017). While clinical trials provide comparisons between the populations receiving the intervention and the control subjects not receiving the intervention (internal validity), they generally do not compare those in the clinical trial to those patients who are likely to receive the treatment in the real world (external validity; Steinberg & Luce, 2005). Consequently, clinical trials have been accused of overstating the effectiveness of the intervention in the real world. John P. A. Ioannidis has published a number of provocative articles questioning the methodology of most clinical research (Tatsioni et al., 2007). Despite their imperfections, clinical trials remain the gold standard.

However, there is growing consensus that a *mixed methods approach* is the one of the most effective ways to evaluate the impacts of policy change, especially in public health. This means that both quantitative and qualitative studies should be used strategically (Schifferdecker & Reed, 2009). For example, think about how one might study the impact of building a new bike path, as described in the RE-AIM discussion in Chapter 8. One might use a combination of interviews and focus groups (qualitative methods) with city council members and neighborhood residents to better understand their motivations for wanting to build a bike path. One would also want to query them about any problems they foresee and potential opposition to the bike path. One can use methods such as "content analysis" and document review to study minutes of city council meetings or check whether the city has a published a Bicycle Plan to better understand the process of adopting and constructing the bike path. One can study records of city expenditures to determine how much money has been allocated. One can use direct observation, engineering devices, or intercept surveys to study ridership before and after the bike path is built. One can collect survey data or obtain secondary data about health behaviors (such as bicycling to work or for leisure) from the target population. One may also collect or obtain secondary data about risk factors and health conditions such as diabetes and heart disease in the surrounding area. One can conduct more interviews and focus groups after completion of the bike path to determine whether there are any barriers to usage or challenges in maintenance. One can use participatory action research techniques such as Photovoice to empower residents to describe their neighborhood environment and their perceptions of the new bike path in their own pictures and words (Wang & Buress, 1997). All of these data sources can be considered together or "triangulated" to gain a composite picture of the success or failure of the bike path. Most of these methods are lower on the hierarchy of studies, but they may be the most useful for your policy analysis.

It is important to understand the strengths and weaknesses of various types of analytical studies. Your analysis will depend on the integrity as well as the types of studies used to support your analysis.

PERFORMING THE ANALYSIS

The role of health policy analysis is more critical today than ever. Technology and the basic sciences have opened more areas of knowledge regarding disease and health. Data sources have expanded, providing greater access to information. Computer systems allow for the analysis of huge quantities of data to provide more precise and sophisticated analytical processes. We will discuss these emerging methods in the next chapter but suffice it to say data sets such as all-payer claims data systems and the increasing use of electronic medical records will expand the opportunity to have more accurate and accessible information on individual medical care that can be aggregated for clinical research. The role of government has been expanded in terms of access to medical care, and the Medicare and Medicaid systems have taken on increased roles in developing new forms of medical care and payment systems, for example, accountability care organizations (ACOs) and insurance exchanges (Centers for Medicare & Medicaid Services, 2021).

The need for health policy analysis has also become greater as the cost of medical care continues to accelerate, requiring an increasing percentage of the country's gross national product for healthcare. The increasing disparities in health experience based on geography, race, ethnicity, and gender all are in need of both investigation and mitigation to create a more equitable healthcare system. The increased focus on the built environment and how it interacts with health status of populations and individuals adds new dimensions to creating the conditions for a healthy population. Health policy analysis is in a position as never before to contribute to the health of individuals and the population.

As mentioned in prior chapters, depending on who you are doing your policy analysis for, you may use data to analyze one or more stages of the policy wheel. Recognizing how data can be used to inform the various stages of the policy process will help you to create a more thorough policy analysis. See **Figure 4.1**. In addition to traditional health policy and social science research tools to those mentioned in Chapter 8, the landscape for conducting analysis is expanding due to larger data systems and flows of data available and more complex and computational tools from the expanding field of data science. It is not uncommon for students, academics, and many workforce analysts to have access to high-power computing clusters, massive local memory and/or cloud storage, and deployable analytical tools using both basic and advanced data science methods. In addition, the very notion of what constitutes "data" has evolved to include anything that is or can be generated by person or machine. No longer are data simply coded numbers and strings structured into spreadsheets of rows and columns. Data include audio files, video files, and free text, in addition to the volumes of numerical data collected yearly. Data science has a broad set of terms that may be unfamiliar to the reader. Many online data science glossaries exist and are updated frequently. One can be found at Springboard (www.springboard.com/blog/data-science/data-science-terms). We encourage you to forge relationships with data science specialists, including epidemiologists, biostatisticians, health economists, and bio-informatics specialists, to guide your policy analysis.

THE DATA ECOSYSTEM

Whereas 25% of the world's data was in digital form in the year 2000, by 2007 that number had grown to 94%. To get a sense of speed, it is estimated that the amount of digital data in the world will nearly double each year. That amounts to 2.5 exa-bytes of data generated each day, or 2.5 billon gigabytes (Balsom, 2022). Of course, much of that is driven by the large, nascent information technology (IT) companies like Google, Facebook, Netflix, and Amazon. Data that are large, fast, and varied are increasingly finding their way into the healthcare field and thus health policy analysis. **Figure 9.1** depicts the evolving data landscape. In 2013 it was estimated that 1.5 exabytes were created from just health system data, a figure likely much larger today (Cottle et al., 2013).

While much of healthcare is still conducted via the tools listed previously (primarily structured data in relational databases such as insurance claims records and patient accounts), the future of health data analysis will involve much broader applications. Patient notes in the electronic medical record, imaging scans, policy

FIGURE 9.1 The evolution of data.

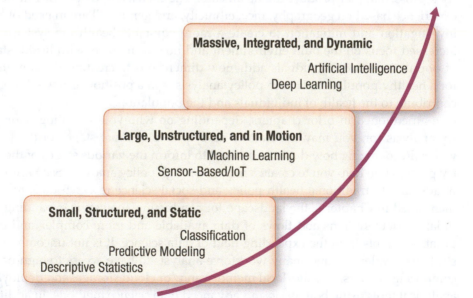

IoT, Internet of Things.

Source: Priestley, J., & McGrath, R. J. (2021). *Closing the analytics talent gap: An executive's guide to working with universities.* Taylor & Francis. Reproduced by permission of Taylor and Francis Group, LLC, a division of Informa plc.

text, advanced geospatial analysis, and more have the potential to expand our understanding of the policy impacts.

In public health, geospatial mapping has garnered particular salience. One only need think of the prevalence and disease spread maps that were used during the COVID pandemic. This type of use is but one example. Geo-mapping, using a combination of geo-tagged data with longitude and latitude coordinates, has begun to inform how the social determinants of health and other related factors are spread and also flow within communities. In one example, researchers utilized person-centered mapping as it relates to the health of a community in Los Angeles California (Douglas et al., 2020). They examined the presence of community assets such as streetlamps and sidewalks and detriments to health such as dark spots and tobacco shops. In doing so, they found relationships and issues that would have been missed by conventional epidemiologic methods.

As these tools and data sources mature, there will be the ability to create policy feedback loops that are near real time. For many health stakeholders, this has equated to an abundance of health-related "data" but a dearth of actual insight into the daily work of healthcare. One cannot make use of all the data, thus the oft heard mantra "data, data everywhere and not an insight had."

Another shift to the analytical process relates to how questions are addressed. The confluence of large amounts of data with high-speed analytical processing power has created the ability to "data mine" for insights where there are no *a priori* hypotheses; one can let the "data tell the story." In data science this is known as *unsupervised learning* (non-hypothesis driven) as opposed to *supervised learning* (data are fed into models in some predetermined way based on some knowledge or hypothesis). We discuss these methods and the need for thoughtful approaches later in this chapter.

Complicating this is that the health workforce remains largely untrained in the methods to collect, store, extract, transform and then reload, not to mention analyze the data. As a consequence, data has been slow to influence strategic decision-making and health policy analysis. For example, one must have the tools, nomenclature, time, and training to have online health professions to collect comparable data.

Massive and comprehensive health data analysis will be a foundational component of health policy formulation, implementation assessment, policy evaluation and policy modification moving forward. Today's thoughtful policy analyst would be wise to understand and explore new tools such as such as data management advances in data lakes and data marts and storage and retrieval tools such as notebooks and online analytical processing (OLAP) software. There have been great advances in multiplatform visualization tools, geospatial and mapping tools, and even deeper programming languages, libraries, and tools to examine social media sentiment. Many, like R and Python, are open-source programs with user-augmented libraries. In addition, each year, new companies emerge to offer prepackaged functions with easier front-end designs. However, no single tool is adept at answering all analytical questions. Because this is meant only to be an overview of general capabilities and considerations, we will keep to a higher-level discussion of analytical functions and how these new tools may aid policy analysis. We also provide guidance as to how to avoid analytical pitfalls such as using the appropriate unit of analysis or using data for which they were not intended. Misuse of data will result in misrepresented findings, overlook discrepancies in the data and analytical output, and sometimes further structural disparities if the analyst is not thoughtful about their methods.

GENERAL ANALYTICAL FUNCTIONS

When looking at the purposes for doing analyses generally, a four-stage model has been widely described by function such as the one in **Table 9.1** developed by Gartner (2022). While these functions pertain primarily to organizational capabilities, and thus value, they are equally suitable for a general discussion of analysis.

In the hierarchy shown in **Figure 9.1**, added value is defined as increasing as the ability to not only describe processes and phenomena well and in a timely way, but to predict and prescribe. A great majority of current analysis falls into descriptive analytics. One could expand this definition from "What happened" to also "What is happening" via point in time estimates or dashboards. COVID-related dashboards illustrate this function well and most vary by ability to examine subpopulations (age, gender, other classifications) or geographic regions.

Diagnostic analysis digs a little deeper and utilizes tools such as correlations, t-tests, chi-square tests, decision analysis, and some economic analyses to assess levels of association or causality. Cluster analysis is an example of useful diagnostic analytics that can then be used for more precise prediction. Predictive analytics is perhaps one of the more quickly growing areas of analysis, where traditional regression models—both linear and nonparametric—have expanded into tools widely termed *machine learning*. Machine learning is not new. It is any analytical function where the computer is making choices based on provided rules parameters. Older programmers will remember this as "IF/THEN" statements. IF an input field or output has a value of (x), THEN take some action. This later has been built into Excel formulas and macros. Now, we use the term *algorithms* to broadly define the breadth of machine learning methods. All of these are simply rules-based criteria directing the computer's actions behind the scenes and all are different forms of artificial intelligence (AI). These machine learning methods include such tools as regression, principal components analysis, decision trees and random forests, gradient boosting methods, support vector machines, and many others. There are dozens of existing machine learning algorithms.

Some machine learning is also used for prescriptive analytics along with other tools such as graph and network analysis, neural network analysis, and others. Prescription can be thought of as simulation and optimization. Being able to run a set of policy variables through a series of model tests (data experiments) to assess the predictive possible outcomes (sensitivity analysis) can be highly useful to social scientists if the data are representative and complete enough. This is often not possible with public use data.

Some of these methods have existed in health research for some time, for example, agent-based modeling (ABM) and system dynamics modeling (SDM; Tracy et al., 2018; Homer & Hirsch, 2006). ABM is a simulation tool that fixes certain characteristics in a system according to prescribed rules and then computationally plays out the interaction of the agents in the model. SDM is a process well known in engineering and computer science and is a similar computational tool for modeling and simulating multiple factors within a proposed system (Homer & Hirsch, 2006). Network analysis, including social network analysis (SNA) is also a useful method in health policy analysis, particularly in terms of analyzing relationships between stakeholders. SNA is discussed further in Chapter 12. There are, in fact, many tools from a variety of fields that are converging under

TABLE 9.1 GENERAL ANALYTICAL FUNCTIONS

FUNCTION	FOCUS
Descriptive	What is happening or has happened
Diagnostic	Why it did happen
Predictive	What will happen
Prescriptive/simulation	What might happen

the umbrella of data science. Many times, different fields may have different names for the same function, thus the simple functional model in Table 9.1 aids in the categorization but also ultimate function of those tools. Another important distinction will be determining whether functions are rules driven (supervised) or not (unsupervised), which is discussed in more detail later in this chapter.

ARTIFICIAL INTELLIGENCE AND BIG DATA

There are many buzzwords in the data science that are not well understood. AI, or artificial intelligence, and Big Data are two such terms. As noted above, AI is any computer-based process that has inherent learning rules within it. Image recognition programs are a good example in which a set of data is fed to a computer with some basic rules and the computer, by virtue of its processing speed, refines the recognition. Inherently, all AI is based on human-fed parameters.

The final term that is widely overused is Big Data. Data have no units of measurement beyond storage size. Tracking pollution from point A to point B can generate petabytes of data. What is big for one analysis may not be for others. What is important is the total amount of data and processing capacity needed to accommodate that volume of data. The data could include time flow or velocity (real time, batched) or differ by the types of data or veracity of the data being examined (standardized fields, text, images, and audio). One would need to evaluate the value of the data given limited resources for analysis (e.g., time and the costs of analytical expertise and computing power).

TOOLS

Here we examine some of the analytical functions as they relate to the policy wheel. We also examine the benefits and trade-offs each provides. Implementing analytics as a strategic process in organizations typically follows what is known as a "stack" (see Figure 9.2). Stacking refers to the general ecosystem necessary to implement an analytics function that is repeatable and updatable given some known time frame. This is often termed a system or set of models that is producible or obtained via a production function.

One example would be disease tracking and migration, where data are populated from multiple sources and models for prevalence are predictively run

FIGURE 9.2 A proposed policy analytics "stack."

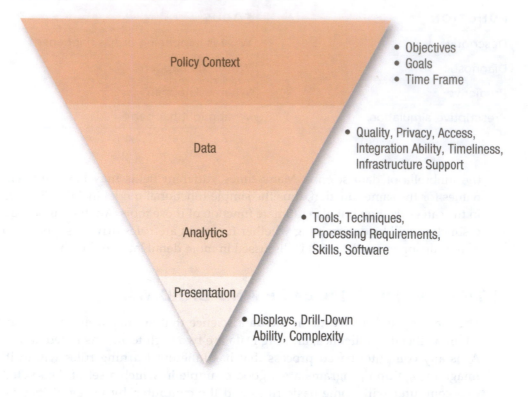

and then results are analyzed and "produced" for consumption at a time stamp (e.g., 7 a.m. each day). Because the system is automated, the time factor becomes integral. The first level of a stack is the policy context, that is, the need to track disease migration in as close to real time as possible. This layer includes the general scope of the policy, who/what the policy affects, the time frame for the policy, and any budgetary considerations or impacts. In level two, data would need to be identified to do this. The second layer is the data layer or what data will inform the analytical inquiry within considerations of data quality, scope, accessibility, privacy and security, and also the ability to link or aggregate data together or over a unit of analysis, for example, from person-level to neighborhood to city, state, or nation. For one country, this would mean that some form of testing is occurring and results or confirmed cases are being reported to a central repository. If not, data may be private, missing, or incomplete. This becomes an issue when attempting to aggregate to a larger geographic area, for example, all of the United States.

The third layer is the analytics layer. This is the primary focus of this chapter. It is concerned with the tools, techniques, processing ability of the systems being used for analysis, the skills of the analyst, and the software being utilized. In this example, level three reporting can occur according to the need and the functions laid out in **Table 9.1** coupled with the nature of the data from level two of the stack. Visual displays are created and, if possible, updated in real time. Predictive models could then be constructed if enough data exist to accurately populate, train, and test them. Ultimately one could then run some form of simulation of spread given other trends in demographics (working from home, shutdowns of travel, etc.). One may also wish to overlay that on a map with socioeconomic and demographic data. Demographic and other population-based data are likely to be available only at a county or perhaps even Census block level. In addition, data may only be released monthly, quarterly, annually, or in 10-year Census intervals. These are all considerations for what type of analysis can be performed.

Once collected and aggregated into an appropriate analytical file, many available software tools can create the geographic overlays relatively quickly if the data are populated and accurate. If, however, you wish to examine near real time sentiment to a policy change that affects access to care via social media, you would need access to such data via an application programming interface (API) or via some agreement with the data host that provides an embedded feed of data to the analytical framework as it occurs. If this first step is possible, then you would need a higher level of computer-processing power; skills in Python, R, or some other programming language; the use of special libraries for conducting the analysis for sentiment analysis; an understanding of natural language processing; and a tool designed to evaluate sentiment in a way that informs policy from the context of the issue being addressed.

The final layer of the stack is the information presentation, which translates the analysis into strategic decisions, hopefully related to the original context. This should be done with some care and caution, especially if output is based on a probabilistic likelihood. Many consumers of your analytical output will not remember their statistical courses or fully grasp what goes into a measure of likelihood. Attempting to contextualize your findings in an easy-to-digest but transparent way will be one of your challenges.

In level four, considerations of how data are consumed and for what purposes come into play. Are these analyses for public consumption, and thus understandable by the lay public? This is to say, if models have parameters of significance or confidence within probabilistic constraints, such are not easily understood or digested and could be misconstrued as more or less important or possible than is the case. Considerations here are the following: Do users understand the information presented? Is it accurate and meaningful? Are end users able to "drill down" for further analysis? Is further analysis even possible? Does the information present actionable insights? An easy example of this concerns looking at weather forecasts. One might look out at a projected week's forecast prior to a vacation and see there is a 54% chance of rain on three of the days. However, this does not include the amount of rain likely. So, if the data point of precipitation amount was added, showing there was only 0.5 cm of rain projected, a very different picture arises, likely altering or reinforcing some decision actions.

Thinking about the policy process, each layer of the stack comes into play at each stage of policy development. Here we are interested in the analytical layer. Table 9.2 examines each level of policy analysis by the analytical function(s) most associated at those levels with examples for each.

TABLE 9.2 THE POLICY PROCESS BY ANALYTICAL FUNCTIONS

POLICY PROCESS	ANALYTICAL FUNCTION	USE EXAMPLE
Policy formulation	Description, data mining (exploration)	Dashboarding, visual display, geospatial display, comparisons
	Prediction	Machine learning/predictive algorithms/simulation
Policy adoption	Description/diagnostic	Statistical comparison
Policy implementation	Description/diagnostic	In addition to descriptive monitoring, sentiment analysis, network analysis
Policy evaluation	Description/diagnostic/ predictive analysis/ prescriptive analysis	Sensitivity analysis, comparing populations or outcomes
Policy modification	Predictive and prescriptive analysis and simulation	Sensitivity analysis or introducing new variables and model testing, sentiment analysis

THE UNINTENDED IMPACTS OF DATA SCIENCE METHODS FOR POLICY ANALYSIS

A health policy analyst will not only need to critically examine academic and think tank policy studies but may also need to design their own analysis to enlighten policy alternatives. In either case, when an analytical file or frame has been developed, new data science tools are rapidly becoming central to the analyst's toolbox.

Data science methods have the potential to improve our knowledge of the health of populations, to chart the prevalence and distribution of diseases, and to simulate policy interventions before they are enacted. The size and scope of current data sets, both health-focused and not, provide the opportunity to develop vastly more complex models for public health analysis. For example, at the individual level, combining health system data (electronic medical records, prescription data, healthcare utilization) with personal heath data (genetics and data from fitness wearables or other online trackers for diet, running, walking, stress, etc.) with other types of data (vehicular driving sensors and risk-taking data, credit card data, geopositioning data from smart phones, internet search and use data) allow an analyst to develop highly individualized predictive models of current and future health status, along with medical care use and costs.

People have two common reactions to this increased linkage of data. One is excitement at the possibilities of individualized medicine, the effective and efficient allocation of resources, the improvement of provider–patient relationships, and the empowerment of individuals for their own care. The other is a concern for the invasion of personal privacy and the potential for this information to be co-opted and monetized and perhaps sold for advertising. From a public health perspective, the information could be used to discriminate or penalize those at higher future health risks and increase and exacerbate current disparities present in the social determinants of health. In fact, one would be correct to experience both reactions because each scenario is likely to occur or has already occurred. As with most advancements, great caution must be taken to optimize the benefit of data analysis while protecting against harm.

DATA GAPS AND THEIR BIASES

Earlier, we gave the example of creating predictive health models based on individually collected data. Obviously, this would require participant consent to collect, combine, analyze, and use that data. That consent may occur once or perhaps not. Consider financial data variables that are used. The individual may have been shopping for a new loan. They decide to use an app that quickly sorts through a variety of lending sources using a predictive tool given the answers to a few questions. They are also asked to consent to the sharing of information. This is a primary consent, but now their data can be used for other purposes, such as solicitation, risk modeling, credit scoring, and others. This is one form of a gap, a consent of use gap.

Many individuals do not realize the downstream uses of their data for practices or policies related to themselves. This problem is exacerbated when taken to more aggregated levels of analysis. At these levels, data are pooled across many individuals, and many different data sets, to attempt to create a broader picture or possibly a predictive model or simulation. Inherent in this type of analysis are the problems of multiple types of gaps, or what are called voltage drops. Think of a simple electrical system: a large battery connected to a bulb. The bulb is bright when the circuit is connected. However, if we place a radio into that circuit, the bulb may dim a bit. Add more bulbs, it dims more. If any one of these connections is imperfectly made or faulty, it dims even more or perhaps the light emitted is now shadowed. If we are using that bulb to understand the contents of a dark room, our picture is muted or flawed at best. These are the voltage drops that occur as we add more complexity to our electrical system.

In conducting an analysis, many conventions can be used to account for missing data. We will not consider ideas of statistical power here, but suffice it to say, each voltage drop could have downstream implications to distort or correctly represent health disparities. A simple example is income. If the population data set has missing values for household income, a standard protocol would be to impute those values. This is typically done by using the median household income for the smallest and most representative group available, for example, a Census block. Of issue, however, is that in some geographic areas there can be widely different incomes within the same Census area. Imputation means that those at lower incomes are raised and those at higher incomes are muted. This may seem better than the alternative of having missing data, but given that some groups are already misrepresented, it potentially serves to skew the disparity when combined with other data. Geist and Samuels (2020) construct a nicely approachable model for considering data gaps of this type and others.

Their typology uses the idea of primary, secondary, and hidden data gaps. The previous example is one of primary gaps, or those of omission either from primary data, or when data from different sources are combined such that some acuity from the original unit of analysis is lost to aggregation.

Secondary and hidden data gaps create even more problematic voltage drops and often have the potential to worsen health disparities through misrepresentation and inherent biases. These are also the most common types of biases that occur when using data science methods for policy analysis. They occur when the models that are created use data from disparate sources that possibly contain missing and/or imputed data, but also data that themselves are inherently biased. This is sometimes because the data were not developed for use in health studies or because the data were inappropriately collected in the first place using flawed mechanisms, or because the phenomenon the data are being collected on already reflect some societal disparity.

One example of this occurred when a commercial healthcare provider attempted to create a model to predict the needs of patients with complex health needs. They constructed an algorithm that was highly predictive, but racially biased (Obermeyer et al., 2019). Population studies have consistently shown that Black patients have poorer health outcomes than White patients in several areas (CDC, n.d.-c). The issue here was that the analysts who developed the algorithm for this health system used healthcare costs as a proxy for overall health. There was a primary gap in analysis due to the imputation method used. The secondary gap was that there already existed a disparity of health status by racial status. Because of unequal access to care, the algorithm predicted fewer Black patients needed complex care provision. Correcting for the bias would have increased the number of Black patients receiving care from 17.7% to 45.6% (Obermeyer et al., 2019). These types of algorithms are routinely employed by large healthcare providers and insurers affecting hundreds of millions of Americans yearly.

A similar bias was found in the Medicare Hospital Readmission Reduction Program algorithm that penalized hospitals acting as safety nets and providing a greater level of care to indigent and racially diverse patients (Joynt Maddox et al., 2019). A voltage drop occurred in this analysis due to a methodological inference bias. Data science methods are often characterized by the inferential method they use, supervised or unsupervised. Some social scientists know this as hypothesis-based or non-hypothesis-based inference. Supervision is simply the idea that the analyst oversees the model construction or methods being used, for example, which variables are included or omitted. This is based on a preexisting hypothesis (as in stepwise regression). Conducting analysis any other way was historically not possible given limited computing power to calculate the number of associations necessary as data sets and the number of variables became progressively large. Today, analysts using laptops can process billions of interactions very quickly in the cloud. In these analyses, data are simply thrown together and the groups that are formed do so based on some rules about how mathematically close together the properties of the variables of those groups are, sans any *a priori* hypotheses. This has led to advances in cluster analysis that has become very useful, but there are also risks of biases.

Data may group together for unknown reasons. Could we compare the birth rate in Croatia to the number of pieces of gum purchased in Ohio? We could if we had data. And if we had data, we could get a statistical comparison with an accompanying significance. But should we do this? This is the major problem of unsupervised data methods. What is lacking here is subject matter expertise, or at least some understanding of the context from which the data arose. A more concrete example might be an analyst who is attempting to model the most prevalent health outcomes for ED visits by the homeless population. When using an unsupervised method, one might find that high blood pressure, heart disease, stress and having a usual source of care are the cluster features. One could then design a predictive model. The problem, of course, is that some of these variables are a function of being homeless (usual source of care and stress) and the others are likely due to lack of access to medication or a healthy diet. The right approach here would be to include variables known to be issues in recidivist homeless populations, for example, loss of digits due to extreme cold, diabetes, and/or substance abuse. Another way to think about this, is ask "does this make sense?" when reviewing unsupervised analytical methods. Having substantive knowledge of the homeless population is critical for an understanding as to which factors are critical.

Another reason for these data gaps and voltage drops is that data science methods rely on testing and training a data set taken from a "real" set of data. Training involves taking a subset of the data that is representative of the frame from which it is taken. The assumption is that the training data represent a level of grounded truth that the algorithms can increase predictability. Models are often compared side by side by the amount of predictive accuracy they have to the "truth." Models may be augmented with variables, or sometimes combined to achieve even higher predictive accuracy. Another way to ground truth models is to work directly with citizens in what is known as "citizen science" approaches. This is an emerging area of research (Alfonso et al., 2022).

If the "truth" of the data already contains structural inequalities or disparities, reflecting those will be the aspirational goal of the model as these disparities will be present in the training data set. This was the case of early facial recognition algorithms that underidentified those as non-White because the training data were skewed toward White person images (Buolamwini & Gebru, 2018). In addition, there may have been a mixing of biases. If the data were originally clustered using unsupervised methods, and not properly vetted by a subject matter expert, inherent misrepresentations could occur even prior to multiple models being run. If the groups were inappropriately formed when the models are run, they will produce some varying levels of predictability.

One other voltage drop stemming from a hidden data gap would be those due to historical inaccuracies, misrepresentative models of theory and thus data collection (think about improperly constructed questions on surveys), and incompleteness of data. One of the premier public health research tools examining health behaviors, the BRFSS, historically faced challenges that required solutions such as complex weighting and data imputation. Gaps in the level of analysis (county level aggregation), changing questions over time, and declining response rates have all combined to create analytical problems.

One final bias that every health policy analyst must consider is that of the lens of the analyst, be it themselves or perhaps the original data purveyor. What biases or perspectives does the analyst or data collector have when examining the issue? There has been a great deal of work done on bias in methodological studies with checklists for consideration (Critical Appraisal Skills Programme, 2022). One's own lens ought also be examined given our potential biases of culture, age, education, income, belief systems, and other factors and attempts made to mitigate those biases where possible (Polit & Beck, 2014).

FINAL CONSIDERATIONS

Analytical methods will no doubt continue to evolve. Data infuses every stage of the policy process, and it should inform the various components of your policy analysis. The goal for public health analysts, however, should be to align with developing and promoting policies that reflect the reduction of health disparities and the improvement of the health of populations. Current and future data collection and analytical methods pose new challenges for analysts wanting to ensure the accuracy of their assessments and the prediction of a policy's impact. These are often rooted in the minutiae of how data were collected and for what purpose; how definitions were developed and whether they remain consistent across platforms; where data and variables were imputed or otherwise constructed; whether data in predictive models were primary or secondary (or tertiary); whether there were issues with the underlying data that could augment underlying disparities or biases, and were there available and thoughtful analytical solutions to those problems. However, it is not completely incumbent upon the analyst to know the specifics of all these issues. Many national agencies are in the process of constructing forward thinking data plans and students of analysis are wise to keep apprised of their parameters, such as the CDC Data Modernization Initiative (www.cdc.gov/surveillance/data-modernization/index.html).

The most beneficial rule for the public health policy analyst is methodological transparency. In an ever-growing complex world, it is important to be thoughtful, but also open and clear as to one's methods to allow others to be able to replicate those methods. Further, public health policy analysts must explain the limitations of their analysis, the limitations of the data, and the potential for further data analysis. In so doing they will not only protect the integrity of their own work, but also limit any future analytical misrepresentation and potential harm to populations.

SUMMARY

Here we have discussed some of the data sources and resources available to the analyst as well as some of the research functions that give rise to help better inform our collective knowledge. We then discussed the various types of analytical functions from description to simulation and what types of methods are useful for what purposes. We ended with a discussion of caveats, data gaps and voltage drops to better assist the analyst.

DISCUSSION QUESTIONS

- Examine one of the public use data sources listed in this chapter and discuss some elements of it that would be important when conducting a health policy analysis.

- Discuss why determining the unit of analysis of a study or analysis is important to consider prior to beginning the analysis.

- Discuss why having an analytical plan is also important to consider before doing the analysis. Relate these ideas to the analytical functions by type.

- Discuss how forms of AI and machine learning could broaden or improve our knowledge base.

- Discuss how forms of AI and machine learning could mislead policy makers and deepen existing disparities of health status and outcomes.

KEY TERMS

analytical bias
analytical functions
analytical studies
artificial intelligence
data gaps
level of analysis

machine learning
National Center for Health Statistics
public use data
qualitative methods
unit of analysis

SPRINGER PUBLISHING CONNECT™

A robust set of instructor resources designed to supplement this text is located at http://connect.springerpub.com/content/book/978-0-8261-8543-3. Qualifying instructors may request access by emailing textbook@springerpub.com.

REFERENCES

Agency for Healthcare Research and Quality. (2022, July). *Healthcare Cost and Utilization Project (HCUP)*. https://www.ahrq.gov/data/hcup/index.html

Alfonso, L., Gharesifard, M., & Wehn, U. (2022). Analysing the value of environmental citizen-generated data: Complementarity and cost per observation. *Journal of Environmental Management*, 303, 114157. https://doi.org/10.1016/j.jenvman.2021.114157

Balsom, P. (2022, February 3). *The surprising things you don't know about big data*. Adeptia. https://www.adeptia.com/blog/surprising-things-you-dont-know-about-big-data

Buolamwini, J., & Gebru, T. (2018). Gender shades: Intersectional accuracy disparities in commercial gender classification. *Proceedings of Machine Learning Research*, 81, 77–91. https://proceedings.mlr.press/v81/buolamwini18a.html

Centers for Disease Control and Prevention. (n.d.-a). *Adolescent and School Health: Youth Risk Behavior Surveillance System (YRBSS)*. U.S. Department of Health and Human Services. https://www.cdc.gov/healthyyouth/data/yrbs/index.htm

Centers for Disease Control and Prevention. (n.d.-b). *Behavioral Risk Factor Surveillance System (BRFSS)*. U.S. Department of Health and Human Services. https://www.cdc.gov/brfss

Centers for Disease Control and Prevention. (n.d.-c). *Minority Health: Impact of racism on our nation's health*. U.S. Department of Health and Human Services. https://www.cdc.gov/minorityhealth/racism-disparities/impact-of-racism.html

Centers for Disease Control and Prevention. (n.d.-d). *National Center for Health Statistics: Classification of diseases, functioning, and disability*. U.S. Department of Health and Human Services. https://www.cdc.gov/nchs/icd.htm

Centers for Medicare & Medicaid Services. (2021, December 1). *Accountable care organizations (ACOs)*. https://www.cms.gov/Medicare/Medicare-Fee-for-Service-Payment/ACO

Cottle, M., Hoover, W., Kanwal, S., Kohn, M., Strome, T., & Treister, N. W. (2013). *Transforming health care through big data: Strategies for leveraging big data in the health care industry*. Institute for Health Technology Transformation. http://c4fd63cb482ce6861463-bc6183f1c18e748a49b87a25911a0555.r93.cf2.rackcdn.com/iHT2_BigData_2013.pdf

Critical Appraisal Skills Programme. (2022, April 26). *CASP checklists*. https://casp-uk.net/casp-tools-checklists

Douglas, J. A., Subica, A. M., Franks, L., Johnson, G., Leon, C., Villanueva, S., & Grills, C. T. (2020). Using participatory mapping to diagnose upstream determinants of health and prescribe downstream policy-based interventions. *Preventing Chronic Disease*, 17, E138. https://doi.org/10.5888/pcd17.200123

Gartner. (2022). *What is data and analytics?* https://www.gartner.com/en/topics/data-and-analytics

Giest, S., & Samuels, A. (2020). 'For good measure': Data gaps in a big data world. *Policy Sciences*, 53(3), 559–569. https://doi.org/10.1007/s11077-020-09384-1

Health Insurance Portability and Accountability Act, Pub. L. No. 104-191, 110 Stat. 1936 (1996). https://aspe.hhs.gov/reports/health-insurance-portability-accountability-act-1996

Homer, J. B., & Hirsch, G. B. (2006). System dynamics modeling for public health: Background and opportunities. *American Journal of Public Health*, 96(3), 452–458. https://doi.org/10.2105/ajph.2005.062059

Joynt Maddox, K. E., Reidhead, M., Hu, J., Kind, A. J. H., Zaslavsky, A. M., Nagasako, E. M., & Nerenz, D. R. (2019). Adjusting for social risk factors impacts performance and penalties in the hospital readmissions reduction program. *Health Services Research*, 54(2), 327–336. https://doi.org/10.1111/1475-6773.13133

Madahian, B., Klesges, R. C., Klesges, L., & Homayouni, R. (2012). System dynamics modeling of childhood obesity. *BMC Bioinformatics*, 13(Suppl. 12), A13. https://doi.org/10.1186/1471-2105-13-s12-a13

Murad, M. H., Asi, N., Alsawas, M., & Alahdab, F. (2016). New evidence pyramid. *Evidence-Based Medicine*, 21(4), 125–127. https://doi.org/10.1136/ebmed-2016-110401

National Cancer Institute. (2022, July 22). *Surveillance, epidemiology, and end results program*. U.S. Department of Health and Human Services and National Institutes of Health. https://seer.cancer.gov

Obermeyer, Z., Powers, B., Vogeli, C., & Mullainathan, S. (2019). Dissecting racial bias in an algorithm used to manage the health of populations. *Science*, 366(6464), 447–453. https://doi.org/10.1126/science.aax2342

Oche, O., Wu, C., Murry, L. T., & Kennelty, K. A. (2021). Research and scholarly methods: Pragmatic clinical trials. *JACCP: Journal of the American College of Clinical Pharmacy*, 5(1), 99–106. https://doi.org/10.1002/jac5.1557

Polit, D. F., & Beck, C. T. (2014). *Essentials of nursing research: Appraising evidence for nursing practice* (8th ed.). Wolters Kluwer Health/Lippincott Williams & Wilkins.

Schifferdecker, K. E., & Reed, V. A. (2009). Using mixed methods research in medical education: Basic guidelines for researchers. *Medical Education*, 43(7), 637–644. https://doi.org/10.1111/j.1365-2923.2009.03386.x

Steinberg, E. P., & Luce, B. R. (2005). Evidence based? Caveat emptor! *Health Affairs*, 24(1), 80–92. https://doi.org/10.1377/hlthaff.24.1.80

Tatsioni, A., Bonitsis, N. G., & Ioannidis, J. P. A. (2007). Persistence of contradicted claims in the literature. *Journal of the American Medical Association*, 298(21), 2517 –2526. https://doi.org/10.1001/jama.298.21.2517

The 21st Century Cures Act, Pub. L. No. 114-225, 130 Stat. 1033 (2016). https://www.govinfo.gov/content/pkg/PLAW-114publ255/pdf/PLAW-114publ255.pdf

Tracy, M., Cerdá, M., & Keyes, K. M. (2018). Agent-based modeling in public health: Current applications and future directions. *Annual Review of Public Health*, 39(1), 77–94. https://doi.org/10.1146/annurev-publhealth-040617-014317

Wang, C., & Buress, M. A. (1997). Photovoice: Concept, methodology, and use for participatory needs assessment. *Health Education & Behavior*, 24(3), 369–387. https://doi.org/10.1177/109019819702400309

Weinfurt, K. P., Hernandez, A. F., Coronado, G. D., DeBar, L. L., Dember, L. M., Green, B. B., Heagerty, P. J., Huang, S. S., James, K. T., Jarvik, J. G., Larson, E. B., Mor, V., Platt, R., Rosenthal, G. E., Septimus, E. J., Simon, G. E., Staman, K. L., Sugarman, J., Vazquez, M., … Curtis, L. H. (2017). Pragmatic clinical trials embedded in healthcare systems: Generalizable lessons from the NIH collaboratory. *BMC Medical Research Methodology*, *17*(1), Article 144. https://doi.org/10.1186/s12874-017-0420-7

Zuidgeest, M. G., Goetz, I., Groenwold, R. H., Irving, E., van Thiel, G. J., & Grobbee, D. E. (2017). Series: Pragmatic trials and real world evidence: Paper 1. Introduction. *Journal of Clinical Epidemiology*, *88*, 7–13. https://doi.org/10.1016/j.jclinepi.2016.12.023

CHAPTER 10

POLICY BACKGROUND SECTION

In the beginning of your policy analysis, it is helpful to provide some background material for the policy issue that you have chosen. The length and depth of this section depend on the intended audience for your analysis. If the intended reader is an expert in this policy area, this section might be quite brief. However, we shall approach this section of your policy analysis as though it is to be read by a general audience. Consequently, it should provide more background information rather than less.

LEARNING OBJECTIVES

To be able to:

- Develop a historical chronicle of the treatment of a health policy issue.
- Develop a statement regarding the significance of a health policy issue.
- Describe the legal basis for a health policy initiative.
- Explain the relationship between one policy initiative and Health in All Policies.
- Develop a rationale for the health policy issue to be placed on the current policy agenda.

HISTORY

It would be highly unusual to explore a policy area where there was no history. In fact, most policy issues and proposals get recycled or have been explored in other states or countries. Most legislation in the United States is based on incrementalism rather than comprehensive policy changes. It is important to recognize successful and unsuccessful past policy initiatives.

For example, health insurance in the United States got its major push after World War II with a tax provision that rewarded employers who provided health insurance to their employees (Starr, 1982). As a result, there is an 80-year history of employer-based health insurance that has become a central characteristic of the

U.S. health insurance system. This is also an important example of how past policy decisions can limit future policy options. As demonstrated by past efforts at national health reform it has been difficult to change the employer-based health insurance market due to the existing stakeholders who have a strong economic interest in maintaining it. Large health insurance companies have developed in the United States because of this initial policy, employee expectations have been built around health insurance as an employee benefit, businesses receive tax benefits, and unions have successfully negotiated generous health benefit packages. Personal and business income tax rulings (e.g., employer health insurance is not counted as taxable income) have been built around employer health insurance. As a result, single payer health insurance system proposals have faced major obstacles from insurance, employer, employee, and union concentrated interest groups wishing to protect the existing health insurance structure. Knowing the history of health insurance is critical to understanding the positions of stakeholders and the resistance to change.

Since your policy area has a history, one of the first things that you should address in this section is a brief history as to how the policy issue has been dealt with over the years. To what extent can you build upon success? What has been the Achilles heel of similar past initiatives? To what extent have circumstances changed to make existing policy less effective? It might be important in this section to demonstrate how other political jurisdictions have dealt with the issue and what lessons one can learn from those experiences. Some of those policy efforts might have been very successful, some dismal failures, and still others a mixed success. There may be very innovative programs in other countries.

While it is important to explore what seems to have worked or not worked in other political jurisdictions, it is important to remember that every geopolitical entity thinks of itself as unique and therefore every policy must be custom fit to its uniqueness. Indeed, given different political cultures, structures, and processes, what works in a European country may not work in the United States. Rivalry between states in the United States may automatically taint a policy in one state as unacceptable. An innovative policy in California may be dismissed just because it evolved from California. Attempting to transplant policies from one political jurisdiction to another is always fraught with the obstacle of convincing policy makers that despite some differences in geopolitics, the policy could work in their state or country.

We have previously discussed the role of the judiciary in the policy process by citing multiple U.S. Supreme Court (USSC) cases influencing public health issues. The history of the Supreme Court's judicial rulings on federal oversight of electoral districts, the right to privacy, the Commerce Clause, and the Second Amendment all have important implications for policy. What is considered "settled law" and what is open to modification or reversal? What is the track record of the political parties on the issue? Executive discretion, or any other topic, is important to discuss. What are the trends of the decisions through time? Where might the Court be headed? What openings does a particular decision provide for additional legislation?

As discussed earlier, due to the political structure of the United States, multiple political avenues are available to those with a concentrated interest to block any piece of proposed legislation. Therefore, legislative proposals are generally constructed to minimize the disruption of the status quo in order gain sufficient political support. This need for compromise diminishes if there is an ideological tsunami or one political party dominates all the political levers of power (e.g., both houses of Congress, the presidency, and the Supreme Court). Divided government (where one political party controls one branch and the other party controls another branch) at the national level has been the recent norm. Some states may have a tradition of one-party domination. Knowing the history of legislative and judicial actions are critical in understanding the parameters of potential change for your policy.

Legislative policy changes can and do occur, but they typically come slowly. Legislative policy adoption takes patience. However, there have been periods in our political history when change has come quickly. Executive orders and judicial rulings can quickly change the policy environment. If you are in such a period, you might be able to take advantage of it. Even if your policy is not in sync with the current political environment, it may be important for it to be a trial balloon to begin a legislative track record and gain support for its eventual adoption.

One of the great resources for previous legislation at the federal level is the Library of Congress (www.loc.gov/index.html). It provides online and in-person services. If you are physically located in the Washington, DC, area, you should attempt to obtain a library card to have full access to its resources. To find current congressional activity, visit the Library of Congress site (www.Congress.gov).

The federal legislative history section of the Library of Congress site (www.loc.gov/law/help/leghist.php) provides a tool to investigate legislative history. For you to use it, you will generally need to know some of the specific legislation in the past. From your knowledge of the policy area or from an introductory article, you might have the public law citation (e.g., P.L. 113-101). If you do not know the statute number or public law number, you might have a reference regarding a proposed piece of legislation that did or did not become law. Another useful reference for finding statutes is Westlaw (Westlaw Professional Legal Research, n.d.). Bills that have been introduced into Congress are cited by using the designation HR or S plus the number of the bill.

Major research universities are designated as depositories for government documents and have reference librarians who are familiar with federal government documents. Government documents are in a separate section of the library. You should make use of these reference librarians since cataloguing government documents is different from normal library cataloguing.

Remember that legislative committee reports are valuable because they contain testimony before one of the congressional committees with jurisdiction over the bill from administrators, proponents, and opponents of the proposed legislation. You must be conscious that the testimony will be tilted since the chair of the committee may have stacked the testimony. They remain a valuable source for gaining insight into the arguments being used by proponents and opponents. They are also frequently useful in attempting to understand the legislative intent of a proposed law.

If you need to access federal regulations as opposed to federal laws a useful website is the U.S. Government Publishing Office's (GPO's) Electronic Code of Federal Regulations (www.ecfr.gov), which includes a search engine for locating relevant administrative regulations. You can also access the daily *Federal Register* by year or date of issue (www.gpo.gov/fdsys/browse/collection.action?collection Code=FR) through the U.S. GPO. Hard copies of the *Federal Register* are usually available in public and university libraries, especially those designated as federal depositories.

At the state level, there is a website for state and local government (www .statelocalgov.net) that allows you to enter the name of a state and access its government web page. For example, if you type in "Oregon," you will see a link to its legislative, executive, and judicial branches in the state. Under the "legislative branch" link, you would see many useful features, including a "Bill Tracker" tab. You can use the Bill Tracker to search for a particular bill by its number, or to search by text. Many states have similar bill tracking features built into their government web pages. If your policy area is child obesity, the Supplemental Nutrition Assistance Program (SNAP; www.fns.usda.gov/snap) as well as legislative efforts such as the Healthy Hunger-Free Kids Act of 2010[1] that was directed at improving child nutrition (www.fns.usda.gov/cn/healthy-hunger-free-kids-act) are useful areas to research.

Another major resource for the legislative/policy history are the people who are familiar with the policy issue. They exist within the bureaucracy as well as the various lobbying groups and nonprofit organizations focusing on that issue. Individuals within those organizations can point you to landmark legislation or current or recent policy proposals. These people can be useful in relating background material as to why legislative proposals failed in the past. If your policy issue focuses on pollution, state and national environmental regulatory agencies and conservation groups may be useful resources. Remember that each federal regulatory agency has a regional office with policy experts attached who are familiar with both state activities within that federal region as well as the national regulations.

There are also many nonpartisan associations such as the National Conference of State Legislatures (www.ncsl.org) that are focused on sharing research and policy ideas adopted by various states. Issue-specific organizations (e.g., your state public health organization, an academic research institute, or a state association of a type of healthcare professional) can sometimes provide information on ongoing legislation within their political jurisdictions. All of these are helpful in finding what is currently being considered or has been recently adopted in your or other political jurisdictions.

There are many nonpartisan foundations that have encouraged the adoption of model programs and conducted extensive evaluations as to their effectiveness, efficiency, equity, feasibility, and other criteria previously discussed. Examples include:

■ Robert Wood Johnson Foundation (www.rwjf.org)
■ The Kaiser Family Foundation (www.KFF.org)

---

1 The most recent reauthorization of the Healthy, Hunger-Free Kids Act, Pub. L. No. 111-296, was signed into law on December 13, 2010. The 114th Congress considered Child Nutrition Reauthorization legislation, but Congress was adjourned in 2016 without passing a final bill. A Position Paper from the School Nutrition Association (SNA) outlines advocacy goals in the absence of a Child Nutrition Reauthorization bill (https://schoolnutrition.org/legislation-policy/action-center/2022-position-paper). More information can be found at https://schoolnutrition.org/legislationpolicy/ federallegislationregulations.

- The Rand Corporation (www.rand.org)
- The Commonwealth Fund (www.commonwealthfund.org)
- The Pew Charitable Trusts (www.pewtrusts.org/en)

THE OBESITY ISSUE

Using obesity as an example, one would need to provide some information on why obesity is a major social problem that should be addressed by policy. This sets the tone in terms of the seriousness of the issue and the need to spend public resources to address the issue. While obesity has occurred throughout the ages, the problem of population-wide obesity is a relatively new phenomenon. What was a human evolutionary advantage, storing fat, has now become a medical diagnosis and an epidemic.

The Centers for Disease Control and Prevention (CDC) has a series of very visual state-based maps tracking the progression of obesity since 1985 (www .cdc.gov/obesity/data/prevalence-maps.html). An Organisation for Economic Co-operation and Development (OECD) study has indicated that the United States has the highest prevalence of obesity among OECD countries (Sassi, 2010). Data suggest that obesity rates in the United States have steadily increased over time. From 1999 to 2018, the prevalence of obesity in the United States increased from 30.5% to 42.4% (Boutari & Mantzoros, 2022; Hales et al., 2020). The prevalence of obesity is 40% among adults aged 20 to 39 years, 45% among adults aged 40 to 59 years, and 43% among adults aged 60 and older. From 2017 to 2020, the prevalence of severe obesity (defined as having a body mass index [BMI] greater than or equal to 40) increased from 4.7% to 9.2%. The annual medical costs associated with obesity in the United States are estimated at $173 billion in 2019 dollars. Among children and adolescents ages 2 to 19 years, the prevalence of obesity in the United States was 19.7% in 2017 to 2020, affecting approximately 14.7 million children and adolescents (CDC, n.d.-c).

These data provide a context for the policy debate concerning obesity in the United States in terms of both its magnitude and its historical context (Hales et al., 2020; Ogden et al., 2012). This is an example of descriptive evidence, or type one evidence as discussed in Chapter 8. If you are focusing on the state level, your state will have its own set of historical data on obesity that could provide a context for policy efforts at the state level. Your state may be in better shape than the national obesity problem or it may be worse.

Pointing to major historical milestones can be important in the development of policy as well as to acknowledge important participants in the development of those policies. This can be important for acquiring supporters for your effort. For example, the concern over obesity in the United States is sometimes dated back to 1952 when the American Heart Association identified obesity as a risk factor for coronary heart disease that could be modified through both diet and exercise (Nestle & Jacobson, 2000). State heart associations or other health groups can be powerful political allies in the support of your proposals.

From an historical perspective, *The Surgeon General's Call to Action to Prevent and Decrease Overweight and Obesity* (Satcher, 2001) is one of the landmark documents in the fight to confront the epidemic of obesity in the United States. Both Dr. David

Satcher and then Secretary of Health and Human Services Tommy G. Thompson under President George W. Bush called for achieving five overarching principles (Satcher, 2001):

■ Promote the recognition of overweight and obesity as major public health problems.

■ Assist Americans in balancing healthy eating with regular physical activity to maintain a healthy or healthier body weight.

■ Identify effective and culturally appropriate interventions to prevent and treat overweight and obesity.

■ Encourage environmental changes that help prevent overweight and obesity.

■ Develop and enhance public-private partnerships to help implement this vision.

One can point to several governors, liberal and conservative, who have pointed out the need to address the obesity problem. There may not be a consensus in terms of the solution to the problem, but there is at least a bipartisan acknowledgment that the obesity problem exists and that some type of public policy must be developed to address it.

The 1980, 1990, and 2000 U.S. Public Health Service national health objectives all recognize obesity as a major national problem. The 1998 National Institutes of Health report, *Clinical Guidelines of the Identification, Evaluation, and Treatment of Obesity in Adults: Evidence Report*, provided extensive evidence-based research on the risks of obesity as well as evidence-based guidelines for treatment by health providers (National Heart, Lung, and Blood Institute, 1998). One of the goals of *Healthy People 2030* is to reduce the proportion of children and adolescents who are obese to 15.5%, by helping people to eat more healthy foods and get recommended levels of physical activity (Office of Disease Prevention and Health Promotion, n.d.-a, n.d.-b).[2]

Children having one or more obese parents are three to four times more likely to be obese due to genetics and unhealthy diets/lifestyles (Sassi, 2010). These data do not include those classified as overweight. These data are important for providing a context for the problem and educating readers as to the growing nature of the problem.

The problem with objectives such as *Healthy People* is that historically there had not been an accompanying list of strategies as to how the targets were to be achieved or a list of agencies/organizations that are accountable for making sure these objectives are met. The 1980, 1990, and 2000 U.S. Public Health Service national health objectives all recognize obesity as a major problem. Historical data are significant in that they provide evidence that despite an early recognition of the policy problem, the past and current efforts have not been successful in reaching established goals. *Healthy People 2030* is beginning to delineate strategies via its "Tools for Action" section (https://health.gov/healthypeople/tools-action).

---

2 For more information, see https://health.gov/healthypeople/objectives-and-data/browse -objectives/overweight-and-obesity/reduce-proportion-children-and-adolescents -obesity-nws-04/data-methodology.

POLICY SIGNIFICANCE

One of the things that you need to remember in the development of a policy proposal is that there are multiple issues struggling to get on the political agenda for consideration. For example, the 112th Congress was presented with 12,299 pieces of legislation; they enacted 284 laws, and passed 721 resolutions (www.govtrack .us/congress/bills/#statistics). There are limits in terms of time and resources that can be expended on any one problem. As a result, the leadership of the various branches of government will establish priorities as to what will be addressed. One of the challenges of any policy analysis is to clearly and concisely explain why this issue should merit being placed on the policy agenda. Does data indicating the extent of the problem, the growth of the problem, the cost of the problem, the number of deaths, the policy window, or other considerations require addressing the issue now?

This is more complicated than it initially sounds. For example, if one measures a problem in terms of the number of deaths, then one can gather mortality data to demonstrate where a disease stands on the list of diseases causing death. However, not all deaths are necessarily equal. Some diseases (pneumonia) strike older adults who are near the end of their natural life span. Other health events (accidents and suicide) strike the young and result in greater loss of life as measured by the number of years of life lost. Presenting data in a meaningful way will help convince policy activists that your issue is critical. Understanding the different ways that disease/disability can be measured will be important in making your case and deflecting critics. Deaths are not the only way to measure the importance of a health issue. Understanding the human impacts of a disease or problem can be another way to demonstrate the importance of an issue. The benefit from the cost to the public sector, for example, the impact of treating obesity for the Medicaid population, can be an effective vehicle for attracting a policy maker's attention to the obesity problem. Refer back to Chapters 8 and 9 on the use of data.

For example, while few people die from obesity, obesity is linked to an increasing number of diseases. Obesity is linked to diabetes, osteoarthritis, cancer, hypertension, stroke, pregnancy complications, asthma, and psychological problems as well as heart disease. As such, it is a major contributor to death and chronic disease in the United States. In 2010, obesity surpassed smoking as the nation's leading cause of preventable death. The shift in the relative impact of obesity and smoking is related to both a reduction in the number of Americans who smoke (coinciding with stricter policies about smoking in the early 1990s) and an increase in the past two decades in the number of people who are obese (America's Health Rankings, n.d.; Boutari & Mantzoros, 2022; CDC, n.d.-f; Danaei et al., 2009).

The level of childhood obesity (which at 19.7% is triple the rate from just one generation ago) is of particular concern since obesity in children tracks to obesity in adults (CDC, n.d.-d). Efforts to reduce obesity in childhood may have a significant impact not only on the reduction of childhood diseases (e.g., adolescent onset of type 2 diabetes) but also a reduction in the incidence of disease later in life. As a result, a great deal of attention has been paid to the increase of childhood obesity in the United States (Singh et al., 2008).

However, children are not the only concern. Older adults can also suffer from obesity. The prevalence of obesity has increased to 43% among adults age 60 and older (Boutari & Mantzoros, 2022; Fakhouri et al., 2012). This increase has major implications for the cost of Medicare. Which area of concern is more important, childhood obesity's cost in the future or obesity's current impact on the cost of Medicare? Again, there is not a simple answer to that question, but it is something that must be addressed in order to build your case for establishing the importance of the problem you are attempting to address and demonstrating its need to be addressed by the political system.

The costs of obesity can be measured in many ways. In 2004, the National Institutes of Health initially indicated that as many as 400,000 deaths and $117 billion in healthcare costs are attributed to obesity (Bassett & Perl, 2004). More recent data suggest that the annual medical costs associated with obesity in the United States are approximately $173 billion in 2019 dollars (Boutari & Mantzoros, 2022).

Costs can also be calculated in terms of indirect costs, such as rising healthcare insurance premiums or increased taxes due to the costs for programs such as Medicare and Medicaid. One study estimated that obesity accounted for 10% of all medical costs (approximately $147 billion) in 2008 and that obese people's medical care spending was $1,429 greater than that for normal-weight people in 2006 (Finkelstein et al., 2009). Obesity-related diseases were cited as being responsible for 27% of the increase in U.S. medical costs from 1987 to 2001 (Thorpe et al., 2004).

There has been a rise in the number of insured people classified as obese and a rise in the number of obese individuals receiving medical care. This has resulted in an increase in the cost of private insurance. In 1987, obese adults with private health insurance spent $272 more per year per person (about 18% more) on healthcare than did normal-weight adults. This raised private healthcare spending by 2%, or $3.6 billion in 1987. By 2002 the relative differences in medical care spending among overweight, obese, morbidly obese, and normal-weight adults had increased substantially. Spending among obese adults averaged $1,244 higher per person (about 56% more) than for normal-weight adults. This raised private health insurance by nearly 12%—more than $36 billion—in 2002 (Thorpe et al., 2005).

The lifespan of an obese person is reduced 8 to 10 years compared to a person of normal weight. While an obese person has higher annual health expenditures, over a lifespan an obese person actually has lower lifetime health expenditures due to an earlier death (Sassi, 2010). While this is logical, it is not readily transparent when talking about the "cost of obesity."

It has been estimated that spending on obesity-related conditions accounted for an estimated 8.5% of Medicare spending, 11.8% of Medicaid spending, and 12.9% of private-payer spending (Cawley & Meyerhoefer, 2012; Finkelstein et al., 2004). This requires either taxation at the state and federal level to support these costs or reduction in coverage for other Medicaid services or clients. Health insurance usually treats being overweight as a behavioral problem and does not typically cover obesity unless it is treated as part of a comorbidity. Medicaid in many states does not cover obesity. For example, states will differ as to whether they cover nutritional counseling or drug therapy for obesity. While not covering preventive measures, most insurance policies and Medicaid do tend to cover bariatric surgery for obesity. Understanding the complexity of existing policies is important background information and a potential reason for the need for a policy analysis.

One of the diseases that has been closely associated with obesity is diabetes in both children and adults (Weiss et al., 2004). Once developed (90% of diabetes is type 2 or adult-onset diabetes), there is no current cure for diabetes; there are merely treatments designed to control it for the rest of that person's life and try to minimize the physical impacts of diabetes. Preventing or delaying the onset of diabetes is an important factor in reducing morbidity, mortality, and the cost of medical care. Diabetes has increased dramatically in the United States. During 1995 to 2010, the age-adjusted prevalence of diagnosed diabetes in the United States increased in all geographic areas with the median prevalence for all states, DC, and Puerto Rico rising from 4.5% to 8.2% (Geiss et al., 2012). More recent data suggest that approximately 1.4 million new cases of diabetes were diagnosed in 2019. Among individuals ages 10 to 19 years, new cases of type 2 diabetes increased for all racial and ethnic minority groups, especially among Black teens (CDC, n.d.-a, n.d.-e, n.d.-f).

Explaining how obesity is related to other diseases could be an important part of the background material. For example, there have been studies of school-based interventions for the reduction in obesity and diabetes (The Healthy Study Group, 2010) and studies linking both diabetes and obesity with socioeconomic status and neighborhoods (Ludwig et al., 2011).

Depending on what aspect of the obesity problem is being addressed, some or all of this data may be important. Access to government statistical data can be gained through web pages of agencies involved with collecting and disseminating such information. For obesity, the CDC (www.cdc.gov) and the U.S. Department of Health and Human Services (www.hhs.gov) would be key resources. Federal data can also be obtained through USAFACTS (https://usafacts.org/data). Access to data collected by the Department of Commerce's U.S. Census Bureau (www.census.gov) will be important for many different policy areas.

If it is clear that the focus of your policy proposal is going to be on childhood obesity, then the data presented and the argument can be more focused. For example, if you were working for the Children's Defense Fund (www.childrensdefense.org) your policy background would most likely be focused on children. However, you will still need to demonstrate why focusing on children is important compared to other subpopulations. If you wanted to focus on adult obesity, a different set of data and laws would be important for the policy background.

LEGAL AUTHORITY/FLEXIBILITY

One of the initial tasks that you need to determine is whether public policy is the appropriate or most useful way to address the problem. Some problems may be adequately or appropriately addressed through private nongovernmental actions. Perhaps voluntary actions taken by an informed public may be sufficient to solve the issue, for example, employers putting exercise equipment at work sites or changing foods available in workplace cafeterias without any government regulation. However, the existence of the problem or the growing scale of the problem itself might be an indicator that past efforts (public and/or private) have not been successful in resolving the issue.

If a public policy approach does seem to be an appropriate, it is also important for you to be knowledgeable as to legal ability of the government to pursue such actions. What statutes provide the authority to act? Remember that Dillion's Rule may prevent county or local governments policy jurisdiction. While certain levels of government have legal authority, do they have the administrative or financial ability to enforce such policies? The federal government might be able to provide money through a grant program to fight obesity in school-aged children, but it may lack authority to initiate specific policies or programs in schools throughout the country. Where does state control of a block grant facilitate or interfere with policy development?

The Constitution's Commerce Clause is the major constitutional provision that provides the federal government with the legal authority to regulate interstate commerce and as a result, healthcare. The federal courts have consistently ruled since the 1940s that the federal government has a clear legal authority in terms of issues involving interstate commerce. Regulation of foods for health and safety and drugs for efficacy and safety are examples of the federal government's legal authority to regulate interstate commerce. However, the federal courts have begun to look more skeptically at federal legislation using the Commerce Clause as its foundation.

If your policy proposal focuses on school-age children, the legal authority might shift to state and governments since they tend to have greater historical and legal authority for dealing with childhood obesity through their control of the public school systems. Because children (preschool to grade 12) are typically within a public school system, a local school board or city government has a great deal of influence over the dietary and exercise patterns of those children within the system. In this case, the federal government can play less of a direct role. Since the federal government traditionally financially supports voluntary childhood and school nutrition programs in state and local communities through the U.S. Department of Agriculture, it can have a greater influence over such programs. However, its legal authority to make specific changes may be more limited than a state's department of education or a local school district that can create mandates.

In dealing with other population segments concerning obesity, legal authority may be less well established. For example, the City of New York's mayor attempted to ban super-size sugary drinks, but it became mired down by legal challenges. In 2013, a New York state appeals court rejected Mayor Michael Bloomberg's attempt to limit the size of sugary beverages sold in the city (*New York Statewide Coalition of Hispanic Chambers of Commerce v. New York City Dep't of Health and Mental Hygiene*, 2013). The court stated that New York's Board of Health "overstepped the boundaries of its lawfully delegated authority when it promulgated the portion cap rule to curtail the consumption of soda drinks … It therefore violated the state principle of separation of powers" (Justice Dianne T. Renwick as quoted in Barclay, 2013, para. 2).

That decision was a setback for the city's Board of Health, which had met significant opposition from the food and beverage industry for years as it attempted to change unhealthy food habits through portion-size regulations. Specifically, Bloomberg intended to require food service establishments to cap sugary beverages at 16 ounces. Mayor Bloomberg described the court's decision as only a "temporary setback" and vowed further appeals, especially since more than half of adults in New York City are obese or overweight. Dr. Thomas Farley, New York's health commissioner, justified limiting soda consumption on the grounds that although eating 17 teaspoons of sugar at a time is difficult, "it's very easy to drink a 20-ounce soda with 17 teaspoons of sugar" (Dr. Thomas Farley as quoted in Barclay, 2013, para. 6). However, we also saw in Breakout Box 2.2 that other localities were able to pass restrictions on sugary drinks. What differentiates these examples?

Different sections of government have different inherent powers. It is important to recognize these differences. For example, the executive branch has the ability to issue or revise "rules and regulations" without having to go through a new legislative process. A governor may or may not have the authority to issue an executive order that will resolve the issue depending on the powers of government spelled out in law or the state's constitution. An attorney general may file suit against another agency or private sector organizations in order to stimulate action. A legislative committee can use its investigative or oversight powers to force various policy issues onto the executive branch. We discuss these topics in greater detail in Chapter 15, Recommendation and Strategies.

In addition to the legal component, there is also a practical side to solving a social problem. Even if New York City had the legal power to control the size of sugary drinks, there is the practical side as to whether a city ordinance would be effective. Would consumers merely go to a neighboring town to get super-sized drinks and skirt the law? New York City has a large population and covers a substantial geographic area. As a result, it might be able to make the case that such a city law could have an impact even though New Jersey is across the river. However, a small town that might wish to limit the sale of sugary drinks to blunt the obesity epidemic in its children might find its ability to have an impact on obesity quite limited and its negative impact on businesses in the town to be substantial. Children or parents could merely go to the next town to buy what their town prohibits. This is where scale (population and geography) matters in policy.

MODEL PROGRAMS/POLICIES

The Robert Wood Johnson Foundation is but one example of a foundation that has initiated community health initiatives throughout the country. The Robert Wood Johnson Foundation (RWJF) has a special focus on childhood obesity (www.rwjf .org/en/our-focus-areas/topics/childhood-obesity.html). It publishes Issue Briefs that summarize what has been learned from its multiple initiatives on childhood obesity throughout the country. Most foundations require an evaluation component built into their grants in order to determine what went well and what needed additional effort or modification. Some foundations such as the Kellogg Foundation have more of a geographic orientation. All national foundations establish priorities of interest that might change from year to year or stay relatively stable for a period of years. It is important to research such foundations for examples of their policy-related initiatives. Many of these projects end up being published in peer-reviewed journals (see Breakout Box 10.1), but many do not, and yet are equally insightful and valuable.

There are also a number of state/community foundations (many financed by the sale of nonprofit healthcare organizations to for-profit investor-owned organizations) that serve as a source of program experimentation at the state/local level. These are generally less well known but may be particularly important because they fund local policy initiatives and therefore have credibility as homegrown

Breakout Box 10.1

OBESITY PREVENTION IN EARLY CHILDCARE AND EDUCATION SETTINGS

Early childhood is a formative period for many important lifestyle behaviors, including diet and physical activity, but little obesity prevention research targeting this age group has been conducted. Early childcare and education (ECE) programs are important settings for obesity prevention because childcare centers provide care for an estimated 30% to 40% of children under the age of 6 years (Ogden et al., 2012; Singh et al., 2008; Ward et al., 2013). Volger et al. (2018) reported that the prevalence of obesity among preschool children in the United States was 13.9%. Children spend, on average, 30 hours per week in these settings. Thus, ECE settings are a promising avenue for interventions targeting young children (birth–age 5), but the limited research provides limited evidence upon which to base policy decisions and practice guidelines to improve healthy eating and physical activity, and ultimately healthy weight development in these settings (Ogden et al., 2012).

Systematic reviews of obesity interventions in ECE settings are available but include only 18 studies that were published in the last decade (Larson et al., 2011). While many of these studies demonstrated positive effects on behaviors, only two out of five studies that assessed weight changes showed positive effects. Two nationally representative studies that have evaluated the nutritional quality of foods offered in childcare settings identified concerns relating to the percentage of energy from saturated fat, average sodium levels, and the number of fruit/vegetables items provided by meals and snacks. With respect to physical activity, only 14% of childcare centers provided the recommended 120 minutes of active playtime, and one-third provided more than 90 minutes. Research suggests that many caregivers may benefit from additional technical assistance and training regarding feeding practices and modeling feeding behavior for children. For example, a recent study found that more than 50% of caregivers received no annual training on nutrition, and only 47% provided nutrition education to children by reading books or playing games with nutrition themes (Robert Wood Johnson Foundation, 2016).

Public and private organizations across the nation are working to encourage adoption of policies for ECE programs that promote healthy eating and physical activity. Two of the most significant examples of recent reports are *Caring for Our Children* and *Preventing Childhood Obesity in Early Care and Education Programs* (American Academy of Pediatrics et al., 2019, 2020); in addition, the Institute of Medicine's (IOM) *Early Childhood Obesity Prevention Policies* examines the evidence and provides guidance on obesity prevention policies for young children (Birch et al., 2011). For example, the IOM recommends that ECE facilities should serve toddlers and preschoolers small, age-appropriate portions and should permit children one or more additional servings of foods that are low in fat, sugar, and sodium as needed to meet the caloric needs of the individual child. Additionally, the IOM recommends that formal nutrition information and education programs should be conducted at least twice per year under the guidance of a nutritionist/dietitian. Head Start facilities are required to provide opportunities for indoor and outdoor active play, adequate space and equipment to promote active play, and opportunities to develop gross and fine motor skills.

In 2011, a panel of experts discussed key issues around measurement of diet and physical activity, policy and environment measurement, intervention approaches, policy research, and capacity development. Following their deliberations, they selected top research priorities for early childhood obesity prevention. The highest-rated priority issues included assessment of the quality of children's meals and snacks, use of financial incentives, interventions that include healthcare providers, the role of screen time, and need for multilevel interventions. The expert panel highlighted the difficulties in measuring policy and environmental change. Instruments like the Environment and Policy Assessment and Observation (EPAO; Ward et al., 2008) and the Wellness Child Care Assessment Tool (WellCCAT; Falbe et al., 2011) have established reliability and validity, but they require intensive training and access to materials. Minority populations, including African Americans, American Indians, and Hispanics, suffer disproportionately high rates of obesity and are important targets for future ECE interventions; however, interventions must be culturally tailored to meet the needs of these populations. Recent interdisciplinary studies have shown promising results in this regard (Holler et al., 2010; Jackson et al., 2021; Volger et al., 2018).

The panel stated that future policy research in the ECE setting would benefit from consensus that traditional study designs and outcome measures may not be appropriate for this age group and setting. For example, randomized trials are often not ethical or feasible in this setting, and high turnover rates of children in ECE can make the traditional cohort design impractical. Cost effectiveness information is also needed. Another recommendation was to use childcare programs as access points to help create linkages to families, pediatricians, and other sources of support for obesity prevention. This type of coordination is recommended in the Affordable Care Act as part of the National Prevention Strategy (National Prevention Council, 2011).

Thought Questions

As a policy analyst, how might you help a policy maker to better understand:

1. The current state of the evidence in ECE settings?
2. Why preventing obesity in ECE settings is important?
3. Why policy and environmental change in these settings is difficult to measure and evaluate?

References

American Academy of Pediatrics, American Public Health Association, National Resource Center for Health and Safety in Child Care and Early Education. (2019). *Caring for our children: National health and safety performance standards* (4th ed.). American Academy of Pediatrics.

American Academy of Pediatrics, American Public Health Association, National Resource Center for Health and Safety in Child Care and Early Education. (2020). *Preventing childhood obesity in early care and education programs* (3rd ed.). American Academy of Pediatrics.

Birch, L. L., Parker, L., & Burns, A. (Eds.). (2011). *Early childhood obesity prevention policies.* National Academies Press.

Falbe, J., Kenney, E., Henderson, K., & Schwartz, M. (2011). The wellness child care assessment tool: A measure to assess the quality of written nutrition and physical activity policies. *Journal of American Dietetic Association, 111*(12), 1852–1860. https://doi.org/10.1016/j.jada.2011.09.006

Holler, D., Messiah, S., Lopez-Mitnikk, G., Hollar, T., Almon, M., & Aqatson, A. S. (2010). Effect of a two-year obesity prevention intervention on percentile changes in body mass index and academic performance in low-income elementary school children. *American Journal of Public Health, 100*(4), 646–653. https://doi.org/10.2105/AJPH.2009.165746

Jackson, J. K., Jones, J., Nguyen, H., Davies, I., Lum, M., Grady, A., & Yoong, S. L. (2021, January 19). Obesity prevention within the early childhood education and care setting: A systematic review of dietary behavior and physical activity policies and guidelines in high income countries. *International Journal of Environmental Research and Public Health, 18*(2), 838. https://doi.org/10.3390/ijerph18020838

Larson, N., Ward, D., Neelon, S., & Story, M. (2011). What role can child-care settings play in obesity prevention? A review of the evidence and call for research efforts. *Journal of American Diet Association, 111*(9), 1343–1362. https://doi.org/10.1016/j.jada.2011.06.007

National Prevention Council. (2011). *National prevention strategy.* U.S. Department of Health and Human Services, Office of the Surgeon General. https://www.hhs.gov/sites/default/files/disease-prevention-wellness-report.pdf

Ogden, C., Carroll, M., Kit, B., & Flegal, K. (2012). *Prevalence of obesity in the United States, 2009–2010* (NCHS Data Brief, No. 82). National Center for Health Statistics. http://www.cdc.gov/nchs/data/databriefs/db82.pdf

Patient Protection and Affordable Care Act, Pub. L. No. 111-148, 124 Stat. 119 (2010). https://www.congress.gov/111/plaws/publ148/PLAW-111publ148.pdf

Robert Wood Johnson Foundation. (2016). *Declining childhood obesity rates—Where are we seeing signs of progress.* https://www.rwjf.org/en/library/research/2016/06/declining-childhood-obesity-rates.html

Singh, A., Mulder, C., Twisk, J., van Mechelen, W., & Chinapaw, M. (2008). Tracking of childhood overweight into adulthood: A systematic review of the literature. *Obesity Reviews, 9*(5), 474–488. https://doi.org/10.1111/j.1467-789X.2008.00475.x

Volger, S., Rigassio Radler, D., & Rothpletz-Puglia, P. (2018). Early childhood obesity prevention efforts through a life course health development perspective: A scoping review. *PLoS One, 13*(12), Article e0209787. https://doi.org/10.1371/journal.pone.0209787. (Correction published 2019, *PLoS One, 14*(1), Article e0211288)

Ward, D., Hales, D., Haverly, K., Marks, J., Benjamin, S., Ball, S., & Trost, S. (2008). An instrument to assess the obesogenic environment of child care centers. *American Journal of Health Behavior, 32*(4), 380–386. https://doi.org/10.5555/ajhb.2008.32.4.380

Ward, D., Vaughn, A., & Story, M. (2013). Expert and stakeholder consensus on priorities for obesity prevention research in early care and education settings. *Childhood Obesity, 9*(2), 116–124. https://doi.org/10.1089/chi.2013.9204

policy responses that are compatible with the local political culture, political structure, political process, demographics, laws, and so forth. Consequently, these experiments may be more politically acceptable to policy makers within that state.

Nonprofit organizations publish useful policy examples. You need to look at the multiple nonprofit associations that are oriented on the issue that you have chosen.

RELATIONSHIPS TO OTHER POLICY ISSUES

Policy issues cannot be thought of in terms of discrete boxes. Due to the nature of policy, policies in one area by their very nature entangle other policies. Transportation policy impacts all types of commercial and social relationships, including health. A highway cutting through a city can separate populations leading to demographic isolation, racial segregation, and loss of services. This has consequences for obesity. The growth of suburbia in the United States is generally attributed to the development of the interstate highway system and banking policies that encouraged single home housing and the growth of suburbia. That in turn has resulted in an automobile-oriented focus that is related to obesity problems. The need to drive for goods and services, the lack of sidewalks, and the lack of frequently scheduled mass transit due to a dispersed population complicate the issue of obesity. The obesity problem cannot be solved without involving many different policy areas, different sectors of government, and cultural perspectives (Marya & Patel, 2021). It is this intersectionality that is important to recognize as one develops any particular policy. To what extent will your policy proposal be made ineffective due to existing policies in transportation, zoning, education, and so forth? Whose perspectives may be overlooked?

As described in Chapter 1, there is a growing international movement to consider "Health in All Policies" (HiAP; CDC, n.d.-b; Collins & Koplan, 2009; Rajotte et al., 2011; World Health Organization, 2010). Refer back to **Breakout Box 1.3**. For example, in the United States, the state of California established an executive order on HiAP. California's Health in All Policies Task Force, established in 2010 by Executive Order S-04-10, comprises 19 different state agencies, departments, and offices. This provides a venue for state agencies and departments to advance multiple goals in order to support healthier and more sustainable community environments (California Executive Order S-04-10, 2010; California Strategic Growth Council, n.d.). The Task Force was charged with identifying

priority programs, policies, and strategies to improve the health of Californians while advancing the goals of improving air and water quality, protecting natural resources and agricultural lands, increasing the availability of affordable housing, improving infrastructure systems, promoting public health, planning sustainable communities, and meeting the climate change goals. (California Department of Justice, n.d., para. 1)

Using the HiAP lens harnesses the power that different government agencies and departments can bring through their diverse areas of expertise. They can identify cobenefits and can bring people from different sectors together to address complex social and environmental issues.

For obesity policy, one would need to examine agricultural policies, food processing policies, food labeling policies, transportation policies, community development policies, educational policies, and recreation policies, among others that play a role in solving the obesity problem for children. In addition, addressing obesity has health insurance and medical cost implications, national defense implications, economic implications, Medicare implications, and so forth. Consequently, any policy is affected by other policies and in turn affects other policies. That, of course, is what makes the development of policy so complex.

One area that is becoming increasingly important for obesity is the built environment. The lack of sidewalks, food deserts, the presence of parks, access to public transportation, and safe walking routes all influence the population level of physical activity in a given geographic population (Aytur et al., 2007; Dixon et al., 2021). The natural environment has its own implications for obesity (Jimenez et al., 2021; White et al., 2019). However, policy decisions that shape the built environment can overcome some of the problems associated with the natural environment. For example, free outdoor community skating rinks may build social capital as well as provide exercise during the winter months. The existence of "food deserts" (the lack of grocery stores providing inexpensive fresh food) in inner cities can be overcome with thoughtful zoning and community development grants (CDC, 2013). These policy areas need to be explored since they provide useful means of attacking the problem in a multifaceted manner. Innovation generally comes from recognizing the synergy between policy areas as well as recognizing unintended consequences and transforming them into intended consequences (e.g., to use existing zoning laws to intentionally eliminate food deserts; see www.healthyfoodaccess.org/policy-efforts-and-impacts-federal).

The synergy between policy areas has its downsides. If everything is connected to everything, one can become overwhelmed with the potential harmful impacts and become paralyzed due to an inability to take everything into account. This also creates difficulties in terms of evaluating policies and demonstrating a significant impact of policies, because so many factors are involved. See **Breakout Box 10.1**. This can lead to policy stalemate, which often leads to deference to the status quo. At some point, one has to draw the line and say that we have considered what we currently perceive are the major policy interactions. If there are others, we will deal with them at a later time.

It is also critical to realize that policies have both intended and unintended outcomes (those not generally anticipated). Unintended consequences can be both positive and negative. There may be some unexpected positive results or some unexpected negative results of the policy/program. If one is focusing on the implications of an education policy (lengthening the school day for increased exercise), one may forget to examine the unintended consequences of that policy on family dynamics and the need for parents to arrange for transportation or alter work schedules. In addition, some policies will have positive impacts for some groups of people and negative consequences for others. Are you sure who is going to benefit and who is going to be disadvantaged by the proposed policy?

POLICY AGENDA

One of the issues that you need to address in this section of your policy analysis is why this issue should reach the policy agenda at this particular time (Baumgartner & Jones, 1991; Kingdon, 1984; Sabatier, 1999). As indicated previously, there are multiple problems to be solved with only limited time and resources available. Why has this issue emerged at the present time? If it is an issue that has been unsuccessfully dealt with on other occasions, why is now the time to act? Has the nature of the problem grown in scale? Have the political dynamics changed to alter the prospect for successful resolution? This is sometimes referred to as the existence of political will or expediency. Sometimes the answer is that an incident (a tragedy or personal experience) has occurred that has generated public interest. For example, an automobile accident killing a young bicyclist might generate public support for finally dealing with the issue of having bicycle paths that are separated from vehicle traffic. A new strain of a deadly virus might increase sensitivity to public hygiene. The major question to answer is, "Why now?" What has changed in the policy environment to place this higher on the policy agenda?[3] Political advocacy coalitions can also shift over time, making a policy proposal more or less viable (Jenkins-Smith & Sabatier, 1993).

This situation is described by Kingdon (1984, 2003, 2010) in his multiple streams theory. Kingdon argues that the convergence of three "streams" (the problem, the policy, and the politics) opens a window of opportunity for change (Kingdon, 2010). He contends that the "art" of policy making involves being prepared to take advantage of windows of opportunity for passing legislation when they occur. Policy "windows" open at particular moments when the timing is right for the problem, the policy, and the politics. This can include such things as sociopolitical factors and budget constraints (Cairney & Jones, 2016; De Wals et al., 2019). Triggers can provide a narrow window of opportunity for a policy proposal to gain traction. However, the window of opportunity can close very quickly. Powerful stakeholders may begin to lobby against any changes in policy and draw attention to the next big event. Policy makers need to be ready to take advantage of the opportunity before the policy window closes.

Reports from the CDC can describe the extent of a health problem, but the general public does not usually read these reports and such data lack a personal connection to make them meaningful to policy makers and voters. Statistical deaths (the number per 100,000) are generally not very persuasive. However, one of the most effective visuals of the obesity epidemic has been the series of CDC maps showing the percentage of obese state by state over time (www.cdc.gov/obesity/data/prevalence-maps.html). Visually, they make a very strong statement as states turn different colors and as old colors disappear and new colors are added as the progression of the obesity epidemic continues. However, it is generally the human face of the problem that makes the problem or the policy much more meaningful to policy makers and voters. In politics, the number of dead or diseased may have less significance than the death of one publicized individual in a local community.

What is it about this time period that makes you to think that your issue is ripe to being addressed now rather than next year or the following year? Has there been a significant shift of public opinion? Has there been an incident that raises the issue's salience to lawmakers or the public? Sometimes the political clock is a determining factor. If the policy is potentially controversial, it may be too close to an election to tackle the problem and make political enemies. That same legislation might be more politically viable right after an election in order to allow time to pass and emotions to cool before the next election. An election that results in the naming of a new chair of an important legislative committee that has blocked previous legislative efforts or the turnover of the party in control of the legislature may be the trigger for promising policy activity. Some state legislatures create a biennial budget and leave general legislation to the second session. Does this create an opportunity for your initiative?

---

3 We encourage readers to learn more about policy theories that are commonly used in public health. A suggested resource for the obesity issue is Clarke et al. (2016).

Policy makers do not always think their policy proposal is ready to pass. Sometimes a legislator may introduce a piece of legislation knowing that it will not pass but hoping that it will stimulate establishing a commission or a special legislative committee report that will stimulate interest in the issue. The introduction of a policy initiative may just be an educational effort to get other policy makers thinking about the issue and alternative solutions. Therefore, policy makers might introduce an idea as a trial balloon, expecting that it will probably be shot down but nevertheless testing the water for political acceptability. Such trial balloons are useful in finding out where major opposition groups might be or what issues might need to be overcome in order to eventually get legislation passed. In addition, some legislators may feel that while there is no possibility for policy action, the issue is so important to them personally that the policy must remain on the political agenda. If there is no bill, there is no possibility of action. A bill can serve as a placeholder until the time when the proposal may be received more positively. The political environment can suddenly change; if a proposed policy/program is readily available, it can respond to that window of opportunity.

The policy agenda is full of competing and complementary policy options. Providing a broad context of the importance of your policy within this agenda provides an important context for your policy makers.

SUMMARY

This chapter focuses on the background of your policy. Since it is unlikely that this public health policy is totally new, you need to familiarize yourself with the political history of dealing with that topic. We discussed various resources to use in order to examine the legislative history. By using the example of obesity, we discussed the various ways in which the significance of the policy issue can be presented to policy makers. You need to take into consideration the legal authority that your decision maker has in dealing with this issue. This chapter also dealt with the importance of examining relationships with other policy areas and model programs. How can your policy issue tag along with other initiatives? Finally, it discusses the importance of getting on the policy agenda and looking for a window of opportunity that is more favorable for your policy initiative. The next chapter focuses on creating a precise statement of the policy issue.

DISCUSSION QUESTIONS

- How has the policy issue of obesity evolved over the years?

- How has the history of abortion evolved over the years?

- Make a case for and against placing gun control on the public health policy agenda for the next year.

- The Supreme Court has been recently narrowing the federal government's use of the Commerce Clause for the basis of federal legislation. Make a case for and against the USSC's direction.

- What health policy issues should be on top of the public health policy agenda for the next congressional term? Defend your choices.

KEY TERMS

Commerce Clause
The Commonwealth Fund
Electronic Code of Federal
    Regulations
Federal Register
Health in All Policies (HiAP)
Healthy People 2030
The Kaiser Family Foundation
Library of Congress
policy agenda

The Pew Charitable Trusts
The Rand Corporation
Robert Wood Johnson Foundation
stakeholders
The Surgeon General's Call to
    Action to Prevent and Decrease
    Overweight and Obesity
U.S. Government Publishing Office
    (GPO)

REFERENCES

America's Health Rankings. (n.d.). *Obesity*. United Health Foundation. https://www.americas healthrankings.org/

Aytur, S., Rodriguez, D., Evenson, K., Catellier, D., & Rosamond, W. (2007). Promoting active community environments through land use and transportation planning. *American Journal of Health Promotion*, 21(4), 397–407. https://doi.org/10.4278/0890-1171-21.4s.397

Barclay, E. (2013, July 30). *Despite legal blow, New York to keep sugary drink fight*. http://www.npr.org/blogs/thesalt/2013/07/30/207026680/despite-legal-blow-new-york-to-keep-up-sugary-drink-fight

Bassett, M., & Perl, S. (2004). Obesity: The public health challenge of our time. *American Journal of Public Health*, 94(9), Article 1477. https://doi.org/10.2105/ajph.94.9.1477

Baumgartner, F. R., & Jones, B. D. (1991). Agenda dynamics and policy subsystems. *The Journal of Politics*, 53(4), 1044–1074. https://doi.org/10.2307/2131866

Boutari, C., & Mantzoros, C. S. (2022, August). A 2022 update on the epidemiology of obesity and a call to action: As its twin COVID-19 pandemic appears to be receding, the obesity and dysmetabolism pandemic continues to rage on. *Metabolism*, 133, Article 155217. https://doi.org/10.1016/j.metabol.2022.155217

Cairney, P., & Jones, M. D. (2016), Kingdon's multiple streams approach: What is the empirical impact of this universal theory? *Policy Studies Journal, 44,* 37–58. https://doi.org/10.1111/psj.12111

California Exec. Order No. S-04-10, Title 3 C.F.R. (2010).

California Department of Justice. (n.d.). *Health in All Policies task force.* Office of the Attorney General. https://oag.ca.gov/environment/communities/policies

California Strategic Growth Council. (n.d.). *California Health in All Policies task force.* https://sgc.ca.gov/programs/healthandequity/hiap/taskforce.html

Cawley, J., & Meyerhoefer, C. (2012). The medical care costs of obesity: An instrumental variables approach. *Journal of Health Economics, 31*(1), 219–230. https://doi.org/10.1016/j.jhealeco.2011.10.003

Centers for Disease Control and Prevention. (n.d.-a). *Diabetes: The facts, stats, and impacts of diabetes.* U.S. Department of Health and Human Services. https://www.cdc.gov/diabetes/library/spotlights/diabetes-facts-stats.html

Centers for Disease Control and Prevention. (n.d.-b). *Healthy places: Health Impact Assessment.* U.S. Department of Health and Human Services. http://www.cdc.gov/healthyplaces/hia.htm

Centers for Disease Control and Prevention. (n.d.-c). *National Center for Health Statistics: Healthy People 2020.* U.S. Department of Health and Human Services. http://www.cdc.gov/nchs/healthy_people/hp2020.htm

Centers for Disease Control and Prevention. (n.d.-d). *Overweight and obesity: Childhood obesity facts.* U.S. Department of Health and Human Services. https://www.cdc.gov/obesity/data/childhood.html

Centers for Disease Control and Prevention. (n.d.-e). *Overweight and obesity: Childhood overweight and obesity.* U.S. Department of Health and Human Services. http://www.cdc.gov/obesity/childhood

Centers for Disease Control and Prevention. (n.d.-f). *Overweight and obesity: Overweight and obesity.* U.S. Department of Health and Human Services. http://www.cdc.gov/obesity

Centers for Disease Control and Prevention. (2013). *A practitioner's guide for advancing health equity: Community strategies for preventing chronic disease* (pp. 66–69). U.S. Department of Health and Human Services. https://www.cdc.gov/nccdphp/dnpao/health-equity/health-equity-guide/pdf/health-equity-guide/Health-Equity-Guide-sect-3-4.pdf

Clarke, B., Swinburn, B., & Sacks, G. (2016). The application of theories of the policy process to obesity prevention: A systematic review and meta-synthesis. *BMC Public Health, 16,* 1084. https://doi.org/10.1186/s12889-016-3639-z

Collins, J., & Koplan, J. (2009). Health Impact Assessment: A step toward Health in All Policies. *Journal of the American Medical Association, 302*(3), 315–317. https://doi.org/10.1001/jama.2009.1050

Danaei, G., Ding, E. L., Mozaffarian, D., Taylor, B., Rehm, J., Murray, C. J. L., & Ezzati, M. (2009). The preventable causes of death in the United States: Comparative risk assessment of dietary, lifestyle, and metabolic risk factors. *PLoS Medicine, 6*(4), 1–23. https://doi.org/10.1371/journal.pmed.1000058

De Wals, P., Espinoza-Moya, M. E., & Béland, D. (2019, June). Kingdon's multiple streams framework and the analysis of decision-making processes regarding publicly-funded immunization programs. *Expert Review of Vaccines, 18*(6), 575–585. https://doi.org/10.1080/14760584.2019.1627208

Dixon, B. N., Ugwoaba, U. A., Brockmann, A. N., & Ross, K. M. (2021, April). Associations between the built environment and dietary intake, physical activity, and obesity: A scoping review of reviews. *Obesity Reviews, 22*(4), Article e13171. https://doi.org/10.1111/obr.13171

Fakhouri, T., Ogden, C., Carroll, M., Kit, B., & Flegal, K. (2012, September). *Prevalence of obesity among older adults in the United States, 2007–2010* (NCHS Data Brief, No. 106). National Center for Health Statistics. http://www.cdc.gov/nchs/data/databriefs/db106.pdf

Finkelstein, E., Fiebelkorn, I., & Wang, G. (2004). State-level estimates of annual medical expenditures attributable to obesity. *Obesity Research, 12*(1), 18–24. https://doi.org/10.1038/oby.2004.4

Finkelstein, E. A., Trogdon, J. G., Cohen, J. W., & Dietz, W. (2009). Annual medical spending attributable to obesity: Payer- and service-specific estimates. *Health Affairs, 28*(Suppl. 1), W822–W831. https://doi.org/10.1377/hlthaff.28.5.w822

Geiss, L. S., Li, Y., Kirtland, K., Barker, L., Burrows, N. R., & Gregg, E. W. (2012, November 16). Increasing prevalence of diagnosed diabetes—United States and Puerto Rico, 1995–2010. *MMWR Morbidity and Mortality Weekly Report, 61*(45), 918–921. https://www.cdc.gov/mmwr/preview/mmwrhtml/mm6145a4.htm

Hales, C. M., Carroll, M. D., Fryar, C. D., & Ogden, C. L. (2020). *Prevalence of obesity and severe obesity among adults: United States, 2017–2018 (NCHS Data Brief No. 360)*. National Center for Health Statistics, Centers for Disease Control and Prevention, U.S. Department of Health and Human Services. https://www.cdc.gov/nchs/data/databriefs/db360-h.pdf

Healthy, Hunger-Free Kids Act, Pub. L. No. 111-296, 124 Stat. 3183 (2010).

Jenkins-Smith, H., & Sabatier, P. (1993). *Policy change and learning: An advocacy coalition approach.* Westview Press.

Jimenez, M. P., DeVille, N. V., Elliott, E. G., Schiff, J. E., Wilt, G. E., Hart, J. E., & James, P. (2021, April 30). Associations between nature exposure and health: A review of the evidence. *International Journal of Environmental Research Public Health, 18*(9), 4790. https://doi.org/10.3390/ijerph18094790

Kingdon, J. W. (1984). *Agendas, alternatives and public policies.* Little, Brown and Company.

Kingdon, J. W. (2003). *Agendas, alternatives and public policies* (2nd ed.). Addison-Wesley Educational.

Kingdon, J. W. (2010). *Agendas, alternatives, and public policies* (updated 2nd ed.). Pearson.

Ludwig, J., Sanbonmatsu, L., Gennetian, L., Adam, E., Duncan G., Katz L., Kessler, R. C., Kling, J. R., Lindau, S. T., Whitaker, R. C., & McDade, T. W. (2011). Neighborhoods, obesity, and diabetes—A randomized social experiment. *New England Journal of Medicine, 365*(16), 1509–1519. https://doi.org/10.1056/NEJMsa1103216

Marya, R., & Patel, R. (2021). *Inflamed: Deep medicine and the anatomy of injustice.* Farrar, Straus, and Giroux Publishers.

National Heart, Lung, and Blood Institute. (1998). *Clinical guidelines on the identification, evaluation, and treatment of overweight and obesity in adults: The evidence report.* Author.

National League of Cities. (2013). *Local government authority.* http://www.nlc.org/build-skills-and-networks/resources/cities-101/city-powers/local-government-authority

Nestle, M., & Jacobson, M. (2000). Halting the obesity epidemic: A public health policy approach. *Public Health Reports, 115*(1), 12–24. https://doi.org/10.1093/phr/115.1.12

New York Statewide Coalition of Hispanic Chambers of Commerce v. New York City Dep't of Health and Mental Hygiene, No. 05505 (N.Y. App. Div., 2013, July 30).

Office of Disease Prevention and Health Promotion. (n.d.-a). *Overweight and obesity.* U.S. Department of Health and Human Services. https://health.gov/healthypeople/objectives-and-data/browse-objectives/overweight-and-obesity

Office of Disease Prevention and Health Promotion. (n.d.-b). *Physical activity guidelines for Americans.* U.S. Department of Health and Human Services. https://health.gov/our-work/nutrition-physical-activity/physical-activity-guidelines

Ogden, C., Carroll, M., Kit, B., & Flegal, K. (2012). *Prevalence of obesity in the United States, 2009–2010. NCHS Data Brief, No. 82.* National Center for Health Statistics. http://www.cdc.gov/nchs/data/databriefs/db82.pdf

Rajotte, B., Ross, C., Ekechi, C., & Cadet, V. (2011). Health in All Policies: Addressing the legal and policy foundations of Health Impact Assessment. *Journal of Law, Medicine, & Ethics, 39*(s1), 27–29. https://doi.org/10.1111/j.1748-720X.2011.00560.x

Sabatier, P. (1999). *Theories of the policy process (theoretical lenses on public policy).* Westview Press.

Sassi, F. (2010). *Obesity and economics of prevention: Fit not fat.* Organisation for Economic Co-operation and Development.

Satcher, D. (2001). *The surgeon general's call to action to prevent and decrease overweight and obesity, 2001.* Office of Disease Prevention and Health Promotion, Centers for Disease Control and Prevention, National Institutes of Health.

Singh, A., Mulder, C., Twisk, J., van Mechelen, W., & Chinapaw, M. (2008). Tracking of childhood overweight into adulthood: A systematic review of the literature. *Obesity Reviews, 9*(5), 474–488. https://doi.org/10.1111/j.1467-789X.2008.00475.x

Starr, P. (1982). *The social transformation of American medicine.* Basic Books.

The Healthy Study Group. (2010). A school-based intervention for diabetes risk reduction. *New England Journal of Medicine, 363*(5), 443–453. https://doi.org/10.1056/NEJMoa1001933

Thorpe, K., Florence, C., Howard, D., & Joski, P. (2004). The impact of obesity on rising medical spending. *Health Affairs, 23*(Suppl. Web Exclusives), W4–W486. https://doi.org/10.1377/hlthaff.w4.480

Thorpe, K., Florence, C., Howard, D., & Joski, P. (2005). The rising prevalence of treated disease: Effects on private health insurance spending. *Health Affairs, 24*(Suppl. Web Exclusives), W5–W325. https://doi.org/10.1377/hlthaff.w5.317

Weiss, R., Dziura, J., Burgert, T., Tamborlane, W., Taksali, S., Yeckel, C., Allen, K., Lopes, M., Savoye, M., Morrison, J., Sherwin, R. S., & Caprio, S. (2004). Obesity and metabolic syndrome in children and adolescents. *New England Journal of Medicine, 350*(23), 2362–2374. https://doi.org/10.1056/NEJMoa031049

Westlaw Professional Legal Research. (n.d.) *How to find statutes*. http://lscontent.westlaw.com/images/content/FindStatutes10.pdf

White, M. P., Alcock, I., Grellier, J., Wheeler, B. W., Hartig, T., Warber, S. L., Bone, A., Depledge, M. H., & Fleming, L. E. (2019). Spending at least 120 minutes a week in nature is associated with good health and wellbeing. *Scientific Reports, 9*, 7730. https://doi.org/10.1038/s41598-019-44097-3

World Health Organization. (2010, April 13). *Adelaide statement on Health in All Policies: Moving towards a shared governance for health and well-being*. World Health Organization & Government of South Australia. https://apps.who.int/iris/handle/10665/44365

CHAPTER 11

STATEMENT OF POLICY ISSUE

The previous section of your policy analysis framework is meant to be fairly general and to provide background material for a macro understanding of the issue and the legal authority and practical considerations to act. In contrast, this section of your analysis is very specific and can be relatively brief. However, this section requires a great deal of thoughtful preparation. It is here that you must narrow the scope of the analysis to one aspect of the policy issue that is going to be addressed. As discussed earlier, your policy issue statement may have already been determined by your policy maker/organization.

LEARNING OBJECTIVES

Be able to:

- Write a policy issue statement.
- Demonstrate the importance of framing.
- Discuss how strategies such as the Public Health Reaching Across Sectors (PHRASES) approach can be used to help frame a public health policy issue.

POLICY ISSUE STATEMENT

Your background section has already explained the complexity of the issue (e.g., obesity) and how it is interwoven with other policy areas. Consequently, while the analysis to date has been on the issue of obesity in general, it is in this section that you will make very explicit choices. Assuming you have a free range of choices, you could focus on childhood, adolescent, or adult obesity; nutrition; diet; exercise; and so forth. There are a multitude of choices that you could make. You might want to focus on the part of the obesity problem that has the greatest impact on disease—reducing diabetes, heart disease, or other diseases (Ogden et al., 2010). Instead, you could concentrate on obesity and its impact on the quality of life. You might choose to focus on obesity and its impact on the cost of medical care in the public sector (Wang et al., 2012). Pursuing obesity from the perspective of the "built environment" or "planetary health" would relate to the wider area of environmental policy. You might want to pursue the obesity issue from a personal interest perspective, for example, bicycle riding, hiking, slow food, or bariatric surgical procedures. You could take advantage of a policy trigger that has pushed a specific aspect of the obesity issue higher on the political agenda. All of these perspectives on the obesity problem are legitimate, and many are interconnected. Since no one policy is likely to solve all aspects of the obesity problem, the task for you is to choose which part of the obesity problem you wish to address. Subsequent policy initiatives can address other equally important aspects.

While the preceding list of options implies wide-open possibilities for focusing the policy, you are more likely to be constrained by the person or agency for whom this policy analysis is being written. For example, the legislator that you are working for may have a special interest in childhood obesity, or the agency that you work for may be focused on the implications of obesity and insurance coverage. A community organization may want to focus on changing the built environment. Working for a nonprofit such as the Robert Wood Johnson Foundation may influence your focus toward community-based programs for childhood obesity. Working for the Kaiser Family Foundation may influence that your policy focus will be on the impact of childhood obesity on the cost of state Medicaid programs.

It is important to remember that there are medical and public health professionals with knowledge and expertise that can assist you in focusing on a particular topic that is ripe for policy action. See **Breakout Box 11.1**. Congressional staffers, organizationally based policy persons, lobbyists, and others might have valuable insights and information that can assist you in crafting a statement of your particular policy issue.

Breakout Box 11.1

THE WASHINGTON STATE "LOCAL FARMS–HEALTHY KIDS" ACT: POLICY ISSUE STATEMENT (STATE LEVEL)

In 2008, Washington State enacted the Local Farms–Healthy Kids (LFHK) Act (2008) in order to increase access to healthy foods and expand markets for local agricultural products (Washington Environmental Council, 2013). Among its many provisions, the LFHK Act established a state farm-to-school program within the Washington State Department of Agriculture to increase procurement of locally grown foods by connecting schools with farmers and providing technical assistance. Funds were appropriated to implement the legislation, including funding to establish a grants program to allow schools to purchase nutritious, locally produced snacks. Additionally, the Act expanded funding for the Women, Infants, and Children (WIC) and Seniors Farmers Market Nutrition Programs and created pilot projects for food banks to purchase fresh food directly from Washington farms. Programs included in the legislation aimed to make it easier for low-income families to obtain Washington-grown food. A Farmers Market Technology Improvement Pilot Program also enabled farmers markets to accept electronic payment cards, including electronic benefits transfers (EBTs) to increase usage of food stamp benefits at farmers markets.

The LFHK Act established Washington State as a national leader in promoting policies to provide healthy, locally grown food to people who need it most. A broad coalition of environmental, farming, education, and public health interests worked together to push the legislation through (Johnson et al., 2013). Through their collaborative efforts, they helped the state legislature to recognize the following principles, which became the foundation of the policy issue statement (Johnson et al., 2013, 176–178):

(1) The legislature recognizes that the benefits of local food production include stewardship of working agricultural lands; direct and indirect jobs in agricultural production, food processing, tourism, and support industries; energy conservation and greenhouse gas reductions; and increased food security through access to locally grown foods.

(2) The legislature finds there is a direct correlation between adequate nutrition and a child's development and school performance. Children who are hungry or malnourished are at risk of lower achievement in school.

(3) The legislature further finds that adequate nutrition is also necessary for the physical health of adults, and that some communities have limited access to healthy fruits and vegetables and quality meat and dairy products, a lack of which may lead to high rates of diet-related diseases.

(4) The legislature believes that expanding market opportunities for Washington farmers will preserve and strengthen local food production and increase the already significant contribution that agriculture makes to the state and local economies.

(5) The legislature finds that the state's existing procurement requirements and practices may inhibit the purchase of locally produced food.

(6) The legislature intends that the LFHK Act strengthen the connections between the state's agricultural industry and the state's food procurement procedures in order to expand local agricultural markets, improve the nutrition of children and other at-risk consumers, and have a positive impact on the environment.

References

Johnson, D. B., Cheadle, A., Podrabsky, M., Quinn, E., MacDougall, E., Cechovic, K., Kovacs, T., Lane, C., Sitaker, M., Chan, N., & Allen, D. (2013). Advancing nutrition and obesity policy through cross-sector collaboration: The Local Farms–Healthy Kids initiative in Washington State. *Journal of Hunger & Environmental Nutrition*, 8(2), 171–186. https://doi.org/10.1080/19320248.2012.761575

The Local Farms–Healthy Kids Act, S.B. 6483 (2008). https://www.washingtonvotes.org/2008-SB-6483

Washington Environmental Council. (2013). *Local Farms, Healthy Kids*. Author. https://wecprotects.org/victories/local-farms-healthy-kids/

WHAT DOES A POLICY ISSUE STATEMENT LOOK LIKE?

This section of the analysis can be relatively brief. Your policy background has provided you with data and information on the history of the problem as well as its significance and potential relationships with other policy areas. The Policy

Background Section should support your narrowing of the policy issue. Your literature section has provided evidence that support the narrowed policy analysis.

First, it should concisely describe the substantive focus of the policy initiative with a brief rationale as to why this is the focus. Second, it also needs to provide a description of the political unit or units that ought to be addressing the issue. The political unit can be the United States, a particular state, a county within a state, or a municipality/political decision-making body within a particular area (e.g., a local school board). You need to make a choice here, because the politics and the legal authority of the level of government will be important in the evolution of the policy proposal.

The statement needs to be brief to bring focus to the rest of the analysis. An important element in the statement is that it should not foreshadow the solution. The problem should not be stated that there is a lack of vaccination sites or the need for additional public health data collection. Vaccination sites may be adequately distributed, but the problem may be a maldistribution of staffing. Additional data collection may be too expensive, and the level of additional specificity obtained from additional data may not be really necessary. A different type of analysis of existing data may be what is needed. The policy problem statement must not make the solution self-evident. The purpose of the analysis is to sort through potential policy alternatives and come up with a recommendation based on data and political considerations.

This statement will have major implications for all the subsequent sections such as developing the criteria for success, the review of policy options, and policy framing covered the remaining parts of your analysis. Although this might be the shortest section, it is perhaps the most critical step in the process.

Let us assume that the policy issue that you or your employer wish to address is "reducing childhood obesity in the United States." See **Breakout Box 11.2** for an example of a policy statement. You have a particular part of the obesity problem (children) as well as a geopolitical area (United States). You could narrow this by targeting school-age children or only elementary school–age children. You could have narrowed the geographic area to a particular state, county, or local unit of government. You could have chosen to focus on a particular school district and its governing board or a state board of education. Instead, you have broadened the geopolitical focus to include the entire country. By selecting the United States, you have consciously taken a bigger geopolitical unit in order to have a potentially greater impact on the problem. Since the federal government does not have direct control of school-age children, you have also complicated the mechanisms by which the policy can be implemented. Federal action is likely to rely upon voluntary state participation with perhaps enticing federal funding to gain adoption. These are all trade-offs that you have consciously made.

Federal influence over school-based programs generally comes by means of federal grants. We discussed the difference between categorical grants and block grants under the discussion of federalism in Chapter 2. The issue of federal leverage over grants to states has become more complicated since the U.S. Supreme Court (USSC) decision in *National Federation of Independent Business v. Sebelius* (2012). Refer back to **Breakout Box 5.3**. Recall that the majority opinion indicated that states could not be forced to adopt the Medicaid requirements of the ACA legislation under penalty of losing all their federal Medicaid monies. This

Breakout Box 11.2

POLICY ISSUE STATEMENT EXAMPLE (NATIONAL LEVEL)

Childhood obesity is a serious public health concern in the United States. Currently, one out of five children in the United States are considered obese (Centers for Disease Control and Prevention [CDC], n.d.). Obesity rates in the United States have increased over time. Among children and adolescents ages 2 to 19 years, the prevalence of obesity in the United States was 19.7% in 2017 to 2020, affecting approximately 14.7 million children and adolescents (Boutari & Mantzoros, 2022). There are disparities in obesity rates across population subgroups. For example obesity prevalence is estimated at 26.2% among Hispanic children, 24.8% among non-Hispanic Black children, 16.6% among non-Hispanic White children, and 9.0% among non-Hispanic Asian children. Thus, obesity remains a serious public health concern for the nation (Robert Wood Johnson Foundation, 2016; Whiteman, 2013). The *Healthy People 2030* goal is to reduce the proportion of obesity among children and adolescents to 15.5% (Office of Disease Prevention and Health Promotion, n.d.).

Obese children are at a much greater risk of chronic disease and cognitive disorders than children of normal weight, resulting in higher care costs (Trasande & Chatterjee, 2009). Because childhood obesity is highly correlated with adult obesity, comprehensive national interventions are necessary to address the epidemic of childhood obesity. The costs associated with childhood obesity are estimated to be $14 billion annually in direct health expenses (Robert Wood Johnson Foundation, 2021; Trasande & Chatterjee, 2009). Enabling people to people access nutritious foods that support their calorie needs and assuring safe places for physical activity can reduce obesity among children and adolescents.

References

Boutari, C., & Mantzoros, C. S. (2022). A 2022 update on the epidemiology of obesity and a call to action: As its twin COVID-19 pandemic appears to be receding, the obesity and dysmetabolism pandemic continues to rage on. *Metabolism, 133*, 155217. https://doi.org/10.1016/j.metabol.2022.155217

Centers for Disease Control and Prevention. (n.d.). *Overweight & obesity: Childhood obesity facts*. U.S. Department of Health and Human Services. https://www.cdc.gov/obesity/data/childhood.html

Office of Disease Prevention and Health Promotion. (n.d.). *Reduce the proportion of children and adolescents with obesity*. U.S. Department of Health and Human Services. https://health.gov/healthypeople/objectives-and-data/browse-objectives/overweight-and-obesity/reduce-proportion-children-and-adolescents-obesity-nws-04/data

Robert Wood Johnson Foundation. (2016, November 30). *Declining childhood obesity rates*. RWJF. https://www.rwjf.org/en/library/research/2016/06/declining-childhood-obesity-rates.html

Robert Wood Johnson Foundation. (2021, October 13). The *state of childhood obesity—Helping all children grow up healthy*. https://stateofchildhoodobesity.org

Trasande, L., & Chatterjee, S. (2009). The impact of obesity on health service utilization and costs in childhood. *Obesity, 17*(9), 1749–1754. https://doi.org/10.1038/oby.2009.67

Whiteman, H. (2013, August 8). U.S. child obesity rates are dropping, says CDC. *Medical News Today.* http://www.medicalnewstoday.com/articles/264548

has allowed states the ability to refuse to participate in the Patient Protection and Affordable Care Act (PPACA) Medicaid expansion without the threat of losing federal money for the other parts of their Medicaid program. While the Court has long recognized the ability of the federal government to put restrictions on the use of federal money by state and local governments, including the threat of the withdrawal of funds, the Court for the first time decided that the threat of losing all Medicaid money crossed the line in terms of a federal "compulsion" of the states to adopt the PPACA Medicaid expansion. However, the Court refused to provide any criteria as to when the line of "compulsion" had been crossed. The issue of when federal requirements become "compulsive" is a whole new arena of policy and court battles. Understanding the political climate of the country, a state, or region is important in deciding which geopolitical unit you feel is most conducive to your policy initiative.

FRAMING

One of the basic techniques of influencing the policy process is called framing the policy issue. Legislation is complex. Any piece of legislation tries to do multiple things. To the public, the legislation can often be confusing. Framing is basically a marketing tool for policy makers to get people to think about the legislation through a particular lens or "frame." It attempts to align a policy with an underlying value or emotion. You want climate change legislation to be framed as protecting the environment for future generations or creating new jobs and not as being anti–fossil fuel or creating job loss. Framing provides the lens through which your proposal is seen. Major opponents of your proposal will attempt to re-frame the policy/program to bring attention to their opposition. The frame is likely to be a simplification of the policy/program and maybe a purposeful distortion of the proposal. For example, the battle over immigration becomes a battle of framing, protecting the border and jobs versus providing the land of opportunity and a refuge for persecuted. If a frame sticks in the public's mind, it will influence how the public and other stakeholders perceive the policy (Wang et al., 2012). The frame will be reinforced by news and social media to send direct and/or subliminal signals as to what the policy/bill is all about. The proposal can be perceived as "protecting our children" or "overreaching big government." The side that wins in the framing battle has an advantage in the rest of the legislative struggle. Issues frequently get reduced to simple phrases such as "right to life," "choice," "pathway to citizenship," "clemency," "big government," "Obamacare," and so forth. One of the major elements in a successful legislative strategy is to be proactive in framing the issue. Breakout Box 11.1 provides an example of framing. Notice how the Washington State legislature framed the issue as strengthening the connections between the state's agricultural industry and the state's food procurement procedures.

When considering policy framing, the role of values becomes critical. Because you have already examined which values are at stake in this policy proposal, you already have an advantage in framing the issue. What values can you build upon? Which values will your opponents use to frame the issue differently? How can your policy issue be framed to draw the support of as many stakeholders as possible or make it more politically difficult to oppose? In framing the issue of childhood obesity, one could use the evidence that children who have more access to exercise have better learning outcomes (CDC, 2014). The frame might then be "academic improvement" rather than "reducing in-class contact time."

Thinking about framing at this stage of the policy process will help your policy maker think about messaging and developing materials to market the proposal to various stakeholders. Political messaging has become quite sophisticated, often involving outside marketing and communications professionals depending on the scope of the policy. Some of it may be very direct and some very subliminal in getting people to support your policy proposal. Stakeholders you previously identified as having deep financial pockets could be important in financing your messaging later in the policy process. Political messaging plays an important role in speech writing, press conferences, campaign strategy, website design, E-blasts, lobbying, and so forth. At this stage, you are not concerned so much with political messaging as with creating a frame for the issue. However, your policy maker's initial press release or news conference may take advantage of your efforts at framing the issue.

In public health, the PHRASES[1] toolkit provides a helpful way to think about framing the issue. PHRASES offers a set of 10 recommendations for effective framing (see Exhibit 11.1). The toolkit also includes a checklist for using clear language that nonexperts are more likely to understand and remember.

There are many other good references about framing and culturally targeted messages (Balls-Berry et al., 2016; Lucas et al., 2021). We encourage readers to access additional references and/or seek the advice of a communications specialist. The FrameWorks Institute (www.frameworksinstitute.org/issues/health) has many publicly available resources about framing public health issues.

EXHIBIT 11.1. PHRASES—RECOMMENDATIONS FOR FRAMING THE ISSUE

Framing tips for public health professionals:

1. Demonstrate your familiarity with the sectors you wish to engage. Refer to the Health in All Policies approach (Chapter 1, **Breakout Box 1.3**) and your stakeholder analysis (Chapter 12) to support this step. Qualitative research methods (e.g., key informant interviews with stakeholders) can also be very helpful if time and resources permit. Examples can be found at www.phrases.org/framing-tools/framing-recommendations-1.

2. Explain the social determinants of health using the foundations of community health metaphor:

   Example 1: Building metaphor: A healthy community is like a building—it depends on a strong and stable foundation. Every sector contributes to laying that foundation, and we all depend on its durability to prop us up. Factors like steady employment, quality education, and safe housing form the base of a functioning society by supporting vibrant communities, strong economies, and long-lasting good health for everyone.

(continued)

---

1 To access the PHRASES (2020) Toolkit, please see www.phrases.org/wp-content/uploads/2020/07/Public-Health-Communications-Toolkit-Final_.pdf.

EXHIBIT 11.1. PHRASES—RECOMMENDATIONS FOR FRAMING THE ISSUE (*continued*)

Example 2: Tree metaphor: A healthy community is like a tree—it depends on strong and stable roots. Every sector contributes to strengthening those roots, and we all depend on the roots to enable use to grow and thrive. Factors like steady employment, quality education, and safe housing form the roots of a functioning society by supporting vibrant communities, strong economies, and long-lasting good health for everyone.
3. Illustrate how the field of public health is changing to meet 21st century needs. For example, think about how the planetary determinants of health (Chapter 1) and the data science methods (Chapter 8) are providing transformative new directions in public health.   Example: "Public health is adapting to meet 21st-century needs, and generating cutting-edge knowledge about how health outcomes are influenced—in both positive and negative ways—by nearly all aspects of social life. For example, public health research has shown that teen suicide rates can be significantly reduced when teachers receive standard professional training in how to support positive mental health for their students, and are able to recognize early signs of mental illness" (PHRASES, n.d.-a, "Framing Can Help").
4. Leverage allies and collaborators working in other sectors, as well as within public health and clinical care, to develop cohesive messages. Refer to Chapter 12, Stakeholder Analysis, to help support this step.
5. Frame collaboration as empowerment. Describe how public health policy proposes to support another stakeholder's mission goes a long way toward helping its professionals see collaboration as an asset.
6. Appeal to the stakeholder values you have identified. For example, appeal to the value of investing in long-term economic gains (see Chapter 15, **Breakout Box 15.1**, The Fresh Food Financing Initiative).
7. Share success stories that connect and reinforce cross-sector collaborations and show progress toward mutual goals. Qualitative research methods such as Photovoice (2007), participatory photo mapping (Dennis et al., 2009), and participatory geographic information systems (GIS) can assist with illustrating success stories.
8. Emphasize health data science expertise. Research suggests that data science expertise can be very enticing to other sectors and stakeholders. See Chapter 8 to support you with this step and/or collaborate with data science professionals.   Example: "Much like a GPS system, public health professionals draw on data to help other sectors plan the best way forward, navigating gridlock when needed and continually responding to new input. We help guide communities to where they want to be by distilling the information that helps them visualize the path ahead, and innovate new visions for what destinations are possible" (PHRASES, n.d.-b, "Framing Can Help").

(*continued*)

EXHIBIT 11.1. PHRASES—RECOMMENDATIONS FOR FRAMING THE ISSUE (*continued*)

9. Keep it positive, while also being scientifically accurate.

   Example: "We know that teachers and administrators care deeply about the health of their students, which is why public health wants to work with the education sector to tackle childhood obesity. We can help garner public support for policies that give young people increased access to nutritious foods and regular physical activity, which would help alleviate numerous health challenges and improve educational outcomes too" (PHRASES, n.d.-c, "Framing Can Help").

References

Dennis, S. F., Jr., Gaulocher, S., Carpiano, R. M., & Brown, D. (2009). Participatory photo mapping (PPM): Exploring an integrated method for health and place research with young people. *Health & Place, 15*(2), 466–473. https://doi.org/10.1016/j.healthplace.2008.08.004

Photovoice. (2007). *Manual and resource kit: Photovoice 2007*. NACCHO. https://www.naccho.org/uploads/downloadable-resources/Programs/Public-Health-Infrastructure/Photovoice-Manual.pdf

PHRASES. (n.d.-a). *10 framing recommendations: Framing receommendation 3*. https://www.phrases.org/framing-tools/framing-recommendations-3

PHRASES. (n.d.-b). *10 framing recommendations: Framing receommendation 9*. https://www.phrases.org/framing-tools/framing-recommendations-9

PHRASES. (n.d.-c). *10 framing recommendations: Framing receommendation 10*. https://www.phrases.org/framing-tools/framing-recommendations-10

SUMMARY

The important aspect for this section is to provide specificity for your policy analysis and protentional initiative. First, you need to decide which part of the larger policy problem that you intend to address through your analysis. In addition, you needed to select a particular geopolitical/political unit for addressing the issue. This involves weighing the legal authority, the geographic area of the political unit, as well as the political climate and culture. Your statement of the problem needs to be specific, but not forecast an obvious solution. Be sensitive to how you are framing the issue throughout the process. The statement will become important in the later stages of the analysis when we develop the criteria for success. How will we determine if or when the policy has been successful? The next sections of your policy analysis will be predicated on a clear and concise statement of the specific policy issue.

DISCUSSION QUESTIONS

- What are the most effective ways of deciding how to frame a policy issue?

- Analyze and critique how Washington State framed the issue of Healthy Kids in **Breakout Box 11.1**.

- Analyze and critique the policy issue statement for childhood obesity in **Breakout Box 11.2**.

- Given current public health issues being discussed, which side has effectively framed the policy issue? Defend your answer. You may draw upon the PHRASES approach or other approaches you may have learned about.

- Using a different current public health issue being discussed, how would you frame the policy issue? Defend your answer.

KEY TERMS

framing
policy issue statement

PHRASES

 A robust set of instructor resources designed to supplement this text is located at http://connect.springerpub.com/content/book/978-0-8261-8543-3. Qualifying instructors may request access by emailing textbook@springerpub.com.

REFERENCES

Balls-Berry, J. E., Hayes, S., Parker, M., Halyard, M., Enders, F., Albertie, M., Pinn, V., & Radecki Breitkopf, C. (2016). The effect of message framing on African American women's intention to participate in health-related research. *Journal of Health Communication*, 21(5), 527–533. https://doi.org/10.1080/10810730.2015.1103333

Centers for Disease Control and Prevention. (2014, May 5). *Health and academic achievement.* https://www.cdc.gov/healthyyouth/health_and_academics/pdf/health-academic-achievement.pdf

Lucas, T., Thompson, H. S., Blessman, J., Dawadi, A., Drolet, C. E., Hirko, K. A., & Penner, L. A. (2021). Effects of culturally targeted message framing on colorectal cancer screening among African Americans. *Health Psychology*, 40(5), 305–315. https://doi.org/10.1037/hea0001073

National Federation of Independent. Business v. Sebelius, 567 U.S. 519 (2012). https://www.supremecourt.gov/opinions/11pdf/11-393c3a2.pdf

Ogden, C. L., Carroll, M. D., Curtin, L. R., Lamb, M. M., & Flegal, K. M. (2010). Prevalence of high body mass index in US children and adolescents, 2007–2008. *Journal of the American Medical Association*, 303(3), 242–249. https://doi.org/10.1001/jama.2009.2012

Wang, Y. C., Orleans, C. T., & Gortmaker, S. L. (2012). Reaching the *Healthy People* goals for reducing childhood obesity. *American Journal of Preventive Medicine*, 42(5), 437–444. https://doi.org/10.1016/j.amepre.2012.01.018

CHAPTER 12

STAKEHOLDER ANALYSIS

In this policy analysis framework, stakeholder analysis becomes an important component of the political feasibility of any policy alternatives. In this chapter we focus on the need to identify the values held by the various people and organizations that are impacted by a specific health policy. Next, we suggest some criteria and tools that can be used to evaluate the potential impact of stakeholders.

THE ROLE OF VALUES

In Chapters 1 and 2, we discuss the centrality of values in the political system. Here you need to be clear what values your policy proposal or program might impact. Values become the basis for support or opposition by various segments of the population. Some policy issues are more controversial and divisive within society than others. Policies may allow individuals freedom to do things, prevent people from doing things, or require people to do things they may not wish to do on their own volition. The COVID-19 pandemic provides a clear example of the acceptance/rejection of vaccination policies based on values. Some people believe that a mandatory vaccination policy provides for the general welfare due to the scientific basis for its effectiveness in minimizing the spread of disease, hospitalization, and/or death. Others believe that the science behind the vaccines is sufficient but that it should not be mandatory. Others believe that the science of effectiveness is not proved or that the vaccine may have significant side effects. Others believe that regardless of the science, mandatory vaccination interferes with individual freedom and is an overreach by the government. Others believe mandatory vaccination of minors weakens parental control. Others believe mandatory vaccinations will lead to exorbitant corporate profits at public expense. One needs to delineate the major values that will probably be impacted by a policy and how widespread and how intensely they are held. Widespread but loosely held values may be less important than intensely held values by a relatively small group. As noted in the description of democratic pluralism, those impacted by intensely held values are more likely to organize and attempt to influence policy process.

By being as clear as possible about the underlying values of a given program/policy, you can begin to understand the potential support and opposition the policy will face (Clark, 2002). It might be useful to list some general values that are important for multiple policy issues. Some of these (in no particular order) might include:

- Physical safety
- Individual freedom
- Freedom from adverse conditions (e.g., freedom from second-hand smoke; freedom from poor air quality; freedom from unsafe school environments)
- Religious freedom
- Family
- Community
- The Second Amendment
- Equity
- Equality
- Efficiency
- Limited government
- Justice
- Reducing social and/or economic disparities
- Education
- Free enterprise
- National security
- Health security
- Privacy
- Parental control
- Healthy communities
- Sustainability

You can add to this list of values. All of these values and many others may be held by various population segments within a geopolitical system and at various levels of intensity. There are periods in which a geopolitical system may reorder its values. For example, after a mass shooting of children there may be a reordering of priorities to allow for the passage of some form of gun legislation. Situations change and so does society's perception of where that balance lies between conflicting values.

EXAMPLE OF STAKEHOLDERS IN CHILD OBESITY

Despite the assumption that having healthy children might be a fairly universal value for a society, it is important not to assume that dealing with childhood obesity in a school setting is without value conflict. If there is a focus on food and obesity in public schools what happens to children who are already obese? Will this new policy lead to more homeschooling to avoid the proposed policy? Will a focus on not being obese have an adverse effect on eating disorders in public schools? Will there be an unintended increase in bullying within the school?

No matter what the policy area you are analyzing, there are value considerations to consider. Often, in public health, more conflict arises around the solution to a problem than the existence of a problem. While there may be relatively widespread consensus that climate change is occurring, people will have very different perspectives on how various proposed solutions will personally affect their lives. Should there be stronger penalties for companies that continue to pollute? Should there be financial incentives for energy conservation or renewable energy sources? It is important to be straightforward in addressing the underlying values of your policy because the penalty will be being surprised by the level and intensity of the opposition to your policy or not taking advantage of natural allies who can assist you in the political process. Either of these can be fatal to the enactment of your policy initiative.

Authority over children is an important aspect of the social system. The political process has already taken away a child's freedom by compelling them to attend a public, private, or home school until they reach a prescribed age or level of education. Mandatory elementary and secondary education is seen as a public good. The state has prescribed a particular curriculum to be covered and sometimes even determines what texts must be used. Both children and parents face penalties for violating these policies.

One of the elements that make childhood obesity an attractive area for policy intervention is that schools already have "control" over the activity of the students during a substantial portion of their weekdays during the school year. Therefore, adjusting this school environment to accommodate a program on obesity could be very incremental and may be a more readily acceptable policy option (National Collaborative on Childhood Obesity Research, 2022).

However, one must recognize that the amount of time in school is already accounted for by current activities. To fight obesity a school could develop a nutrition program. However, that might require reallocating resources or extending the school day, both of which have both positive and negative consequences. The school system might have to find additional competent individuals to teach nutrition or train existing staff in how to apply nutrition lessons. A new nutrition program may result in opposition from teachers and administrators who value focusing on the "basics" in education and oppose spending time on material that they feel parents should be teaching their own children. Opposition might arise from taxpayers due to the increased costs involved. School administrators may not want to lose the money from companies allowed to install their soda/candy machines inside the school.

Increasing the amount of physical exercise within the school day might also raise concerns about the additional costs or potential conflicts with the school's organized sport teams. How are children with disabilities to be accommodated by a policy of increased physical activity in the school day? By addressing these value conflicts, you will begin to see that confronting obesity in the school system is more complex than you initially thought it to be.

In addition, students are only controlled by the school system part of their day. If you focus on a school-based program, will that be sufficient to have a substantial impact on obesity? Outside school, children are subjected to a different variety of influences. They could rush to the convenience store next to the school and minimize any impact of the school's program. They will be influenced by social media advertisements designed to make products appealing to them (Coleman et al., 2022). Fast food chains develop playgrounds and giveaway toys to increase sales volume. As children age, they acquire their own purchasing power. Large and small stores will resist laws restricting marketing practices in the name of free enterprise, corporate profits, and loss of jobs. These values will prompt some to resist social regulations/laws infringing on their ability to sell their products and services to children. Some of these claims will be legitimate and some of these claims may have little substance. Which of these legitimate claims can be overcome through accommodation or compromise?

STAKEHOLDER ANALYSIS

Stakeholders are those that are intensely interested in the outcome of policy debates for that policy area. They are the prime actors in democratic pluralism. Stakeholders only have political power if they aggregate and create organized groups. As you learned in Chapter 4, those groups that are large and more tightly organized tend to have more political power because they can focus their resources (time, money, political action, lobbying, etc.) at critical points in the political policy process. Some groups might have vast resources to spend on mass media campaigns for or against a policy proposal. Other groups might have an effective communication network by which e-mails can deluge a legislator's office in a matter of hours.

Some stakeholders, especially those with great resources, will be actively monitoring legislative initiatives submitted to legislative committees and will become aware of any efforts that might impinge on their activities. Technology has allowed these monitoring activities to engage in almost instantaneous and daily communication with identified supporters. Some organizations have extensive policy sections with people hired either on retainer or who are full-time employees who will readily assist policy makers to write legislation, provide data, or lobby key political participants. Other stakeholders may initially be more passive about the issue, but when prompted by others will act. Some may not consider the issue to be of critical importance but be willing to reciprocate support to a group that has supported their causes in the past. Coalitions of stakeholders might be briefly created over a particular issue and then fall apart once the issue has been resolved. Other coalitions may be more permanent.

Some individuals may be so moved by the policy issue that they will create a new grassroots organization specifically for that issue. It may appear as a genuine voice of the citizens. Alternatively, some organizations may be created to look like grassroots organizations of local constituents but are funded by large commercial organizations to look like a genuine grassroots organization (AstroTurf organizations). One of the characteristics of the current political climate is the rise of Internal Revenue Service Section 501(c)(4) "social welfare" groups that gain tax exempt status but that can actively lobby and support political causes during elections but are not under any obligation to report who has provided financial support to that organization. These are just some examples of the types of stakeholders who exist or will emerge as the policy process evolves (Malloy et al., 2022; see Appendix for additional examples on climate change and environmental justice). Since most policy proposals have been introduced before, some of these groups will have previous working relationships with each other.

The task in stakeholder analysis is not to become overwhelmed by potential obstacles, but rather to recognize where potential opposition and support may develop as you move through the policy process. Qualitative research methods (described in Chapter 9) and social network analysis (SNA; Otte & Rousseau, 2002) can be helpful in conducting a stakeholder analysis. For example, Friedrichs et al. (2022) utilize a case study approach to describe organizing a coalition of interdisciplinary healthcare stakeholders to address the health impacts of climate change in the state of New Hampshire.

All stakeholders are not equal. You may have millions of individual stakeholders in support of your policy, but one small but highly organized and politically connected stakeholder could derail or support your policy's progression. In the Friedrichs et al. (2022) example, healthcare professionals are a very important stakeholder group because research suggests they are among the most trusted messengers of information about climate change (Kreslake, 2019). National companies and organizations with large resources can quickly overwhelm a school district, county, state, or even the federal government.

As you will remember from democratic pluralism, the first characteristic of stakeholder power is the nature of its organization. To be effective stakeholders must be well organized. Health policy issues frequently impact older adults, but it is due to organizations such as AARP and National Committee to Protect Social Security and Medicare that their voice becomes meaningful in policy debates. Similarly, the poor and disenfranchised, although large in number, are frequently left out of policy debates due to their lack of organization and resources.

There are some questions you might want to answer regarding your group of stakeholders. When an organization purports to represent a given constituency, what percentage belong? What is the organization's ability to quickly mobilize its members for action? What is the organization's ability to fund a continuous lobbying activity? What is the reputation of the organization regarding the credibility of its past statements and positions? Can the organization fund or conduct its own research and policy analysis? What technology capability does it have to assist in a policy debate? What personal political connections does the organization have with existing policy makers? What is the organization's ability to punish politicians (e.g., campaign contributions) who disagree with its positions?

Stakeholders will come to the policy debate with a different set of resources. Some may have data. Some may have money. Some may have personal political contacts. Some may have a substantial number of members located in key legislative districts but not have a great deal of money. All of these characteristics impact their ability to influence the policy process. In short, what value does this stakeholder's support or opposition provide? In developing a policy initiative, it is important to understand who these important stakeholders might be and how they will respond to your policy analysis.

There is one set of stakeholders that is more important than others, those that potentially can block your policy initiative. Their importance is due to the previously described structure, process, and culture of the U.S. political system. Defeat in one legislative committee within one chamber of the legislature may be sufficient to end your policy proposal. Unlike you, your opponents need only one chamber or one powerful committee chair to win the policy debate. Strategies that can help you get your policy proposal adopted are discussed in Chapter 15.

Given multiple interests, stakeholders will prioritize their issues and the policy arenas in which they are prepared to defend those interests. While a local or state policy initiative that may initially appear to be relatively insignificant nationally, it can attract opposition of significant national organizations. They may want to defeat even a minor policy initiative in a small state to prevent it from gaining a foothold of political legitimacy and be copied by other jurisdictions. On the other hand, a stakeholder may devote token resources, but not an extensive amount of resources, to any particular issue. There are some large interest groups representing a very eclectic membership that are differentially impacted by the same policy. That stakeholder may be unwilling or unable to take an active position on that issue due to a division of opinion among its membership.

The advocacy coalition theory (Jenkins-Smith & Sabatier, 1994; Sabatier & Jenkins-Smith, 1993) can be useful when thinking about how stakeholders organize around policy issues. Advocacy coalitions comprise groups of stakeholders and policy actors who may interact to work toward shared policy goals or to advance shared values. Additionally, as described by Malloy and Ashcraft (2020), coalitions can sometimes be expanded to include latent actors, such as members of disadvantaged groups, who may not be as organized or mobilized compared to groups with more wealth or power. The authors provide an example of implementing socially just climate adaptation policies and plans (Malloy & Ashcraft, 2020). Expanding advocacy coalitions to include communities affected by environmental justice concerns can be an important outcome of a well-constructed Health Impact Assessment (HIA) process as described in Chapter 7.

You will need to carefully consider the values that are being impacted by your policy and then identify critical stakeholders. One of the values we identified earlier was parental control. This value may be closely aligned with values associated with individual freedom. At the local level, some issues and parents may be very influential people within the community as seen with the politicization of Critical Race Theory. There is a national group (Parental Rights Foundation, 2022) that is proposing a constitutional amendment on parental rights. One would want to evaluate the potential impact of such an amendment, its likelihood of passing, and what this organization's position might be regarding obesity. There are groups such as the National Parents' Rights Association (2015) as well as other groups who may decide to take a position on childhood obesity. Alternatively, there are organizations such as the World Health Organization that feel childhood obesity is an important public health issue and have specific policy recommendations on that topic (World Health Organization, 2016). You want to evaluate the political sophistication and power of potential stakeholders.

The mandate by the Patient Protection and Affordable Care Act (PPACA) to require menu nutrition information has increased the political attention of fast-food chains and their political organizations. They have monetary resources as well as a geographically diffuse group of local franchise owners that can be politically activated very quickly. Farmers assisted by federal corn subsidies will not want those subsidies impacted because of an attack on corn syrup. Convenience store owners will resist attacks on their ability to sell profitable items or be located near schools. Major soft drink manufacturers and local distributors will also resist policies that might lead to a reduction of sales. Local farmers and public health advocates may be able to form coalitions and craft compromises with potential opponents, thereby garnering enough political support for policy adoption (as was the case in Washington State). Major grocery chains might support subsidies to reduce "food deserts" in inner cities, as was the case in the Pennsylvania Food Financing Initiative. All of these stakeholders will have a concentrated interest in the outcome of the policy debate on childhood obesity (Rincón-Gallardo Patiño et al., 2020).

Put yourself in the position of as many stakeholders as you can (Vanderlee et al., 2016). This will help you understand the complexity of the policy issue as well as areas of potential compromise, as well as levers for incentivizing cooperation rather than political opposition. Which of these stakeholders, or set of stakeholders, are the most critical for the particular childhood obesity policy being advocated?

Given the limitations of your time and resources, it may be impossible for you to develop an exhaustive list of all stakeholders and complete an analysis of each of their strengths and weaknesses. However, going through the exercise of stakeholder analysis will provide you with insights to the coming political struggles. It is good to take one's best guess at the involved stakeholders to assist in constructing a childhood obesity policy that stands a chance in the political process. It is important to note that additional stakeholders might be added to your current list of stakeholders as the policy expands or contracts due to political compromises. Compromise is a core component of incremental policy making. New grassroots organizations may emerge, and existing stakeholders may create new temporary coalitions.

TOOLS FOR STAKEHOLDER ANALYSIS

Various tools and templates are available to help you organize and analyze information about stakeholders (Brugha & Varvasovszky, 2000). For example, the Centers for Disease Control and Prevention (CDC) Healthy Brain Initiative has a practical qualitative template (see Table 12.1). The CDC POLARIS website also has many helpful tools and resources (www.cdc.gov/policy/polaris/policy process/policy_analysis.html). Brugha and Varvasovszky (2000) provide additional practical guidance.

Developing a Stakeholder Impact Matrix might be useful in terms of quantitatively summarizing the power of major stakeholders, both those tending to favor and those who may oppose a policy initiative on childhood obesity. See Table 12.2. This can also be done informally as part of your writing process. To do this, you would first need to create a list of criteria to measure the political power of

TABLE 12.1 STAKEHOLDER ANALYSIS TEMPLATE (QUALITATIVE)

STAKEHOLDER NAME AND AFFILIATION	CONTACT PERSON (EMAIL, PHONE)	IMPACT: HOW MUCH DOES THE POLICY OR ACTIVITY IMPACT THEM? (LOW, MEDIUM, HIGH)	INFLUENCE: HOW MUCH INFLUENCE DO THEY HAVE? (LOW, MEDIUM, HIGH)	WHAT IS IMPORTANT TO THEM?	HOW COULD THEY CONTRIBUTE TO SUPPORT THE POLICY OR ACTIVITY?	HOW COULD THEY HINDER THE POLICY OR ACTIVITY?	STRATEGY FOR ENGAGING THE STAKEHOLDER

Source: Adapted from Centers for Disease Control and Prevention. (2019, October 24). *Planning for action: Initial steps for implementing the Healthy Brain Initiative road map.* https://www.cdc.gov/aging/healthybrain/pdf/Planning-Guide-HBI-Road-Map-508.pdf

an organization. One could use the size of membership, the amount of financial resources, the level of intensity of the issue for the organization, the ability of the organization to rally its members (unity), its technology capability, the level of ongoing lobbying activity, its ability to inflict punishment on legislators, or other characteristics that you feel measure the power of a stakeholder.

A matrix is only a blunt tool, so the more honestly you construct the tool, the more useful it can be. The matrix is more important as a tool to make you think through the relative importance of various stakeholders than to give you an absolute score. Each measure would need to be scored, perhaps on a scale of 1 to 10. A stakeholder having more members would get a higher membership score. Having a larger budget for lobbying or having a full-time lobbyist would give it a higher score. Having other people in the policy field rate these groups according to your criteria will add some external validity to the index. Even with that, this will not be a precise measure and it will be based on many subjective judgments (e.g., ability to inflict punishment on legislators voting against their positions) as well as more objective facts (e.g., financial resources). For example, you could create categories for financial resources for lobbying with 1 representing $0 to $5,000, 2 representing $5,001 to $20,000, and so forth. These lobbying resources would have to be adjusted based on the geopolitical unit; $2,000 for lobbying a local school board might be a great deal of money while the same amount for lobbying Congress would be inconsequential. The intent is to take one's best estimate of the forces supporting and opposing your policy alternative and to measure them all by the same criteria.

Table 12.2 provides an example of a Stakeholder Impact Matrix that can be used to evaluate stakeholders. Note that some of the criteria that are used are numerical and relatively objective (financial and number of members) while others are more subjective (intensity and unity). An individual author or a group consensus model can be used to evaluate these. The intent is to construct a useful summary of the impact of stakeholders. One would list those that appear to be the most critical supporters or opponents and the most critical characteristics.

Notice in Table 12.2 that Organization A has the highest total score since it has the highest level of financial resources (financial) and a fairly large number of members (members) and feels relatively intense (intense) about this issue area or values. You could also conclude by looking at the organization's history that it has been able to get its members to actively support its policy positions (unity) by getting members to contact legislators or the executive branch. Organization B has a large membership, and it feels intensely about the policy issue. It also has relatively large resources but has historically not been able to mobilize its resources for action.

TABLE 12.2 STAKEHOLDER IMPACT MATRIX (QUANTITATIVE)

ORGANIZATION	FINANCIAL	MEMBERS	INTENSITY	UNITY	TOTAL
A	10	8	8	8	34
B	8	10	10	4	32
C	10	5	2	2	19
D	8	4	8	6	26
E	10	10	4	2	26

Organization C has a great deal of financial resources but scores poorly on other elements in the matrix. Although it has great financial power, it is not likely to engage in this issue perhaps due to it being a low priority on its current legislative agenda or being a divided eclectic organization unable to unite its members on this policy issue. Therefore, it has the least political power of the stakeholders listed.

The Stakeholder Impact Matrix in Table 12.2 assumes that all the elements of the political power index of stakeholders have equal weight. However, you may need one particular stakeholder's asset more than another. You could construct the matrix so that financial resources weigh twice as much as membership or membership weighs 1.5 the value of financial resources. One could do separate Stakeholder Impact Matrices for likely supporting stakeholders and likely opponents. It is less important to have an exact measure of the power index of various stakeholders than it is to begin to evaluate where supporters and opponents of the policy are likely to come from and that general comparisons can be made.

Since this matrix is not an exact measure, the credibility of your analysis will rest on your honesty and objectivity. The intent of a policy analysis is to not only make a recommendation for a policy that is the most effective, efficient, or equitable in solving the policy problem but to also recommend a policy that also has some chance of political success. Most likely you will not put this Stakeholder Impact Matrix in your final document. Indeed, you may merely do this informally and not commit it to paper. However, going through the exercise of evaluating stakeholders either subjectively or objectively is an important step in the analysis.

Another quantitative method that can be used in stakeholder analysis is SNA. In a policy context, SNA is the study of the relationships among stakeholders and the resulting effect on the policy process. SNA can be used to identify connections between stakeholders and to map the flows of information and resources flow between them. The value of SNA is the ability to assess how stakeholders or coalition members influence one another over time. Relationships can be described in terms of the number, length, and strength of social ties; the quality of connections among the network members; and the types of resources exchanged (Varda et al., 2012). Changes in social and political capital can be measured via standard SNA domains such as connectivity, density, centrality, trust, and reciprocity (Gilbert et al., 2022; Sherchan et al., 2013). SNA utilizes mathematical algorithms to analyze these factors and visually represent them in the form of a network map. For example, Brinkley et al. (2021) used SNA to map local food systems and to reveal locations where marketing networks were aligning with concurrent social movements. SNA can also be used evaluatively to identify the conditions and reasons for the varying effectiveness of a coalition's efforts, and to plan, manage, and iteratively improve their process accordingly (Varda, 2011). SNA often requires special software and training in data science methods. A growing body of literature discusses SNA in policy analysis (Smit et al., 2020).

EXAMPLES OF STAKEHOLDERS IN POLICY

As an example of the importance of stakeholders, Breakout Box 12.1 describes the Local Farms–Healthy Kids (LFHK) Act that was passed in Washington State in 2008. It examines the policy development process and how various stakeholders came together to pass the legislation. Breakout Box 12.2 examines another local policy, the menu-labeling regulations in Seattle/King County, to compare and contrast the stakeholder interests and advocacy groups involved. In each case, a diverse group of stakeholders came together as allies. Values and goals had to be clarified, and compromises had to be forged. Breakout Box 12.3 highlights a federal regulation, the U.S. Department of Agriculture (USDA) Smart Snacks in School rule. Once again, pay attention to the inherent value conflicts, the compromises that are reflected in the policy, and the way that scientific information can be used to bridge barriers.

Breakout Box 12.1

LOCAL FARMS–HEALTHY KIDS POLICY DEVELOPMENT IN WASHINGTON STATE

The LFHK policy development process was especially noteworthy because only 9 months elapsed from the first discussion of the idea to the LFHK bill's passage (Johnson et al., 2013). A broad coalition of public health, environmental, farming, and education interests formed a coalition to push the legislation through. The process began when a statewide antipoverty advocacy group convened the first meeting in July 2007 to discuss ways of supporting farm–to–food bank programs. The diverse group of attendees represented advocacy groups, a social service organization, and a large metropolitan health department. As dialogue progressed, the group's focus broadened beyond food banks to bringing local food to institutions, particularly schools. At a second meeting, the group solidified their focus on farm-to-school efforts. The policy director of the Washington Environmental Council (WEC) volunteered to present the issue to the Environmental Priorities Coalition (EPC), a coalition of leading environmental advocacy organizations in the state, for consideration as one of their priority issues for the state's upcoming legislative session.

Because the WEC and EPC had historically focused on issues related to climate change, land use, and water rights, there had occasionally been tension with the interests of farmers. However, the WEC policy leader immediately recognized a way to find common ground. Specifically, the policy director noted that the farm-to-institution effort offered a way to collaborate on an issue that was broadly popular and less contentious. The EPC approved the farm-to-school issue as one of its four priority issues for the 2008 legislative session.

For the remainder of 2007, stakeholders from multiple sectors worked together to draft the legislation. Advocates made a strategic effort to identify and address concerns of potential opponents during the writing process. For example, bill authors struck or negotiated politically sensitive terms (e.g., "organic," "conventional") and made sure to reference all key stakeholders. The final bill included a broad array of strategies designed to benefit vulnerable populations as well as the environment and local farms.

In January 2008, state policy makers introduced an LFHK bill in the Washington State Legislature, where it was assigned to the Senate Committee on Agriculture and Rural Economic Development. Messaging efforts highlighted the bill's benefits for Washingtonians in terms of improving economic vitality for farmers while increasing access to healthy foods for children. Primary responsibility for promoting the bill was given to two experienced lobbyists. The lobbyists recruited a lead legislator for the bill in each legislative chamber and made a successful push to recruit a considerable number of legislators from both Republican and Democratic parties as cosponsors. Advocates secured 51 cosponsors in the House (out of 98 total members) and 33 (out of 49) in the Senate. The LFHK bill passed in March 2008 with only one dissenting vote.

Reference

Johnson, D. B., Cheadle, A., Podrabsky, M., Quinn, E., MacDougall, E., Cechovic, K., Kovacs, T., Lane, C., Sitaker, M., Chan, N., & Allen, D. (2013). Advancing nutrition and obesity policy through cross-sector collaboration: The Local Farms–Healthy Kids Initiative in Washington state. *Journal of Hunger & Environmental Nutrition, 8*(2), 171–186. https://doi.org/10.1080/19320248.2012.761575

Breakout Box 12.2

MENU-LABELING POLICY DEVELOPMENT IN KING COUNTY, WASHINGTON

In the United States, some local health departments have rulemaking authority to regulate restaurants and other food environments (Pomeranz, 2011). For example, in King County, Washington, the Board of Health passed a menu-labeling regulation that required chain restaurants with 15 or more locations nationwide to provide information about calories, saturated fats, carbohydrates, and sodium to customers starting January 1, 2009. King County was the second jurisdiction to require menu labeling (New York City was the first).

To examine the policy processes associated with the passage of restaurant menu-labeling regulations, researchers at the University of Washington utilized qualitative research methods such as document review and key informant interviews with 12 key stakeholders (Johnson et al., 2013). Participants included a representative of the Washington Restaurant Association, three public health practitioners, four members of the Board of Health, and four restaurant owners.

The researchers found that stakeholders could be grouped into two main categories or advocacy coalitions: a public health coalition and an industry coalition. *Advocacy coalitions* are groups of policy actors brought together by their common values and beliefs to advocate for a common policy outcome (Sabatier & Jenkins-Smith, 1993). For example, within these two coalitions, the researchers identified shared values and beliefs about the appropriate role of governmental regulation in protecting population health and the need for environmental change. Policy actors in both coalitions generally shared concerns about the increasing prevalence of obesity and diabetes. They recognized that approximately one third of total calories consumed in the United States come from food eaten away from home, and they also recognized the need for restaurants to be profitable.

However, the process was adversarial at times, as national and state restaurant associations strongly opposed the initiative initially. Industry coalition members believed that menu-labeling regulations may harm the economy, that voluntary mechanisms are more appropriate than regulations, and that it is unfair to "single out" restaurants. In contrast, public health coalition members believed that it is appropriate to use regulations when necessary to protect the health of the community, that population health is a priority, that environmental change is needed to make it easier for people to make healthy choices, and that citizens are entitled to nutrition information.

Value conflicts played out in three major areas: industry freedom versus the consumer's right to know; educational versus regulatory approaches; and the importance of environmental change versus a reliance on individual responsibility make healthy food choices. Representatives of both coalitions came together to hear each other's point of view, and eventually they were able to reach compromises on parts of the regulation (e.g., details about the public display of menu information, and the scope of the requirements). Over time, members of the two coalitions learned from each other and began to trust one another. Members agreed that establishing trust and building relationships throughout the process was a key factor in the policy's ultimate success. Public health staff played a key role in developing scientific briefing papers and providing technical assistance about policy implementation issues. The Board of Health and the restaurant association worked together and eventually developed a menu-labeling policy that was acceptable to both sides. Subsequently, members continued to collaborate in order to revise the regulations so that they would comply with national menu-labeling legislation under the PPACA.

The PPACA Section 4205 requires that standard menu items at qualifying chain restaurants and vending machines have proper nutrition labeling. Although the ACA was signed into federal law in 2010, menu-labeling requirements were not implemented until May 7, 2018, having been delayed several times by the U.S. Food and Drug Administration. The menu-labeling requirements fall under Title IV of the ACA: Prevention of Chronic Disease and Improving Public Health (The White House, 2015).

References

Johnson, D. B., Cheadle, A., Podrabsky, M., Quinn, E., MacDougall, E., Cechovic, K., Kovacs, T., Lane, C., Sitaker, M., Chan, N., & Allen, D. (2013). Advancing nutrition and obesity policy through cross-sector collaboration: The Local Farms–Healthy Kids

Initiative in Washington state. *Journal of Hunger & Environmental Nutrition, 8*(2), 171–186. https://doi.org/10.1080/19320248.2012.761575

Patient Protection and Affordable Care Act, Pub. L. No. 111-148, 124 Stat. 119 (2010). https://www.congress.gov/111/plaws/publ148/PLAW-111publ148.pdf

Pomeranz, J. L. (2011). The unique authority of state and local health departments to address obesi*ty. American Journal of Public Health, 101*(7), 1192–1197. https://doi.org/10.2105/ajph.2010.300023

Sabatier, P., & Jenkins-Smith, H. (1993). *Policy change and learning.* Westview Press.

The White House. (2015). *Title IV. Prevention of chronic disease and improving public health.* https://obamawhitehouse.archives.gov/health-care-meeting/proposal/titleiv

Breakout Box 12.3

SMART SNACKS IN SCHOOL

Children consume up to half of their calories at school each day. On June 27, 2013, the USDA (2013) issued a set of nutrition standards called the Smart Snacks in School rule. It applies to foods and beverages sold in public schools. The last time the USDA updated snack and a la carte food standards was 1979. Congress directed the USDA to update the standards as part of the bipartisan Healthy, Hunger-Free Kids Act of 2010, which requires the USDA to establish nutrition standards for all foods sold in schools beyond the federally supported meals programs.

Because kids have access to less healthy snack food and beverage options, improving school snack foods could have a dramatic effect on their diets. Once implemented, the standards are intended to ensure that snacks in vending machines, school stores, a la carte lines, and snack bars are healthy. A food must be a fruit, a vegetable, protein, dairy, or whole grain; have fewer than 200 calories; and be low in fat, sodium, and sugar. The standards apply to all foods sold before, during, or up to 30 minutes after the school day. Research conducted by the Pew Charitable Trusts shows that the majority of U.S. secondary schools currently do not sell fruits and vegetables in stores, snack bars, or vending machines (The Pew Charitable Trusts, 2013; Donze Black, 2013; Taber et al., 2012).

However, there will be some exceptions to the rule. The standards apply to food sold during the school day, not to food sold during evening or weekend activities such as football games or band concerts. The rule gives states the authority to make exemptions for infrequent fundraiser events, so state leaders will need to make those determinations. If parents, teachers, and students want some occasional departures from the standards, state and local leaders have the option of allowing that. However, some schools have found that they can make just as much money, if not more, with nonfood fundraisers. Schools or districts could choose to apply the standards to all after-school activities, but that is not required by the USDA.

A barrier for many school districts in implementing the standards is the concern that there may be a negative impact on school budgets. However, a recent HIA (Barnes et al., 2021; Health Impact Project, 2012) found that schools that implemented healthier standards for snack and a la carte foods generally broke even or increased food service revenue. This allowed a more acceptable framing, namely, when fewer unhealthy snacks are available, students are more likely to purchase a school meal—a change that benefits both children's health and school budgets. Additional research has demonstrated that students in states with strong school nutrition standards gain less weight than those without such guidelines (Chriqui et al., 2020; Rosenfeld et al., 2016; Taber et al., 2012). Policy Toolkits have also been developed for practitioners (see www.fns.usda.gov/tn/guide-smart-snacks-school and www.fns.usda.gov/tn/local-school-wellness-policy-outreach-toolkit).

References

Barnes, C., McCrabb, S., Stacey, F., Nathan, N., Yoong, S. L., Grady, A., Sutherland, R., Hodder, R., Innes-Hughes, C., Davies, M., & Wolfenden, L. (2021). Improving implementation of school-based healthy eating and physical activity policies, practices, and programs: A systematic review. *Translational Behavioral Medicine, 11*(7), 1365–1410. https://doi.org/10.1093/tbm/ibab037

Chriqui, J. F., Lin, W., Leider, J., Shang, C., & Perna, F. M. (2020). The harmonizing effect of smart snacks on the association between state snack laws and high school students' fruit and vegetable consumption, United States—2005–2017. *Preventive Medicine, 139*, Article 106093. https://doi.org/10.1016/j.ypmed.2020.106093

Donze Black, J. (2013, July 18). *7 questions about smart snacks in school standards.* https://www.pewtrusts.org/en/research-and-analysis/articles/2013/07/18/7-questions-about-smart-snacks-in-school-standards

Health Impact Project. (2012). *Health Impact Assessment: National nutrition standards for snack and a la carte foods and beverages sold in schools.* The Pew Charitable Trusts. https://www.pewtrusts.org/en/search?q=HIA%20food%20a%20la%20carte&sortBy=relevance&sortOrder=asc&page=1

Healthy, Hunger-Free Kids Act, Pub. L. No. 111-296, 124 Stat. 3183 (2010).

The Pew Charitable Trusts. (2013, February 19). *Financial impacts of nutrition standards for snacks sold in schools.* https://www.pewtrusts.org/en/research-and-analysis/articles/2013/02/19/financial-impacts-of-nutrition-standards-for-snacks-sold-in-schools

Rosenfeld, L. E., Cohen, J. F., Gorski, M. T., Lessing, A. J., Smith, L., Rimm, E. B., & Hoffman, J. A. (2016). How do we actually put smarter snacks in schools? NOURISH (nutrition opportunities to understand reforms involving student health) conversations with food-service directors. *Public Health Nutrition, 20*(3), 556–564. https://doi.org/10.1017/s1368980016002044

Taber, D. R., Chriqui, J. F., Perna, F. M., Powell, L. M., & Chaloupka, F. J. (2012). Weight status among adolescents in states that govern competitive food nutrition content. *Pediatrics, 130*(3), 437–444. https://doi.org/10.1542/peds.2011-3353

U.S. Department of Agriculture. (2013, June 27). *Agriculture secretary Vilsack highlights new "smart snacks in school" standards; will ensure school vending machines, snack bars include healthy choices* (Report No. 0134.13). Author. https://www.usda.gov/media/press-releases/2013/06/27/agriculture-secretary-vilsack-highlights-new-smart-snacks-school

SUMMARY

Because the political system determines winners and losers in the contest of values, it is important to understand how your policy will fit with different values and how those values are tied to participants in democratic pluralism. Understanding the value conflicts underlying your proposal will allow you to identify the potential major stakeholders for and against your policy proposal. Knowing the important stakeholders generally comes from political experience and knowledge. Much of this analysis is going to depend on your background and knowledge of the issue and the political power brokers within a particular political setting. Stakeholder analysis is quite subjective. There are tools available to organize your assessment. However, understanding the history of the policy in the past or how it fared in other political jurisdictions will help considerably in gaining insight as to the important stakeholders. If you lack that knowledge directly, access knowledgeable partners who are familiar with the political actors and influencers in your geographic area. These partners can often be found in academic institutions, research consulting firms, and nonprofit organizations.

DISCUSSION QUESTIONS

- Discuss why a stakeholder analysis is critical in health policy development.
- Discuss the pros and cons of quantitative versus qualitative approaches to stakeholder analysis.
- Analyze and critique the handling of stakeholders in the menu labeling example in **Breakout Box 12.2**.
- Using the Smart Snacks example in **Breakout Box 12.3**, list the important stakeholders in your community. Which would be the most important?
- Identify a current issue in public health in your state and list the critical stakeholders.
- Given the stakeholders you just listed, evaluate them in terms of their ability to influence any policy action.

KEY TERMS

advocacy coalition theory
POLARIS
social network analysis

stakeholder impact analysis
stakeholder matrix

A robust set of instructor resources designed to supplement this text is located at http://connect.springerpub.com/content/book/978-0-8261-8543-3. Qualifying instructors may request access by emailing textbook@springerpub.com.

REFERENCES

Brinkley, C., Manser, G. M., & Pesci, S. (2021). Growing pains in local food systems: A longitudinal social network analysis on local food marketing in Baltimore County, Maryland and Chester County, Pennsylvania. *Agriculture and Human Values, 38*(4), 911–927. https://doi.org/10.1007/s10460-021-10199-w

Brugha, R., & Varvasovszky, Z. (2000). Stakeholder analysis: A review. *Health Policy and Planning*, *15*(3), 239–246. https://doi.org/10.1093/heapol/15.3.239

Clark, T. W. (2002). *The policy process: A practical guide for natural resources professionals*. Yale University Press.

Coleman, P. C., Hanson, P., van Rens, T., & Oyebode, O. (2022). A rapid review of the evidence for children's TV and online advertisement restrictions to fight obesity. *Preventive Medicine Reports*, *26*, Article 101717. https://doi.org/10.1016/j.pmedr.2022.101717

Friedrichs, P. E., Thompson, E., Madison, M., Aytur, S., & Thyng, D. (2022). Case study: The rapid growth of an interdisciplinary statewide climate and health movement. *The Journal of Climate Change and Health*, *7*, Article 100165. https://doi.org/10.1016/j.joclim.2022.100165

Gilbert, K. L., Ransome, Y., Dean, L. T., DeCaille, J., & Kawachi, I. (2022). Social capital, Black social mobility, and health disparities. *Annual Review of Public Health*, *43*(1), 173–191. https://doi.org/10.1146/annurev-publhealth-052020-112623

Jenkins-Smith, H. C., & Sabatier, P. A. (1994). Evaluating the advocacy coalition framework. *Journal of Public Policy*, *14*(2), 175–203. https://doi.org/10.1017/s0143814×00007431

Kreslake J. M. (2019). Perceived importance of climate change adaptation and mitigation according to social and medical factors among residents of impacted communities in the United States. *Health Equity*, *3*(1), 124–133. https://doi.org/10.1089/heq.2019.0002

Malloy, J. T., & Ashcraft, C. M. (2020). A framework for implementing socially just climate adaptation. *Climatic Change*, *160*(1), 1–14. https://doi.org/10.1007/s10584-020-02705-6

Malloy, J. T., Ashcraft, C. M., Kirshen, P., Safford, T. G., Aytur, S. A., & Rogers, S. H. (2022). Implementing just climate adaptation policy: An incremental analysis of recognition, framing, and advocacy coalitions in Boston, U.S.A. *Frontiers in Sustainable Cities*, *4*, 1–13. https://doi.org/10.3389/frsc.2022.928230

National Collaborative on Childhood Obesity Research. (2022, June 7). *Tools*. https://www.nccor.org/nccor-tools

National Parents' Rights Association. (2015). *Know & protect your legal rights as parents*. http://www.npra.info

Otte, E., & Rousseau, R. (2002). Social network analysis: A powerful strategy, also for the information sciences. *Journal of Information Science*, *28*(6), 441–453. https://doi.org/10.1177/016555150202800601

Parental Rights Foundation. (2022, August 9). *Protecting children by empowering parents*. https://parentalrights.org

Rincón-Gallardo Patiño, S., Zhou, M., Da Silva Gomes, F., Lemaire, R., Hedrick, V., Serrano, E., & Kraak, V. I. (2020). Effects of menu labeling policies on transnational restaurant chains to promote a healthy diet: A scoping review to inform policy and research. *Nutrients*, *12*(6), 1544. https://doi.org/10.3390/nu12061544

Sabatier, P., & Jenkins-Smith, H. (1993). *Policy change and learning*. Westview Press.

Sherchan, W., Nepal, S., & Paris, C. (2013). A survey of trust in social networks. *ACM Computing Surveys*, *45*(4), 1–33. https://doi.org/10.1145/2501654.2501661

Smit, L. C., Dikken, J., Schuurmans, M. J., de Wit, N. J., & Bleijenberg, N. (2020). Value of social network analysis for developing and evaluating complex healthcare interventions: A scoping review. *BMJ Open*, *10*(11), Article e039681. https://doi.org/10.1136/bmjopen-2020-039681

Vanderlee, L., Vine, M. M., Fenton, N. E., & Hammond, D. (2016). Stakeholder perspectives on implementing menu labeling in a cafeteria setting. *American Journal of Health Behavior*, *40*(3), 371–380. https://doi.org/10.5993/ajhb.40.3.9

Varda, D. M. (2011). Data-driven management strategies in public health collaboratives. *Journal of Public Health Management and Practice*, *17*(2), 122–132. https://doi.org/10.1097/phh.0b013e3181ede995

Varda, D., Shoup, J. A., & Miller, S. (2012). A systematic review of collaboration and network research in the public affairs literature: Implications for public health practice and research. *American Journal of Public Health*, *102*(3), 564–571. https://doi.org/10.2105/ajph.2011.300286

World Health Organization. (2016). *Report of the commission on ending childhood obesity*. Author. https://www.who.int/publications/i/item/9789241510066

CHAPTER 13

CRITERIA FOR SUCCESS

This chapter focuses on the importance of understanding and explaining exactly what the intended consequences of your policy are to be. This is critical in terms of gaining supportive stakeholders as well as potentially deflecting opposing stakeholders. Such criteria will be important in the future evaluation as to whether the policy has achieved its goals or there is need for policy, administrative or financial adjustments.

LEARNING OBJECTIVES

Be able to:

- Discuss how various stakeholders may define the "success" of a policy in different ways.

- Identify criteria regarding the intended short-term, medium-term, and long-term consequences of your policy.

- Identify specific measurements for your criteria for success.

- Discuss how different stakeholders may view the relative importance of the criteria differently.

- Describe ways to evaluate the effectiveness of a policy.

This topic can normally be briefly covered in your written policy analysis compared to other sections. However, brevity is not related to importance. The basic question that this section seeks to answer is, "What do you want to accomplish by this policy?" This will help you later to answer a corollary question, "How will you know to what degree this policy has been a success or a failure?" These considerations relate to "Policy Evaluation" portions of the policy wheel in Chapter 4. It is important to think about how the policy's success could be evaluated not just after its implementation. Statements of the policy's success in the absence of measurable and preferably agreed-upon outcomes open themselves to subjective interpretation and debate based on rhetoric rather than evidence.

Childhood obesity continues to be a major problem in the United States and globally, but eating disorders (EDs) are also on the rise. Among children and adolescents ages 2 to 19 years, the prevalence of obesity in the United States was 19.7%

in 2017 to 2020, affecting approximately 14.7 million children and adolescents. Research suggests that the prevalence of obesity is also rising rapidly in low- and middle-income countries. However, EDs are also important conditions to address, and the prevalence of both EDs and obesity have been increasing, suggesting that the conditions may share some common risk factors. The policy examples in this book are intended to promote access to healthy foods and safe places for physical activity that support a healthy weight for persons of all ages. Communication science, messaging, and clinical interventions for EDs are evolving, but outside the scope of this text. Recent studies are beginning to examine the effectiveness of integrated prevention approaches that address obesity and EDs simultaneously, often via school-based or psychosocial interventions, but no systematic reviews have been completed at the time of this writing. More research is needed to provide a better understanding of the mechanisms and risk factors that underly these conditions in order to provide tailored and timely treatment (Centers for Disease Control and Prevention [CDC], n.d.-a; Leme et al., 2018; Stabouli et al., 2021).

DEFINITION OF SUCCESS

One must always be careful in attributing causality when dealing with complicated social policies. The increase in obesity rates in the United States is likely to come from several factors in the environment. Attacking one element may have only a marginal impact on a multifactor public health problem. Consequently, your policy may help in solving the problem but not eliminate it. Nonhealth initiatives such improving the economy or a reduction in income disparity may have the most dramatic impact on obesity rates. These macro changes may have little relationship to your proposed policy. However, it is important to provide measures that can focus on the degree that your policy can contribute to the overall solution of this public health problem (Namba et al., 2013). At this stage of the policy analysis process, you need to select a set of methodological data and tools that will help to demonstrate the impact of your proposed policy.

Your proposed measures of success are probably not going to demonstrate causality unless you have developed a rigorous study design with sophisticated analytical models as described in Chapter 9. However, at a minimum, you need to provide some parameters that indicate your policy is having an impact as intended. See **Breakout Box 13.1**. You may be able to assess statistical associations from observational studies or from the literature that support the relationships between the policy and the outcome (Kerr et al., 2013). Short-term goals can facilitate buy-in from stakeholders to support your proposed policy. In addition, they can be used to demonstrate early success or to make a quick adjustment in the implementation phase. Different stakeholders may have different visions as to the definition of success.

One thing that you need to consider in selecting goals for your policy proposal is to remember that policy makers are not known for having a long-term perspective. A politician's time frame tends to be until the next election. Given the need for fund raising for the next election, the time frame can be quite short. Due to their 6-year term of office, U.S. senators generally have the luxury of being able to think further into the future and take more political risks. However, even if a particular politician is not up for re-election, adverse electoral results for their political party may result in a change in legislative leadership and committee chairs. However, short-term returns on public health policies can be problematic since the interactive nature of the exosome may take many years to play out.

Due to policy makers' relatively short-term perspective, a policy that will demonstrate an outcome 10 years from the policy's passage is a harder political sell than one that demonstrates more immediate results. Enacted policies that show immediate positive results can be used to gain political capital. Policy makers in the bureaucracy are less impacted by the election cycle and have a longer policy lens. These differing perspectives have been demonstrated throughout the COVID-19 pandemic (Nayak et al., 2022).

What is important at this stage of your analysis is that you understand what concrete results are expected from your proposed recommended program/policy. The implementation phase will involve writing new regulations or establishing a new set of institutions and/or hiring of additional personnel. The Patient Protection and Affordable Care Act (PPACA) was enacted in 2010. While some elements of the policy were implemented rather quickly after its passage, the enforcement of the individual mandate and the insurance exchanges were designed to take effect 4 years later in January 2014. The actual impact of its major provisions is still being debated. When will concrete outcomes begin to appear and how can they be measured so that your policy maker can claim credit for improving public health?

Some outcomes of programs addressing childhood obesity may not occur until adolescence, adulthood, or even old age. However, you cannot expect people to wait 50 years to see the consequences of your policy proposal. This is especially true during difficult economic times when attempts to cut programs that are underperforming will be high on the legislature's cutting block. Consequently, you need to be explicit as to your policy objectives in the short term, medium term, and long term.

Breakout Box 13.1

MENU LABELING EXAMPLE

Menu labeling has been a recent policy approach intended to help people make more informed choices about the foods they eat. But does it work? New York City implemented the first calorie-posting law in 2008. Philadelphia added a law in 2010 requiring sit-down chain restaurants to list saturated fats, trans fats, carbohydrates, sodium, and total calories beside every menu item. The restaurant industry initially fought hard against menu-labeling laws, but eventually backed a uniform national rule that would preempt all local ordinances. The federal calorie-posting rule, which was part of the 2010 Affordable Care Act, is weaker than what some states had proposed. Intense lobbying about which restaurants/products would be affected has since delayed a final rule. In fact, implementation was not finalized until 2018.

Several research studies have been conducted to evaluate the success of menu-labeling initiatives (Krieger et al., 2013; Liu et al., 2020). For example, researchers in Washington State examined the impact of a menu-labeling regulation in King County, Washington, on calories purchased and awareness and use of labels at 6 and 18 months after policy implementation (Krieger et al., 2013). Although the researchers found no significant changes in calories purchased in the short term (e.g., 6 months after implementation), they did find a modest decrease in the calories purchased after 18 months, particularly among women and patrons of certain types of food chains. The researchers found that the average number of calories per purchase at chain restaurants fell by 38 calories, from 908.5 to 870.4 calories (at coffee chains, the average decrease was 22 calories, from 154.3 to 132.1 calories). After implementation of the policy, food chain customers who reported using calorie information purchased fewer calories (143 calories less) compared to those who reported seeing but not using the information and those who reported not seeing the information at all (135 calories less). Customer awareness of calorie information increased in food chains (18.8%–61.7%) and in coffee chains (4.4%–30%).

In another study (Roberto et al., 2010) the researchers assessed the impact of restaurant menu calorie labels on food choices and food intake. They randomly assigned 303 participants in a study dinner to one of three conditions: (1) a menu without calorie labels (no calorie labels), (2) a menu with calorie labels only (calorie labels only), or (3) a menu with calorie labels and an informational label stating, "The recommended daily caloric intake for an average adult is 2000 calories" (calorie labels plus information). Food choices and intake during and after the study dinner were measured. The researchers found that participants in both calorie label conditions (Groups 2 and 3) ordered fewer calories than those in the no calorie labels group (Group 1). Groups 2 and 3 (combined) consumed 14% fewer calories than the "no calorie labels" group. However, individuals in Group 2 (calorie labels only) consumed more calories after the study than those in both other groups. When calories consumed both during and after the study dinner were combined, participants in the "calorie labels plus information" group (Group 3) consumed an average of 250 fewer calories than those in the other groups. The researchers concluded that calorie labels on restaurant menus did affect food choices and intake and adding a recommended daily caloric requirement label increased this effect.

A more recent study (Liu et al., 2020) assessed the impact of menu labeling in the United States 10 years after the federal policy was adopted. The authors used a microsimulation model to estimate changes in cardiovascular disease (CVD) events, diabetes cases, quality of life, costs, and cost-effectiveness of the menu calorie labeling intervention, accounting for potential industry reformulation. The impacts were assessed over 5 years and a lifetime from healthcare and societal perspectives. The authors found that, between 2018 and 2023, implementation of the federal restaurant menu calorie labeling law helped to prevent 14,698 incident CVD cases (including 1,575 CVD deaths) and 21,522 new cases of type 2 diabetes, gaining 8,749 quality-adjusted life years (QALYs). Over a lifetime, this accrued to 135,781 new CVD cases (27,646 CVD deaths), 99,736 type 2 diabetes cases, and 367,450 QALYs. Under the assumption of modest restaurant item reformulation (e.g., a net 5% calorie reduction in meals), both health and economic benefits were found to be twofold larger than that predicted by consumer response alone.

Thought Questions

1. How do these examples use different study designs and research methods to study different parts of the policy process?
2. Think about the RE-AIM framework. Which of the RE-AIM functions (Reach, Effectiveness, Adoption, Implementation, Maintenance) does the information from these studies contribute to? In what ways?
3. How might a conservative policy maker frame these results differently from a liberal policy maker?

References

Krieger, J. W., Chan, N. L., Saelens, B. E., Ta, M. L., Solet, D., & Fleming, D. W. (2013). Menu labeling regulations and calories purchased at chain restaurants. *American Journal of Preventive Medicine, 44*(6), 595–604. https://doi.org/10.1016/j.amepre.2013.01.031

Liu, J., Mozaffarian, D., Sy, S., Lee, Y., Wilde, P. E., Abrahams-Gessel, S., Gaziano, T., & Micha, R. (2020). Health and economic impacts of the national menu calorie labeling law in the United States. *Circulation: Cardiovascular Quality and Outcomes, 13*(6), Article e006313. https://doi.org/10.1161/circoutcomes.119.006313

Patient Protection and Affordable Care Act, Pub. L. No. 111-148, 124 Stat. 119 (2010). https://www.congress.gov/111/plaws/publ148/PLAW-111publ148.pdf

Roberto, C. A., Larsen, P. D., Agnew, H., Baik, J., & Brownell, K. D. (2010). Evaluating the impact of menu labeling on food choices and intake. *American Journal of Public Health, 100*(2), 312–318. https://doi.org/10.2105/ajph.2009.160226

Short-term policy goals are often linked to "process" evaluation metrics. For example: Was the policy implemented as intended? Were all students tested for obesity? Was a standardized protocol used for testing obesity and was the test conducted by a trained person? Did public awareness of the problem increase? If a menu-labeling policy was adopted, what percentage of restaurants complied with posting the labels, and were customers aware of seeing the labels when they visited a restaurant? You might set having 100% of elementary public schools screened for obesity within 2 years. You might set a goal of having fresh fruits and vegetables accounting for x% of the calories of school lunch programs in the United States by a given year. Alternatively, or conjointly, a criterion might be to increase the efficiency of the same program by reducing the cost per meal by 10% by a given year. Your goal could also include the elimination of a program over time, for example, the removal of snack/soda machines in all public schools. What is important is that you have reliable, valid, and practical data (either using available data or facilitating additional data collection) pertaining to the policy and the outcome.

Medium-term policy goals are often linked to "impact" evaluation metrics that can include such things as changes in knowledge, beliefs, or attitudes (e.g., students reporting that they prefer fresh fruit over French fries) or customers reporting selections of healthier menu items and behaviors (students buying more fresh fruit compared to French fries in the cafeteria or customers consuming more healthy food and changing caloric intake). Long-term outcomes refer to actual changes in health conditions (e.g., decreased obesity rates or decreased prevalence of diabetes).

There are several different criteria that you could use. Some of these include:

- *Effectiveness,* for example, increasing the number of individuals covered or the comprehensiveness of interventions so as to change rates of obesity (or other disease outcomes) in a positive manner; aligned with *Healthy People 2030* targets.
- *Efficiency,* for example, improving the ratio of input costs to outputs.
- *Equity,* for example, assuring that minority populations have the same or even more access to healthy choices as more affluent populations.
- *Feasibility,* for example, the practical operational factors associated with a policy's adoption and implementation.
- *Flexibility,* for example, allowing local variation in the administration of the program.
- *Ideology,* for example, supporting local and parental control or strict federal standards for local communities to follow.
- *Sustainability*, for example, focusing on policies that emphasize balancing environmental, economic, health, and social justice goals.
- *Budget/fiscal principles and longevity,* for example, focusing on strategies that enable the policy to be maintained over time.
- *Politics,* for example, gaining the support of a powerful stakeholder to score points against the other political party or politician so as to gain political advantage; building coalitions for an upcoming election.

This is not an exclusive list. However, you need to be explicit in terms of what you are attempting to accomplish by your policy proposal and how you plan on demonstrating the policy is meeting its goals.

Of course, you can have more than one criterion for success. You can design a nutrition program for children that would be effective, efficient, equitable, and politically advantageous. One would want to have measures of success for each. However, your proposal might also increase the government's budget at the national, state, or local levels.

To maximize the reduction of obesity in children in the United States, effectiveness might be the major or only indicator of success. Cost, efficiency, and equity may be secondary. However, having the most effective program may also be expensive. Where is the trade-off between cost and effectiveness? Alternatively, decreasing the disparity of obesity rates among various subpopulation groups in the United States might be your primary goal and other criteria might fall away. If not losing a powerful supportive stakeholder (e.g., major beverage manufacturers) becomes a key criterion for success, then perhaps effectiveness and efficiency might become less important. Compromises with powerful stakeholders during the policy process to make it more politically viable may alter your original criteria for success.

These criteria for success should be drafted before you have completed your review of policy alternatives. Your criteria for success should be front and center as you review various alternative policy/programs. You might want to revisit your criteria after you have completed your review but using the same criteria for policy alternatives keeps your analysis more objective. Developing the criteria after you have selected your policy/program is stacking the deck in favor of a predetermined solution. Each policy/program is going to have both its strengths and weakness in meeting your criteria for short-term, medium-term, and long-term success. You are probably going to have to make a recommendation at the end of your review of alternatives. Honestly appraising the alternatives gives your readers greater confidence in the option you have selected.

MEASUREMENT

Having criteria is only one step in the process. You will need to have data that are valid (an accurate measure of what you are attempting to measure), reliable (the ability to get the same measure time after time), and practical (a relatively inexpensive and easy set of data to obtain or initiate). One acronym that is frequently used is SMART goals, goals that are Specific, Measurable, Attainable, Realistic, and Timely (CDC, n.d.-b).

If you have selected national level as your geopolitical unit, you have both complicated and eased your ability to obtain data. On one hand, you need measures that reflect progress toward your goals for all 50 states. You could use data that are collected the same way in all 50 states, or alternatively you could use a statistically representative sample of the school-age population that reflects the nation as a whole. You will also need data that are collected and available over time at the appropriate geographic scale so that you can measure progress in the short term, medium term, and long term. As described in Chapters 8 and 9, data coverage can be spotty and inconsistent in the United States. It can be difficult to find publicly available data at scales smaller than the county level, particularly for rural places.

By selecting a national program, you have also made your evaluation task easier since the federal government is the largest collector of health data. If your geopolitical unit is a state or a local community, you might be more limited in what data are available. However, if data are available, such information might be more detailed. States vary greatly in the amount and quality of their data. What is the reputation of your geopolitical system's data collection efforts? Is there regional data available to compare your state's progress against neighboring states?

The question of the frequency of data collection is also critical. You will want to use a measure that is collected frequently enough so you can demonstrate trends over time in a standardized manner. While the U.S. Census has a wealth of detailed data, it is collected once every 10 years. There are inter-Census estimates for some Census data, but not all. Release of the Census data typically takes a year or two. Therefore, make sure that you have measures that correspond to your short-, medium-, and long-term goals for your policy proposal.

Many states and school districts have their own obesity-related data. However, there are many different protocols used in testing. In some jurisdictions a nurse might take the measurement of height and weight using a standard medical scale. In other jurisdictions a teacher may do the measurements using a bathroom scale and tape measure. When and how frequently the measurements are taken on children can also be important. If some data are collected in the fall and some in the spring, there is an 8-month difference in data collection. Does this matter? Unless there is some standardization of the process of measurement, it is difficult to determine if a change is the result of the policy or a result of better/poorer measurement or merely maturation.

One could set up a nationally representative sample of schools (elementary and secondary) and have a standard yearly measurement of childhood body mass index (BMI). That, however, takes additional money, staffing, protocols, and organization. It also requires a consistency in funding and state collaboration so that data are collected on a regular basis. Funding for data collection is frequently one of the first things to be cut during difficult budget times. New data sets that have not demonstrated their utility may be especially vulnerable.

Policies have both intended consequences (results that we anticipate and desire) and unintended or indirect consequences (consequences that are by-products of our policy and may not initially be intended). Unintended consequences can be both positive and negative.

Given the example of childhood obesity, an adverse consequence might be increased stigma of obese children and/or the increase in the incidence of EDs as a result of testing children's BMI. This is a real possibility given the serious consequences of EDs (e.g., bulimia nervosa and anorexia nervosa) in youth. On the other hand, a potentially positive yet unintended consequence of your policy might be new federal funding for bike and walking paths. With increased bike paths, children as well as adults will have increased ability to exercise and use a mode of transportation that helps to control weight as well as protect the environment. While that would increase access to exercise, it may also result in more injuries both in short-term and long-term results. There will likely be increased bicycle collisions and falls. There may be increased wear and tear on joints that will lead to costly knee and hip replacements in 50 years. Some of these adverse consequences could be avoided if bicycle/walking paths were made of composite materials that were more forgiving for falls. In cities, one would want to assure that bicycle and pedestrian paths follow appropriate design guidelines, such as those developed by the American Association of State Highway and Transportation Officials (AASHTO). Some adverse consequences can be foreseen, and some may be less obvious.

You may decide to also have indicators for some potential adverse consequences. For example, you could systematically collect information about bicycle/auto collisions using estimates of the increase in bicycle traffic (Kerr et al., 2013). One might hope for a decrease in the number of automobile/bicycle collisions given the intentional design of the bike paths, but one would want to see a decrease in the rate of such events.

You may wish to consult with researchers at a local university as to how to identify and measure these potential intended and unintended consequences. The major advantage of beginning to think about these potentially adverse consequences of your policy proposal is that you can make modifications to it even before enactment to minimize adverse consequences. By thinking about these and measuring them, you can deflect potential criticism of your policy.

This section of your policy analysis would be a relatively brief discussion of the variables that one would use to measure the short-term, medium-term, and long-term success of your policy. This would include specific goals with time frames. You would identify measures that are available, valid, reliable, and accepted. You would want to make sure that the data are available in sufficiently frequent intervals to demonstrate the policy's impact over time.

Ideally, such data sources should come from respected public sources of data. The perennial problem is that such public data probably will have been collected for a different purpose than demonstrating the success of your policy. The data may not be the most precise measure for your policy, but it may a suitable compromise between "ideal" data elements and those that are available.

SUMMARY

Policies are enacted for multiple purposes, and they have both intended and unintended consequences. We would prefer policies that have positive, intentional consequences and minimal adverse unintended consequences. Developing criteria for success makes the intentions explicit. These will include process measures for immediate impact and then measures of efficiency, effectiveness, equity, political expediency, cost benefit, and so forth for longer term results. Trade-offs will undoubtedly have to be made due to stakeholders, data availability, staffing costs, and available expertise. These criteria should be initially established prior to the analysis of alternative policies so that you evaluate policy alternatives on a common set of desired outcomes. You may then want to adjust them for your specific policy proposal.

One needs to have knowledge and access to data that can measure "success." Data that are public and commonly accepted as valid and reliable are generally better indicators than new data created for a particular policy/program. Short-term, medium-term, and long-term goals with accompanying data points need to be identified. You also need to remember that most policy makers have relatively short time frames or perspectives since election and re-election are the primary measure of a politician's success.

DISCUSSION QUESTIONS

- Using COVID-19 as an example, describe the intended and unintended consequences of your state's health policy.

- Using the menu labeling example in **Breakout Box 13.1**, how would you define and measure success?

- Given a current public health problem in your state, how would you define success?

- What measurements of success would you use to indicate short-term, medium-term, and long-term success?

- Discuss how different stakeholders may view the relative importance of the criteria for success differently. How would you resolve this?

KEY TERMS

budget/fiscal longevity

efficiency

effectiveness

equity

feasibility

ideology

intended consequences

policy success

policy sustainability

politics

process evaluation

unintended consequences

A robust set of instructor resources designed to supplement this text is located at http://connect.springerpub.com/content/book/978-0-8261-8543-3. Qualifying instructors may request access by emailing textbook@springerpub.com.

REFERENCES

Centers for Disease Control and Prevention. (n.d.-a). Overweight & obesity: *Childhood obesity facts*. U.S. Department of Health and Human Services. https://www.cdc.gov/obesity/data/childhood.html

Centers for Disease Control and Prevention. (n.d.-b). *Public Health Professionals Gateway: Develop SMART objectives*. U.S. Department of Health and Human Services. https://www.cdc.gov/publichealthgateway/phcommunities/resourcekit/evaluate/develop-smart-objectives.html

Kerr, Z. Y., Rodriguez, D. A., Evenson, K. R., & Aytur, S. A. (2013). Pedestrian and bicycle plans and the incidence of crash-related injuries. *Accident Analysis & Prevention*, *50*, 1252–1258. https://doi.org/10.1016/j.aap.2012.09.028

Leme, A. C. B., Thompson, D., Lenz Dunker, K. L., Nicklas, T., Tucunduva Philippi, S., Lopez, T., Vézina-Im, L. A., & Baranowski, T. (2018). Obesity and eating disorders in integrative prevention programmes for adolescents: Protocol for a systematic review and meta-analysis. *BMJ Open*, *8*(4), Article e020381. https://doi.org/10.1136/bmjopen-2017-020381

Namba, A., Auchincloss, A., Leonberg, B. L., & Wootan, M. G. (2013). Exploratory analysis of fast-food chain restaurant menus before and after implementation of local calorie-labeling policies, 2005–2011. *Preventing Chronic Disease*, *10*, E101. https://doi.org/10.5888/pcd10.120224

Nayak, S., Maehr, N., & Reynolds, M. E. (2022, May 13). *How has Congress responded to issues surrounding vaccinations?* Brookings. https://www.brookings.edu/blog/fixgov/2022/05/13/how-has-congress-responded-to-issues-surrounding-vaccinations

Patient Protection and Affordable Care Act, Pub. L. No. 111-148, 124 Stat. 119 (2010). https://www.congress.gov/111/plaws/publ148/PLAW-111publ148.pdf

Stabouli, S., Erdine, S., Suurorg, L., Jankauskienė, A., & Lurbe, E. (2021). Obesity and eating disorders in children and adolescents: The bidirectional link. *Nutrients*, *13*(12), 4321. https://doi.org/10.3390/nu13124321

CHAPTER 14

REVIEW OF POLICY OPTIONS

This chapter describes the culmination of your research in terms of the history of the policy area and the quantitative and qualitative evidence regarding various policy options in furthering progress on your previously determined criteria for success. Here, too, is where you must decide on the political aspects of your proposal. To what extent is the political expediency of incrementalism countered by the need to be innovative and potentially better able to meet your criteria for success? Finally, we briefly discuss when your research phase is over.

LEARNING OBJECTIVES

Be able to:

- Describe different types of evidence used in the policy process.
- Describe the precautionary principle.
- Synthesize the evidence gathered.
- Determine the political viability of policy options.
- Discuss the advantages and disadvantages of an incremental approach to policy change.

Here it is critical to go back to check the specifics of your assignment for the policy analysis. Based on the evidence you have gathered your assignment might be to recommend one policy over other alternatives. Your analysis may lead you to conclude that one policy is less effective but more politically acceptable or more effective but has more political challenges. On the other hand, your assigned task may be to present alternative policies with the strengths and weaknesses of each. Presenting the trade-offs associated with several viable policy alternatives can be very important. This will impact how you structure this section. Either way, you must build the best evidence you can from the material that you have accessed. At this stage you also need to reflect back on Chapter 4 regarding the strengths and weaknesses of incrementalism or building the basis for a major policy change.

Any policy changes within the business environment (including healthcare) tend to realign factors that advantage some stakeholders and disadvantage others. Business organizations typically prefer predictable environments, even if there are some elements within that environment that are not particularly favorable to them. Existing stakeholders have survived, and some have thrived within the status quo; disruption leads to uncertainty. Especially in areas where policies are synergetic and interconnected, a small change is more predictable and less threatening than a large change. A requirement for certain restaurants to post nutrition information becomes more acceptable, especially if it can deflect the call for more dramatic changes.

By adopting incrementalism, one is merely tweaking the existing policy/program and the risk of failure is lessened. In addition, a small change can more easily be reversed if it appears as though that change may have too many unintended adverse consequences. In addition, incremental changes tend to be less costly, at least in the short term, if not for the long term. It is also worth noting that the political process can facilitate incrementalism (e.g., a policy could become an amendment to a budget bill).

The existing policy/program already has an organizational structure and staff; it might merely need some minor support or additional funds. It should also be remembered that politicians tend to have short-term perspectives (Brownson et al., 2009). Incremental policy changes (even if small) may be more immediately visible and result in positive public reaction.

With all these advantages, it is sometimes hard to argue against an incremental policy. However, there are also disadvantages to incrementalism. One of the major criticisms of incrementalism is that it places a premium on coming to an agreement among existing stakeholders rather than solving the social problem. Getting existing stakeholders to reach a compromise is not necessarily the same as solving the problem. This is especially true since not all stakeholders have equal power. Those stakeholders with the most power may prefer the status quo. There are times when major policy changes need to be made and when incremental changes are not going to have a sufficient impact on the problem. Incremental policy changes are likely to result in small changes in the social problem. If a problem such as obesity is escalating very rapidly but the proposed solution is incremental, there is likely to be a widening gap between social/health goals and what actually occurs. Incremental solutions may not be sufficient to make headway in such instances. For example, getting restaurant chains to post the calorie content of their existing entrees (a relatively inexpensive policy option for restaurants to implement) was shown to be only marginally effective in actually changing consumer product selection (Krieger et al., 2013). More recent systematic reviews and meta-analyses have also reported mixed results (Fernandes et al., 2016; Grummon et al., 2021).[1]

---

1 Grummon et al. (2021) examined the calorie content of menu items at large chain restaurants before and after implementation of federally mandated menu calorie labels from 2012 to 2019. This covered the time period before and after the implementation of the federal menu-labeling policy in 2018. Changes in menu items' calorie content after restaurant chains implemented calorie labels were estimated, adjusting for prelabeling trends. Results suggested that, after the implementation of menu labeling, there were no statistically significant changes in mean calorie content for all menu items or continuously available items. However, new items that were introduced after the menu-labeling policy was implemented did show a lower mean calorie content than items introduced before labeling. Thus, menu labeling was associated with the introduction of lower-calorie items but not with changes in continuously available or removed items.

Perhaps one of the most significant disadvantages of incrementalism is also one of its advantages; it protects the status quo. As a result, those who are disadvantaged by the current system (e.g., poor minority consumers living in food deserts) will remain disadvantaged, although perhaps marginally less so. One of the problems for inner cities is that there are areas where the only practical choice for inexpensive meals is a fast-food chain or readily available prepared foods. Mass transit often does not go to outlying inexpensive grocery stores. Making fresh and nutritious food available to those in such food deserts requires more than posting nutrition and calorie information. Eliminating food deserts is likely to require important zoning changes, supporting multimodal transportation or extending mass transit service, limiting the number of fast-food chains, developing farm-to-institution legislation, providing subsidies for vendors of fresh foods, changing restrictions on the use of SNAP (Supplemental Nutrition Assistance Program) benefits, allowing customers to use electronic benefit transfer (EBT) cards at farmers markets, and so forth. These more comprehensive changes will generally tend to be more politically controversial.

Nonincremental policies are certainly possible, as we saw with the Local Farms–Healthy Kids Act, and may be more effective in solving the public health issue. However, one must recognize that in many jurisdictions, such policies may also be more politically challenging to pass. We talk about this further in Chapter 15, Recommendation and Strategies. There is a common political aphorism stating that the perfect is often the enemy of the good (Redman, 2001). Sometimes striving for the ideal solution creates too many political enemies and rather than having something less perfect enacted, nothing gets passed. There is a political trade-off here: doing what is more feasible rather than attempting to accomplish the ideal.

The Overton Window developed at the Mackinac Center for Public Policy maintains that there is narrow group of policy solutions that are politically viable at a given point in time (Russell, 2006). The political climate limits the number of acceptable policy choices along an ideological continuum that can be considered by policy makers and still win re-election. A disruptive policy may cause pre-election anxiety among voters without providing sufficient time to demonstrate any positive feedback. Policies outside this window may be more optimal in solving the problem, but they are not politically viable at the time. COVID-19 mask policies may be scientifically beneficial, but mask fatigue may prevent their adoption unless there is a dramatic change in mortality risk. A change in circumstances may allow the window to shift to include policy options that might not have been previously politically viable. School shootings, *E. coli* outbreaks, environmental disasters, or a viral outbreak can widen the window of policy opportunity.

Your examination of peer-reviewed literature and meta-analyses may lead you to a policy approach that you had previously not considered. Frequently, policy areas become locked into a particular paradigm or become fixated on a type of approach that has been used in the past. Stepping back and examining the public health problem from a new perspective is a valuable exercise. Sometimes you can borrow something from another policy area and apply it to climate change, obesity, mental health, and so forth. This is an opportunity to be creative and to shift the thinking about how a public health policy issue can be addressed. This creativity may open your policy proposal to potential funding by a foundation that is looking for innovative policy approaches to the policy problem. Your policy may lay the foundation for a pilot program in one community that can be duplicated by other communities. With innovation comes the task of (1) demonstrating that this innovation may produce favorable results and (2) that it is politically viable.

You should not limit your thinking to only an incremental policy. Nonincremental policy proposals may well stimulate debate and move policy discussions in a different direction. Typically, policies have a long history of evolution; your policy could start the evolutionary process. By advocating a major policy change, one is at least putting it on the policy agenda for discussion and potential future action. Major change cannot come about without (1) an advocate and (2) a proposal. Compromises might have to be made to make it politically viable, but it can provide a new framework for solving a public problem.

EVIDENCE

At this point of your analysis, you should remember several things from Chapters 7, 8, and 9. Type two evidence is very different in nature from the type one evidence you used in Chapter 10 to describe the policy background or in Chapter 11 to create the statement of the policy issue. For that you needed mostly descriptive data (type one evidence), such as incidence rates of childhood obesity, to demonstrate that a problem existed. Now, however, you need to go beyond that and provide evidence to convince policy makers that a particular program or policy is associated with positive impacts on the obesity problem. This is a different level of evidence (type two evidence), which considers statistical relationships and causal inference, which can be assessed using the analytical methods described in Chapter 9.

Your political or lay audience may not have a great understanding of the importance and differences in the types of studies and methodologies that are used, so you will probably need to assist them to appreciate the weight given to any individual study or data-driven models. This is a heavy responsibility. Your understanding of statistics and data analysis becomes important because you are going to be making an assessment as to which program/policy has the greatest level of evidence demonstrating that it is effective, cost-efficient, equitable, or otherwise meets the criteria of success you have established. If you are not confident about your analytical skills, you need to seek assistance.

Because obesity is a multifaceted problem with potential genetic, biological, and social causal factors, it is going to be difficult to determine the appropriate strategy to reverse the obesity trend in the United States. In fact, there is no definitive single solution to the problem. If there were, it would probably have been proposed and adopted in multiple communities or states with clear indicators of success. Consequently, your policy initiative is not likely to "solve" the problem of obesity in the United States, but it may provide a partial response to the growing obesity epidemic.

Because the success of your policy/program proposal is not a given, you will need evidence to support its adoption. You need to provide potential supporters with evidence to support the policy and you need to provide evidence to counter the skeptics. The evolution of evidence-based medicine/public health was discussed in Chapters 7 to 9. In this section of the policy analysis, you will focus on the development of a rational case for your policy.

Here you should recall the difference between efficacy and effectiveness as discussed previously. Efficacy is basically whether the proposed policy or program can work at all; this is typically under ideal circumstances. Remember that a randomized clinical trial (RCT) is such a test of efficacy. However, whether or not the policy or program will work in a real-life setting is a much different question. There are issues of political acceptability, varying values and cultures, legal and ethical questions, or mere practicality that might undermine a potentially efficacious program. In health policy we are more concerned about the "real world" with all its complications than we are in the ideal world. Therefore, external validity becomes very important in policy analysis (Rao & Anderson, 2012; Thomson & Thomas, 2012). This does not mean that internal validity (the degree of certainty that the intervention being studied is associated with the effect) is not important. However, if your policy proposal is unlikely to work in the real world, it has limited utility as public policy.

It becomes complicated and ethically problematic to do RCTs outside clinical settings, although group-randomized (quasi-experimental) designs are frequently used in public health (Hollar et al., 2010). A policy or program is usually developed for a particular geopolitical unit, and some type of formal or informal evaluation will be conducted to assess its impact. For example, if you are assessing a school nutrition policy intervention, sometimes there is a "before and after" evaluation in schools exposed to the intervention. Alternatively, there might be an evaluation comparing schools using the intervention to schools in which the intervention was not used. Sometimes there may be a "natural experiment" in which certain jurisdictions adopted a policy before others and you can compare the effects over time. Refer back to the menu-labeling policies described previously. Sometimes there will be multiple cases with some type of random or nonrandom selection according to geography or setting. There might be a rigorous qualitative evaluation of the policy development process (see the nutrition policy examples from Washington State in Chapter 12). Sometimes there will be no formal evaluation, but merely subjective opinions by participants as to the degree of the policy/program success. Programs and policies funded by external sources (e.g., foundations or government agencies) tend to require formal evaluations. However, keep in mind that people/organizations do not like to be associated with a "failed" program or policy, so that any evaluation designed and conducted by the managers of a program may be slanted toward a positive outcome. Evaluations conducted by external evaluation experts tend to carry more weight.

The hierarchy of evidence we discussed in Chapters 7 and 8 should not be taken too dogmatically. A well-designed single case study (which is at the bottom of the traditional hierarchy) may be a very useful study for a policy proposal because it can reveal details about the process of adopting or implementing a policy. Such case studies are important to provide guidance as to which factors may be most important to policy work in the real world by examining the contextual factors of a policy's development (Yin, 2009). Qualitative research is a very valuable tool for policy analysis, especially for studying policy formulation and implementation (Sofaer, 1999). Cross-sectional studies can also be very useful, as the national data surveillance systems we mentioned previously (e.g., BRFSS [Behavioral Risk Factor Surveillance System], NHANES [National Health and Nutrition Examination Survey]) lend themselves to this type of analysis. As mentioned previously, qualitative and quantitative data can be used in a complementary manner as part of a mixed-methods design.

A study describing the implementation of a child nutrition program in an elementary school in New Jersey will tend to discuss in detail the types of things that worked well and those that did not work well. Of course, such single case studies suffer from a potential lack of generalizability or external validity, that is, the success of that program might be totally unique and not replicable elsewhere. The extent to which a policy can be replicated elsewhere is a critical issue. However, if you were developing a policy for the state of New Jersey or a county in New Jersey, this single case study might be very valuable since the case exists within the same value/political/legal culture of New Jersey. However, if your policy/program is to be at the national level, the example from New Jersey provides some evidence, but it is less persuasive that it will work in New Mexico where a different set of value/political/legal variables will be at play. This does not mean that the case study in New Jersey is not important in your discussion for a national policy. The program may have been established as part of a demonstration program funded by a large organization and undergone careful external evaluation. For example, the Alliance for a Healthier Generation (2012) has done a study on its "healthy schools" program. A particular program might be very innovative and worth funding as a federal demonstration project in other states.

Another caveat is that many states have considerable "divides" in terms of their value/political/legal cultures, often along urban/rural or north/south or east/west geographic areas. California and Virginia have had multiple proposals for dividing their respective states.

What is important from the analytical side is that you are aware of the strengths and weaknesses of various types of studies supporting and opposing various policy options. Potential opponents to your policy proposal will indeed point to the weaknesses of the evidence that you select, so you need to be prepared to defend the evidence that you have.

This analytical process can be quite frustrating since the role of science has become politicized in policy debates. There have always been skeptics of science, sometimes based upon religion, conspiracy theories, and/or politics. Much of the debunking of science has revolved around vaccines. Perhaps the most celebrated example was the study published and later withdrawn by *Lancet* that involved only 12 children and made a link between measles, mumps, and rubella (MMR) vaccinations and autism in children. The study has been discredited and subsequent studies such as a study involving 537,303 children born in Denmark from 1991 to 1998 indicated that there was no increased risk of autism from MMR vaccination (Madsen et al., 2002). Despite this and many subsequent studies debunking the author and the article, anti-vaxer groups seized on the study to oppose public health vaccination campaigns. The incident caused an outbreak of childhood disease and fueled vaccine skepticism across the world.

Regulation of secondhand smoke in the early 2000s led to an industry led to advocates for "sound science." This was an effort by industry and public relations firms to stop the adoption of local and state antismoking laws (Ong & Glantz, 2001). Advocates for "sound science" frequently pointed to one study or a few studies (no matter their evidentiary strength) that questioned the preponderance of evidence presented by the scientific literature. One study of questionable quality was sufficient to derail the adoption of a health policy since the science was not settled. According to advocates of "sound science," any evidence that raised doubt was sufficient to oppose policy adoption until the science was unanimous. This argument was based on a misunderstanding of the essence of science, the continual process of reexamination of facts, and the use of the scientific method using standard methods of analysis. Unlike the laws of nature, there are few things in the complicated multifactorial world of health and social science that can be demonstrated to be true 100% of the time. Even within very successful clinical trials, the intervention rarely works 100% of the time. "Sound science" was a marking tool used by political opponents of antismoking legislation to make it appear their position was scientifically based.

Vaccine skepticism has returned with the COVID-19 epidemic. A significant proportion of the U.S. population remains unvaccinated for a variety of reasons. As previously noted, this has resulted in more preventable deaths than in Australia with a more trusting population. Scientific skeptics and politics have again joined forces in opposing public health initiatives. As public health experts gained more experience with COVID-19 and its variants, this has led to reassessment of previously recommended public health policies. This is to be expected as the science evolves. However, this has also led to organized threats of violence against public health officials and a subsequent loss of public health leaders (Freeman, 2022). How this will impact public health policy recommendations in the future is uncertain.

Scientific studies vary as to the populations covered, the research designs used, data and variables selected, and the analytical methods applied. Any of these elements might lead to differing results. A policy analyst needs to be able to know the difference in the credibility of studies. Health communication is a field in its own right; partnering with a communication science expert is recommended to enhance your policy analysis. It is wise to be familiar with those studies that provide contrary evidence to your policy because opponents will quickly use those studies to attempt to discredit the evidence that you have presented.

Public health professionals have recognized precautionary principle as one important consideration for policy advocacy (Goldstein, 2001). This principle contends that the burden of proof for deliberating potentially harmful actions rests on the assurance of safety, and that when the health of the public or the environment is at risk, it is not necessary to wait for scientific certainty before policy action is taken to limit potential harm. Public health policy makers use this principle to justify decisions in situations where there is the possibility of harm from not acting. This principle maintains that there is a social responsibility to act if there is probable concern for the safety of the population. Refer back to the Breakout Boxes in Chapter 12 to see how this was reflected in the policy examples from Washington State. The adopted policy can be changed if subsequent scientific studies reveal different outcomes or unintended consequences.

The important thing to remember is to be honest and straightforward in the presentation of the evidence available. You are preparing this analysis for someone else. You do not want to have their credibility questioned or set them up for failure. You are collecting evidence and trying to assemble the best information available. No individual study is ever decisive, especially in a social/policy setting. If you rest your case on one study, opponents only have to find flaws in that one study to undermine your policy. What you need to do is to decipher what the preponderance of the evidence shows and what the highest quality studies suggest regarding impacts and outcomes of your policy recommendation in a real-world setting. This is not an easy task.

WHEN TO CALL IT QUITS

You may have started to get overwhelmed by the material you have discovered. You could probably continue for months. However, your policy maker has undoubtedly given you a deadline and the policy agenda window of opportunity may be closing. At some point you need to be sufficiently comfortable that you have covered the critical available evidence. If you have discovered a recent systematic review of the literature that may help. However, at some point you will discover that you keep seeing the same sources being cited in peer-reviewed literature. Grey literature is another story since there is an abundant of different sources of grey literature and so there is probably more out there to be discovered. However, even here the same examples tend to be repeated. You should make sure that you have covered the positions of significant stakeholders, especially those that might be critical of your analysis, and have the means to mount political opposition. Here it would be helpful to interview experts in the field. State administrators attend conferences of professional associations where they hear presentations of innovative policies or programs are being tried around the country. These formal and informal networks predate the existence of grey literature and peer-reviewed literature.

SUMMARY

This is going to be one of the longest sections to write in your policy analysis. Here is where you are going to be collecting evidence as to what might work or what has been tried in the past or in other geopolitical units. Depending on your expertise of the policy area, your search may require a great deal of effort and time. Accessing experts in the field, systematic reviews, and meta-analyses will help you get an overview of the important studies that have been completed. Accessing electronic databases for both peer-reviewed and grey literature (government and private organizations) will be important in finding important policies and programs. You will need to be critical of the studies by examining the data and methodologies used, the logic of the conclusions derived from the data, and evaluating internal and external validity. Deciding when you have explored major alternatives and have sufficient evidence will be a key factor in terminating this portion of your analysis. This section will require the application of all your analytical skills that you have acquired.

DISCUSSION QUESTIONS

■ Review the scenario of "Susan" presented at the end of Chapter 1. Discuss different policy options at the federal, state, or local level that may be leveraged to improve the health of Susan's community.

■ In weighing evidence for your policy, how would you decide which is more persuasive, peer-reviewed literature or grey literature?

■ How much weight should your public health department place on the importance of incrementalism for the next viral pandemic?

■ Describe the strengths and weaknesses of a clinical trial in the context of policy.

■ Describe a missed window of opportunity for the introduction of a public health policy in your state.

KEY TERMS

incrementalism

political viability

precautionary principle

type one and type two evidence

 SPRINGER PUBLISHING CONNECT™

A robust set of instructor resources designed to supplement this text is located at http://connect.springerpub.com/content/book/978-0-8261-8543-3. Qualifying instructors may request access by emailing textbook@springerpub.com.

REFERENCES

Alliance for a Healthier Generation. (2012, October). Technical assistance matters: Schools need support to become healthier. Robert Wood Johnson Foundation. http://www.rwjf.org/content/dam/farm/reports/issue_briefs/2012/rwjf402203

Brownson, R. C., Chriqui, J. F., & Stamatakis, K. A. (2009). Understanding evidence-based public health policy. *American Journal of Public Health, 99*(9), 1576–1583. https://doi.org/10.2105/ajph.2008.156224

Fernandes, A. C., Oliveira, R. C., Proença, R. P., Curioni, C. C., Rodrigues, V. M., & Fiates, G. M. (2016). Influence of menu labeling on food choices in real-life settings: A systematic review. *Nutrition Reviews, 74*(8), 534–548. https://doi.org/10.1093/nutrit/nuw013

Freeman, L. T. (2022). Unanticipated pandemic outcomes: The assault on public health. *American Journal of Public Health, 112*(5), 731–733. https://doi.org/10.2105/ajph.2022.306810

Goldstein, B. D. (2001, September). The precautionary principle also applies to public health actions. *American Journal of Public Health, 91*(9), 1358–1361. https://doi.org/10.2105/ajph.91.9.1358

Grummon, A. H., Petimar, J., Soto, M. J., Bleich, S. N., Simon, D., Cleveland, L. P., Rao, A., & Block, J. P. (2021). Changes in calorie content of menu items at large chain restaurants after implementation of calorie labels. *JAMA Network Open, 4*(12), Article e2141353. https://doi.org/10.1001/jamanetworkopen.2021.41353

Hollar, D., Messiah, S. E., Lopez-Mitnik, G., Hollar, T. L., Almon, M., & Agatston, A. S. (2010). Effect of a two-year obesity prevention intervention on percentile changes in body mass index and academic performance in low-income elementary school children. *American Journal of Public Health, 100*(4), 646–653. https://doi.org/10.2105/ajph.2009.165746

Krieger, J. W., Chan, N. L., Saelens, B. E., Ta, M. L., Solet, D., & Fleming, D. W. (2013). Menu labeling regulations and calories purchased at chain restaurants. *American Journal of Preventive Medicine, 44*(6), 595–604. https://doi.org/10.1016/j.amepre.2013.01.031

Madsen, K. M., Hviid, A., Vestergaard, M., Schendel, D., Wohlfahrt, J., Thorsen, P., Olsen, J., & Melbye, M. (2002). A population-based study of measles, mumps, and rubella vaccination and autism. *New England Journal of Medicine*, 347(19), 1477–1482. https://doi.org/10.1056/nejmoa021134

Ong, E. K., & Glantz, S. A. (2001). Constructing "sound science" and "good epidemiology": Tobacco, lawyers, and public relations firms. *American Journal of Public Health*, 91(11), 1749–1757. https://doi.org/10.2105/ajph.91.11.1749

Rao, J. K., & Anderson, L. A. (2012). Examining external validity in efficacy and secondary articles of home-based depression care management interventions for older adults. *Preventing Chronic Disease*, 9, E172. https://doi.org/10.5888/pcd9.120110

Redman, E. (2001). *The dance of legislation: An insider's account of the workings of the United States Senate*. University of Washington Press.

Russell, N. J. (2006, January 4). *An introduction to the Overton window of political possibilities*. Mackinac Center. https://www.mackinac.org/7504

Sofaer, S. (1999). Qualitative methods: What are they and why use them? *Health Services Research*, 34(5 Pt. 2), 1101–1118. https://www.ncbi.nlm.nih.gov/pmc/articles/PMC1089055

Thomson, H. J., & Thomas, S. (2012). External validity in healthy public policy: Application of the RE-AIM tool to the field of housing improvement. *BMC Public Health*, 12, Article 633. https://doi.org/10.1186/1471-2458-12-633

Yin, R. K. (2009). *Case study research: Design and methods* (4th ed.). Sage.

CHAPTER 15

RECOMMENDATION AND STRATEGIES

In this chapter we discuss making a recommendation as well as recommending strategies to get the policy adopted. These two parts of your analysis can be treated separately or together. This will probably depend on the expectations of your organization, your target audience, or a specific policy maker. You might wish to focus more on your recommendations and then follow up on strategies in an accompanying document or an appendix. We discuss proposed legislative, executive, and litigation strategies.

LEARNING OBJECTIVES

Be able to:

- Evaluate your analysis of peer-reviewed literature and grey literature to a provide a policy recommendation based on the best scientific evidence available.

- Evaluate your previous analysis to make a recommendation as to which policy alternative fits your criteria for success and is the most politically viable.

- Utilize your knowledge of the political structure, process, and culture to recommend legislative, executive, and/or litigation strategies for getting the policy adopted.

- Recommend a legislative, executive, or litigation strategy to facilitate the adoption of your recommendations.

- Discuss and defend which elements of your recommendations are core and which are negotiable.

RECOMMENDATION

This section of your report is the culmination of all your previous work. It is important at this stage to review your work to make sure that the recommendations are supported by each section of your analysis and that they tie together. For example, in the policy issue statement, you narrowed the area of concern to a specific policy topic and to a specific geopolitical system. Are your potential recommendations consistent with your policy issue statement? In establishing your criteria for success, you defined what a successful policy might look like and how you might be able to measure its progress. Do your recommendations align with those criteria? Your criteria for success might be more complicated than previously thought, or the data needed to measure success might have to change. In doing the review of policy options, you may have evolved in your thinking from your original perception of the problem. That is a positive sign. Have you developed a solid evidence-based rationale for your recommendation? Your policy analysis is an iterative process. You will likely write and rewrite many of its sections, perhaps multiple times.

Certainly, one of the measures of success you could use is the potential for your policy proposal to improve the public health problem you have targeted. Hopefully your analysis thus far has provided you with a good idea as to which proposal(s) may work best in your geopolitical system.

Your recommendation may also be influenced by the gain or expenditure of political capital. Remember that politicians generally want to gain political capital (public support, party leadership, major endorsements, or monetary contributions) for their re-election campaign or passage of other pieces of legislation. Policy makers frequently trade favors with other policy makers on a quid-pro-quo basis to gain support for their own proposals. Which of these alternative proposals increases your policy makers' political capital? Given your understanding of the political structure, process, and culture, how much political capital do you think your policy maker and allied stakeholders are willing to spend to get this policy adopted?

The role of political ideology will also play a role in your recommendation. Given the current ideological division in the United States, it is important to be aware of how your policy might be impacted by these divisions. Which is the most effective proposal in attaining success? Which is the most cost-effective proposal? Which recommendation addresses any equity gap? This is where your weighting of social and political values and the stakeholder analysis undergirding your policy proposal come into play.

It is unlikely that there is one policy option that is so outstanding that it would be unanimously accepted by everyone. However, your choice among the policy alternatives may have long-lasting consequences. Every policy has "winners" and "losers," or persons who benefit more than others. Your recommendation may cut off future policy options. Remember how eliminating the public option from the Patient Protection and Affordable Care Act (PPACA) improved its political acceptability but eliminated the possibility for Medicare-for-All. While the PPACA successfully expanded healthcare coverage for low-income persons, premiums for persons who made ≥400% of the federal poverty level went up in some markets.

Since your policy maker(s) will likely have to defend your recommendation, you need to provide them with what you believe are both its strengths and potential weaknesses. This section needs to not just sell the recommendation but also warn your policy maker where the proposal is most vulnerable to attack. A recommendation that is artificially positive may make it difficult for your policy maker to deflect early criticisms from opponents. Policy makers need to be forewarned as to what problems or issues might arise and where potential opponents may focus.

If there is evidence from your Review of Policy Options section that strongly supports one alternative over others, then that needs to be stated and reinforced in the recommendation section. If there is consistency of the evidence, you need to use that to make your case stronger. Is there a pattern that demonstrates that studies with methodological rigor reinforce studies using different methodologies and different populations? Do newer studies reinforce or contradict older studies? Do studies with different population samples lead to similar results? Does the evidence supporting your proposal rest upon one major study whose results have not been supported by other studies? What you are looking for is a pattern within the evidence that tends to support one alternative, or a narrow set of alternatives. Remember that your busy policy makers may have skipped over or only skimmed your Review of Policy Options. The Recommendation section needs to directly but concisely state the strength of the evidence for your recommendation. Remember that appendices can be used to provide additional details and references.

The level of evidence for many policy interventions is likely to be mixed (some studies may have found a positive impact in certain populations, but other studies may have found no significant impact). Different measures, populations, or analyses used in the studies may point to different levels of success, as we saw with the menu-labeling policies in **Breakout Box 13.1**. You may not be able to find a randomized or group-randomized trial to rigorously evaluate your policy. The lack of a sophisticated study design is frequently used as a political tactic to stall the adoption of policy by pointing to the need for more scientific evidence. However, you are unlikely to ever have absolute certainty about the impacts of many policies in public health, making it necessary for policy makers to proceed with decision-making in the face of uncertainty.

Recall from our policy process diagram (**Figure 4.1**) that policy making is iterative. As new data come to light, policies can be terminated or revised. Due to the severity and complexity of many public health problems, we do not always have the luxury of waiting for more research to accumulate before acting. When the consequences of inaction are great, action in the absence of perfect knowledge may be preferable. Delaying the implementation of a proposal may result in increasing economic costs, additional years of life lost, or other adverse effects. Delaying action may also result in the loss of the window of policy opportunity.

Since positive results are not a given, what is the probability that they will materialize? To what extent will people and/or entities cooperate to support of the policy and thus avoid costly enforcement? What is the likelihood that business interests will file suit to delay the implementation of your proposal? What, if anything, is necessary for the 50 states to enact to implement your federal policy proposal? What is the probability that states will comply? Are there sufficient incentives for state action?

Be clear how you are determining the probabilities of success. Most likely, this will be a subjective assessment based on personal knowledge or the knowledge of your collaborators/stakeholders. This is fine but know that areas of subjectivity are also areas where your analysis will likely be challenged. Also realize that as your policy expands its impact, the likelihood of adoption and successful implementation might decline due to opposition from additional stakeholders and increased disruption to the status quo. Is a pilot or demonstration program more likely to be politically acceptable?

Every policy choice has intended and unintended consequences. Those consequences that are intended will generally be clearly stated in your policy proposal since those will align with your Criteria for Success. There may be collateral positive impacts as well. These are often called cobenefits or multisolving approaches (Multisolving Institute, 2022). Positive cobenefits of a school-based obesity policy might be the increased sale of locally grown foods that boosts the local economy, the development of new safety equipment, the development of child activity centers, the increase in construction of bike paths, or the increase in parental physical activity due to increased child activity.

There are also unintended consequences to policy choices. These are consequences that are unforeseen or less probable. You may be able to highlight some unintended consequences, but you may have missed some. Policies focusing on obesity and body weight may increase the problem of eating disorders (Bacon & Aphramor, 2011). An unintended consequence of increasing the duration and intensity of exercise for children is the potential for increased physical injuries, or exposure to poor air quality in urban areas. Some of these unintended consequences might be minor and others could result in serious individual health programs, especially for politically disadvantaged groups. The likelihood of these negative unintended consequences may not be quantified but should be thoughtfully considered. One can use historical trends, case studies, published scientific studies, and other data to make some estimates on what the impact might be.

Preventive actions might be built into the proposal to mitigate some of these known potential negative unintended consequences (e.g., funding the best examples of the built environment to minimize injuries; providing culturally appropriate messaging; implementing trauma-informed approaches), but some negative impacts may nevertheless occur. Some of these unintended consequences may shift costs both to individuals and/or society. Can lower-income families afford the costs of safety equipment or bicycles to fully participate in increased physical activity, or are disparities likely to arise or even widen? Is there be sufficient support to shift resources to build and maintain bicycle paths? One can never fully account for all the unintended consequences (positive and negative) that will occur, but to the extent that one can be aware of potential adverse consequences, the less surprise there will be regarding the net impact of the program (Sawin, 2018).

Due to these unintended consequences, it is good to have various checkpoints for the progress of the program/policy. Most programs/policies are not perfect; they generally need some tweaking, especially if they are innovative. One type of program evaluation called "developmental evaluation" emphasizes that one should continuously engage in evaluative thinking during the policy process and not just at the end of implementation (Patton, 2010). Sometimes goals themselves need to be adjusted as the context changes over time; this should be documented. If your policy is not meeting its targets for specific time frames, it may be necessary to make modifications in the program or alter the measures for determining its success. You should attempt to estimate how long after the implementation of your policy you can start to measure progress toward its stated goals. Refer to the study by Krieger et al. (2013) in **Breakout Box 13.1** about the menu-labeling policy in King County.

To put this all into perspective, you could create a table or matrix that could be part of the document, compiled into an appendix, or simply used as a tool to organize your thoughts during the writing process. Any matrix is merely a tool that can help you structure your own decision-making. As such, it is only useful if you use it honestly. As in the matrix for the stakeholders, one could develop a scale (e.g., from 1 to 10, with 10 being the highest). Much of this will be somewhat subjective, but what the matrix forces you to do is to measure each of the alternatives using the same criteria. You gain nothing by not being forthright in your analysis. Table 15.1 is a hypothetical example; it is not based on any actual analyses and is intended merely to demonstrate how such a table might be developed. The Centers for Disease Control and Prevention (CDC) POLARIS website offers some other helpful resources and templates for creating tables and matrices for policy analysis (www.cdc.gov/policy/opaph/process/analysis.html, Tables 1 and 2). Other examples can be found in the Health Impact Assessment (HIA) literature (Harris et al., 2009).

As seen in the Recommendation Matrix in Table 15.1, the various policy options have different strengths and weaknesses. The evaluations in Table 15.1 are fictitious and are meant to only illustrate the process. For example, the Healthy Kids Nutrition Program and the Federal Menu Labeling Requirements are evaluated as being the most incremental. The Federal Complete Street Funding option is evaluated as the having the lowest political acceptability. One can change the criteria being used (the columns). One can total the rows to get a total score for each of the options. Table 15.1 treats all the criteria (Effectiveness, Incremental, etc.) as equals. However, you could weight the criteria differently with Effectiveness being 1.5 compared to 1 for Incremental. What is important is that you do not treat the matrix as an absolute, but rather as a tool to help you think through how the various options compare.

While the matrix will probably not appear in your report, developing it might help you write your narrative concerning the strengths and weaknesses of your recommendation. Given that most of the table is based upon subjective evaluations, one would not want to interpret the numbers too literally. If one had a panel of experts judge the alternatives, the values might have more meaning. However, since this is just your opinion, you would not want the matrix to be misinterpreted by your reader to mean anything other than its representation of your evaluation. If one alternative is clearly a winner on one criterion, this might tip the balance in terms of your recommendation and be the focus of your narrative in defense of that alternative.

Policy makers who may be familiar with the HIA process may prefer a presentation of policy alternatives with qualitative and/or quantitative information about the pros and cons of each alternative (Cole & Fielding, 2007; Farhang et al., 2008; Health Impact Project, n.d.).

You may be torn between two policies or you may feel uncomfortable recommending one over the other, particularly when the underlying scientific evidence is mixed. As an alternative to providing one recommendation, you could list the alternatives in priority order. In this case you are indicating that one alternative may be better than others, but you are leaving other options on the table. In this situation, you should probably explain the potential situations that would give rise to one alternative rising above the others. Under different circumstances, Policy Option B might supplant Policy Option A. For example, if an upcoming election is likely to change control of one of the branches of government, then perhaps the whole political landscape might change after the election, thus making a different

TABLE 15.1 RECOMMENDATION MATRIX

POLICY ALTERNATIVE	EFFECTIVENESS	INCREMENTAL	COST EFFECTIVE ANALYSIS	POLITICAL ACCEPTANCE
Healthy, Hunger-Free Kids Nutrition Program	6	9	6	8
Federal Supplemental Physical Fitness Program	7	5	Not available	4
Federal Menu Labeling Requirements	4	9	Limited cost data available in some states	9
Federal Complete Street Funding	6	6	Not available	3
Healthy Food Financing Initiative	8	7	9	9

alternative more politically viable. To make your analysis more useful you should be as direct and specific as possible.

LEGISLATIVE STRATEGIES

Your policy recommendation will have little impact unless you begin to think about how such a policy/program could be both adopted and then implemented by the political system. The "best alternative" may not be politically viable. However, there are different strategies that can be used to increase the chances of success. The policy strategies that you recommend may be the most important contribution of your analysis. This is where your understating of the political structure, process, and culture becomes critical (see **Breakout Box 15.1**). You have already begun strategizing by addressing the policy framing the issue. A thoughtful policy analyst will continue to be mindful of framing in developing their policy recommendations and alternatives. Your policy maker's initial press release or news conference may take advantage of your efforts at framing the issue.

Breakout Box 15.1

THE FRESH FOOD FINANCING INITIATIVE

In 1999, a nationally recognized nonprofit called The Food Trust partnered with the Philadelphia Department of Public Health and researchers at University of Pennsylvania to conduct a study on food access and found that low-income residents are less likely to live near a full-service supermarket and more likely to suffer from diseases related to a poor diet. The Food Trust is "dedicated to ensuring that everyone has access to affordable, nutritious food, and information to make healthy decisions" (Nutrition Incentive Hub, n.d., para. 1). In 2004, the State of Pennsylvania allocated $30 million over 3 years to create the Fresh Food Financing Initiative (FFFI) to help lower the costs associated with opening and operating grocery stores in urban areas. The Reinvestment Fund (TRF), a Philadelphia-based community development financial institution, leveraged the state's investment with private funds and tax credits to build a $120 million fund. The FFFI became a collaboration between TRF, the Food Trust, and the Greater Philadelphia Urban Affairs Coalition. TRF manages the financing and grant program, distributing funds that can be used for predevelopment costs, land assembly and other capital expenses, preopening costs, and construction expenditures. Applicants are eligible if their project demonstrates a benefit for an underserved area (defined as a low- or moderate-income Census tract), an area with supermarket density that is below average, or an area with a supermarket customer base with more than 50% living in a low-income Census tract. The Food Trust coordinates with supermarket developers to match community needs with FFFI resources and promotes the fund through a statewide marketing campaign.

As of June 2010, FFFI had approved 93 applications for funding, totaling $73.2 million in loans and $12.1 million in grants since its inception in 2004. In addition to increasing access to healthy and fresh foods at affordable prices, the new and expanded stores have had a substantial economic impact on their neighborhoods. The funded projects created or retained 5,023 jobs throughout the state (TRF, 2022). A recent study of selected supermarkets in the Philadelphia region demonstrated that 75% of part-time jobs (84% of all positions) were filled by local residents who lived within 3 miles of their workplace (Goldstein et al., 2008). Furthermore, over 400,000 residents have benefited from increased access to healthy food (Giang et al., 2008). The CEO of TRF framed the issue in a way that appealed to many stakeholders: "These markets provide economic anchors for communities across Pennsylvania, attracting jobs to the community. These investments can drive the health and economic vitality of these communities, particularly during difficult economic times" (Jeremy Nowak as cited in "National Healthy Food Financing Initiative," 2010, para. 15). Framing the issue of food deserts as an opportunity for economic development and job creation broadens the potential coalition and prevents the issue from being framed as providing handout food for the poor.

The FFFI has been recognized as one of the Top 15 Innovations in American Government and by the CDC for its impact on public health (The Food Trust, 2022a; 2022b). The FFFI demonstrated that, through a public-private partnership, grocers and other healthy food retailers could overcome the higher costs associated factors such as infrastructure, risk management, and workforce development that can affect businesses in underserved communities (The Food Trust, 2022a; 2022b).

The project was so successful that a federal Healthy Food Financing Initiative (HFFI) was launched in 2009 through a national campaign led by Policy Link, The Food Trust and Reinvestment Fund, with stakeholders from across the country. The aim was to create a comprehensive federal response to address the inequitable access to healthy foods in low-income communities in both rural and urban areas. The effort coincided with Michelle Obama's "Let's Move" campaign to reduce childhood obesity.

Since its launch, the HFFI has awarded almost $200 million to Community Development Financial Institutions (CDFI) and Community Development Corporations through the CDFI Fund at the U.S. Department of Treasury and the Office of Community Services at the Department of Health and Human Services. More than 100 organizations, representing a wide variety of stakeholders, voiced their support for a national solution to address the lack of access to healthy food. The collaborative effort resulted in the inclusion of HFFI in the Agricultural Act of 2014 (the 2014 Farm Bill), where it was authorized for up to $125 million at U.S. Department of Agriculture (USDA). In January 2017, Congress appropriated $1 million to the HFFI program at USDA in its fiscal year 2017 omnibus spending package.

Thought Questions

1. Compare the initial framing reflected in the Food Trust's mission to the framing presented by the CEO of TRF. Which is likely to resonate with both conservative and liberal voters?
2. Although the FFFI is a success story, there are several characteristics of the Philadelphia context that helped to ensure success. In what ways might this serve as a national template? In what ways might it be unique?

References

Agricultural Act, Pub. L. No. 113-79, 128 Stat. 649 (2014). https://www.govinfo.gov/content/pkg/PLAW-113publ79/pdf/PLAW-113publ79.pdf
Giang, T., Karpyn, A., Laurison, H. B., Hillier, A., & Perry, R. D. (2008). Closing the grocery gap in underserved communities: The creation of the Pennsylvania fresh food financing initiative. *Journal of Public Health Management and Practice, 14*(3), 272–279. https://doi.org/10.1097/01.phh.0000316486.57512.bf
Goldstein, I., Loethen, L., Kako, E., & Califano, C. (2008, August 1). *CDFI financing of supermarkets in underserved communities—A case study*. The Reinvestment Fund. https://www.reinvestment.com/insights/cdfi-financing-of-supermarkets-in-underserved-communities-a-case-study
The Food Trust. (2022a). *Healthy food financing initiative*. https://thefoodtrust.org/who-we-are/people/hffi
The Food Trust. (2022b). *Special report: HFFI impacts the nationwide success of healthy food financing initiatives, a proven, economically sustainable solutions*. https://thefoodtrust.org/wp-content/uploads/2022/07/HFFI-Impacts-Report.pdf
National Healthy Food Financing Initiative gets budget funding. (2010, February 22). CSP Daily News. https://www.cspdailynews.com/foodservice/national-healthy-food-financing-initiative-gets-budget-funding
Nutrition Incentive Hub. (n.d.). *The Food Trust*. https://www.nutritionincentivehub.org/about/partners/partner-detail/the-food-trust
The Reinvestment Fund. (2022, March 19). *The economic impact of supermarkets on their surrounding communities*. https://www.reinvestment.com/insights/the-economic-impact-of-supermarkets-on-their-surrounding-communities

Using the legislative process for policy approval is the typical strategy that one would follow to adopt a new program/policy. Given your understanding of the legislative process as described in Chapters 4 and 5, here are some strategic questions that you may wish to address in developing strategic options:

- Preliminary
  - What is the most desirable scope of decision makers involved?
  - Is the window of opportunity right for the introduction of this bill?
  - Is your issue framing appropriate for the bill?
  - Is this to be a trial balloon proposal, incremental, or major policy proposal?
  - Who are the major stakeholders for this policy?
  - Is there a coalition of stakeholders that can be created or reactivated?
  - Which bureaucratic agencies can lend support? Which ones will oppose?

- What resources (money, lobbyist, public relations) do the different stakeholders possess?
- Can the policy be implemented by a budgetary change instead of authorization bill?

■ Bill proposal
- Is party leadership concentrated or divided?
- What personal connections exist with key legislators and/or staff?
- Which legislative staffs/offices can provide technical support?
- What procedural legislative rules or traditions can be used to advantage?
- Is bipartisan support for the bill desirable or even possible?
- Can this proposal be merely attached to another bill?
- What should be the name of a freestanding bill?
- Who should be the sponsors of the bill?
- Which committees and subcommittees are critical for passage?
- Does the policy require both authorization and appropriation?
- Can the proposal be written in such a manner that a more favorable committee will be given jurisdiction?
- Who will shepherd the bill through each chamber?
- What knowledge do we have of legislators' and/or spouses' careers or personal interests that can be leveraged to change their opposition to being neutral if not supportive of the bill?
- Which legislators will not be seeking re-election and/or are willing to expend political capital on the bill?
- What ideological hot buttons are raised by the bill?
- Which lobbyists are going to oppose the legislation?
- What portions of the bill are non-negotiable, and which can be negotiated?
- When is defeat preferable to additional compromise?

■ Alternative strategy
- If you expand the scope to the general public does this increase your chances for success?
- What messaging might assist in its adoption?
- Do you have the legal structures for an initiative or referendum?
- Do you and other allied stakeholders have the requisite resources to win an initiative or referendum?

It is not expected at this stage that you will determine this legislative strategy yourself. Much of the legislative strategy will change as the policy works its way through the legislative process. You may be able to reach out to legislative staffers, legal analysts, or some of your identified stakeholders to seek advice as to the best legislative strategies to pursue. However, to the extent possible, you should provide your policy maker with some idea as to how this policy could work its way through the legislative process. At this stage, you merely need to be cognizant of the major political forces, personalities, and value orientations involved (Clark,

2002). The legislative process is a long, circuitous, and frustrating process intentionally designed to weed out legislative proposals. Most legislative bills do not become law.

As indicated earlier, an alternative to using the normal legislative process is using state-specific statutes for an initiative or referendum as described in Chapter 3. This bypasses an unreceptive state legislature and/or executive. However, this process will require gaining a sufficient number of voter signatures to qualify it being placed on the ballot. By expanding the scope of the decision-making process, you are gambling that popular support is on your side. Are there any public opinion polls to support your position? Defeat at the polls may be a decisive end to any chance of your proposal being adopted. Following the specifics of your state's process will be critical. The proposal on the ballot needs to be expertly written to be clear, unambiguous, and avoid unintended consequences. Legislative bills are generally examined by many legal experts to find implications of a policy for existing laws. Who will do this for your proposal to avoid potential litigation? Here policy framing might be critical in how the proposal is seen among various groups of voters. How will you mobilize supporters? You will need substantial resources to publicize the issue in statewide media. Can you access the resources to support such an effort?

Administrative Strategies

Generally, when we think about the policy process, we think about the legislative process as has been described. That is, indeed, where much policy is made. However, it is not the only place. As previously discussed, the executive branches at the national and state levels can make policy through writing both executive orders and writing rules and regulations. For a president or governor facing an antagonistic legislature, this can be one way to change or influence policy without having to go through the legislative process. While executive orders cannot be contrary to existing law, they can guide the interpretation and enforcement of existing laws by agencies within the executive branch. As a result, getting your policy adopted may be as "easy" as getting the executive to issue an executive order. Of course, this assumes that the executive supports your proposal. An executive order has less permanence since it can be reversed by the next executive. It is likely to have a limited but potentially important policy impact. Is an executive order an appropriate strategy for your proposal?

We discussed the importance of rules and regulations in Chapter 5. Since regulations have the impact of laws, this may be a sufficient strategy for your proposal. This again assumes that you have a sympathetic executive branch including a receptive agency administrator. The administrative procedure law regarding issuing regulations may be complicated and time-consuming, but it offers an important alternative for getting policy adopted. Bureaucrats will be careful not to alienate powerful legislative committees that control their future budget requests. Key stakeholders will be cognizant of any changes in regulations and will lobby to make their interests prevail. Can you win in a bureaucratic battle or are you more likely to win by expanding the scope of decision-making through a more public process?

Litigation Strategy

Rather than go the legislative or administrative policy routes, another strategy is to pursue a litigation strategy. Existing laws may provide justification for a lawsuit and a legal remedy. Class action suits or legal action taken by the attorney general might be an alternative to get your policy implemented. In some states, attorneys general are elected positions and they may not be of the same party as the governor. Are the attorney general and the chief executive linked or independent? Attorneys general can be very useful in consumer-related cases. If you do not have the support of the attorney general, the cost of litigation will be borne by the litigants; that may be prohibitive for your nonprofit public health organization. What resources do you have to pursue a litigation strategy? Is there an organization that will financially back your case or take it on a pro bono basis? Are there organizations that will file an amicus brief in support of your case? In which state or which state court will you file your case to get a favorable initial ruling or favorable appellate court ruling?

One of the major reasons to take a litigation strategy to policy is that the legislative and/or executive branches either refuse or are unable to make a policy decision when lives or important individual rights are at stake. Those subject to a policy may be powerless in the legislative process even as their lives are being impacted by that policy. For example, in the 1960s people committed to mental institutions lacked political power and were deprived of their liberty without receiving appropriate mental health therapy that would allow them to regain their freedom. In many states, the courts stepped in to direct the political system (the legislatures and executives) to solve the policy issue. Sometimes courts issued direct orders to administrative agencies. Patients' rights, de-institutionalization of mental health, community mental health programs, and other policy changes emerged from these court orders.

The courts have been especially important regarding tobacco and behavioral/mental health issues at both the federal and state levels. The Tobacco Master Settlement Agreement (MSA) resulted in seven tobacco companies paying states $206 billion dollars as a result of 46 attorneys general filing suit (Public Health Law Center, 2010). Some advocates see the tobacco settlement as a model for resolving other types of policy issues such as obesity (*Pelman v. McDonald's Corp.*, 2003). A more recent area where courts have been active is forcing states to address past and present sexual abuse and violence in juvenile detention centers and provide compensation for the victims of abuse. The courts can be a resource for policy change when the political branches refuse or are unable to act.

Another major advantage of the litigation route is that courts can issue an injunction to immediately stop further damage to potential victims. The legislative process may take years; an injunction can prevent further injury from happening. For example, a court order could immediately stop the spread of a pollutant causing environmental damage or a threat to human health. Once an injunction is issued, you can then advocate a legislative or administrative strategy to propose a longer-term solution to the pollution problem.

Another advantage of a litigation approach is that the cost of solving the policy problem can be shifted from the public's general tax base to those who are deemed responsible for the adverse impacts. As in the tobacco case, money is still being paid to states by the tobacco companies as compensation for the past health impacts of smoking on their Medicaid programs. Some states have used this money to support new smoking prevention activities and others have merely put the money back into their general funds. In either case, some of the costs of tobacco usage have been shifted from public treasuries to the tobacco companies. Economic awards can create a deterrent effect in the private sector. Companies might change their behavior if there is a threat of civil or criminal litigation. Corporate public relations may also encourage a change in behavior to avoid lengthy and costly litigation or adverse publicity.

One major disadvantage of litigation is that the decision regarding a particular court case may initially apply only to the specific litigants of the suit. Consequently, multiple lawsuits might need to be filed in multiple court jurisdictions to have a widespread policy impact. One way for litigation to have a larger policy impact is to file a class action suit or to raise a constitutional or broader legal issue. Under a class action suit, one of the litigants represents a class of people (e.g., consumers) and the resulting decision applies to all such litigants or consumers. Another way for the lawsuit to have more of a policy impact is to have the case appealed to an appellate court (state or federal). If the case is accepted for appeal, a more general ruling may result in a wider application. If the litigation is successfully appealed to a federal appellate court, it has potential to impact the entire country. However, the U.S. Supreme Court (USSC) has made several decisions that have limited the ability to file a class action lawsuit (*American Express Co. v. Italian Colors Restaurant*, 2013; *AT&T Mobility LLC v. Concepcion*, 2011).

However, this brings up another problem with litigation; litigation takes a great deal of time and money with potentially limited results. Cases may take years to work their way through the system. It may require hiring lawyers with expertise in constitutional law or who are admitted to the bar to argue cases before the USSC. Appellate courts have various degrees of discretion as to which cases they will review and which cases they will ignore. Litigation remains an important political strategy to change policy, especially if the political process appears to be a dead end. However, litigation should not be seen as a quick and easy strategy. Organizations with few resources are at a disadvantage compared to those organizations that can afford to hire the best lawyers and prolong the litigation for years. Is litigation a viable strategy for your policy maker? Are there favorable legal precedents for your case? Are judges popularly elected and perhaps more responsive to the electorate?

You have different strategies available to you. At this stage, the strategy cannot be described in detail because much of it will change as the political process unfolds. However, in making your policy recommendation to your policy maker, it is important for you to understand how different strategies might influence your recommendation. Unless you are proposing to be a trial balloon, you probably do not want to propose a policy that is dead from the very beginning. Perhaps the most important strategic element you should ask your policy maker is how much political capital they are willing to expend to make this proposal a reality.

SUMMARY

This section is the culmination of all the other sections of your policy analysis. As such, it is the most important and visible section of your analysis. It is what most people will focus upon when reading your analysis. However, its acceptance rests on how well the other sections have been developed. You need to understand what your policy maker or organization wants in terms of recommendations: one alternative, a list of alternatives in priority order, or a list with the strengths and weaknesses presented for each alternative. You will need to ensure that the previous sections such as your analysis of policy alternatives support your policy recommendations. You may need to revisit some of those sections.

Since your policy recommendation is unlikely to be universally acclaimed, you may wish to provide the strengths, weaknesses, and trade-offs you have made in your recommendation. What aspects of your recommendation are non-negotiable and which elements can be used to bargain for gaining the core elements of success? You cannot make a recommendation and then just let your policy makers ad lib a defense for the policy proposal. They need the details that will help sell the policy proposal to friendly stakeholders and help to withstand counterarguments from likely opponents.

Your recommendation is going to impact multiple stakeholders. Some of these people may be well represented in the political process and some of these people may not be represented or underrepresented. Some powerful stakeholders may be marginally impacted. Some stakeholders may pay with their lives or livelihoods but have little influence in the political process. Remember that you are making a value-laden decision that has real and important consequences for multiple groups of human beings. In making your recommendation, put yourself in the position of multiple stakeholders. How would you feel about this policy if you were poor? How would you feel about this policy if you were a member of a minority group? How would you feel about this policy if you were CEO of an impacted business? How would you feel about this policy if you were governor of a state being impacted by a federal policy? Place yourself in as many positions as you can so that you can begin to appreciate the impact of your policy proposal.

Every policy proposal will have to go through some type of political process for its approval, funding, and implementation. While you cannot control all the variables in the political process, you must understand the dynamics of what is likely to occur and to propose responsible strategies so that the policy can be adopted and result in public health improvement. For this proposal to gain traction, your policy maker will need to expend political capital (time, money, staff, and political trades). Your policy makers may have to oppose powerful interest groups that have supported them in the past. Your policy maker may gain public or new political capital. What is the political cost of this proposal? Are the costs outweighed by the benefits (votes for an upcoming re-election, campaign contributions, providing a partial solution to the problem)? Remember that solving the policy issue is only one of the potential benefits to your policy makers.

Aspects of the political process may determine the fate of your proposal. Therefore, you may need to reframe the proposal so that it attracts supporters and deflects opponents. Framing begins the marketing process of your policy proposal. It provides the lens with which the proposal will be perceived by the press and major stakeholders in the political process. In addition, you can start to think about messaging, the words and phrases that will be used to describe the proposal in press releases, press conferences, policy literature, advertising, and other documents. What would a press release look like for your proposal?

There are multiple strategies that can be used to turn your policy proposal into policy. Will you chose a legislative, executive, or judicial strategy? Depending on your policy maker's position, an executive order or new rules and regulations may be sufficient to actualize the proposal. Understanding which strategies are possible and the strengths and weaknesses of each will add credibility to your proposal. Once you have completed this section, it is time to write your executive summary as discussed in Chapter 7.

Policy analysis is not for the faint of heart. It is a challenging process that requires clarity of values, analytical capacity, imagination, empathy for those impacted, clarity in writing, and a knowledge of the political system. It can be very intimidating and challenging but seeing a policy/program enacted that has the ability to impact the lives of thousands or millions of people becomes the ultimate reward.

DISCUSSION QUESTIONS

- Given the Fresh Food Financing Initiative in **Breakout Box 15.1**, describe ways in which your approach would be similar and/or different in terms of your recommendation and/or strategy.

- Review the scenario of "Susan" presented at the end of Chapter 1. Describe your recommendation and/or strategy to improve the health of Susan's community.

- Regarding a public health policy on obesity, which elements of the recommendation would be core and which elements of your recommendation are you willing to compromise as it goes through the policy process?

- Given a specific public policy issue in your state, how would you decide between pursuing a legislative, executive, or litigation strategy?

- Regarding the above issue in your state, which elements would be core and which elements would be open for compromise?

KEY TERMS

executive strategies	POLARIS
intended consequences	positive cobenefits
legislative strategies	recommendation matrix
litigation strategies	unintended consequences

A robust set of instructor resources designed to supplement this text is located at http://connect.springerpub.com/content/book/978-0-8261-8543-3. Qualifying instructors may request access by emailing textbook@springerpub.com.

REFERENCES

American Express Co. v. Italian Colors Restaurant, 57 U.S. 228 (2013). https://supreme.justia.com/cases/federal/us/570/228

AT&T Mobility LLC v. Concepcion, 563 U.S. 333 (2011). https://supreme.justia.com/cases/federal/us/563/333

Bacon, L., & Aphramor, L. (2011). Weight science: Evaluating the evidence for a paradigm shift. *Nutrition Journal*, 10(9), 2891–2901. https://doi.org/10.1186/1475-2891-10-9

Clark, T. W. (2002). *The policy process: A practical guide for natural resources professionals*. Yale University Press.

Cole, B. L., & Fielding, J. E. (2007). Health Impact Assessment: A tool to help policy makers understand health beyond health care. *Annual Review of Public Health*, 28, 393–412. https://doi.org/10.1146/annurev.publhealth.28.083006.131942

Farhang, L., Bhatia, R., Scully, C. C., Corburn, J., Gaydos, M., & Malekafzali, S. (2008). Creating tools for healthy development: Case study of San Francisco's eastern neighborhoods community Health Impact Assessment. *Journal of Public Health Management and Practice*, 14(3), 255–265. https://doi.org/10.1097/01.phh.0000316484.72759.7b

Harris, E. C., Lindsay, A., Heller, J. C., Gilhuly, K., Williams, M., Cox, B., & Rice, J. (2009). Humboldt County general plan update Health Impact Assessment: A case study. *Environmental Justice*, 2(3), 127–134. https://doi.org/10.1089/env.2009.0018

Health Impact Project. (n.d.). *Health Impact Project*. The Pew Charitable Trusts. https://www.pewtrusts.org/en/projects/health-impact-project

Krieger, J. W., Chan, N. L., Saelens, B. E., Ta, M. L., Solet, D., & Fleming, D. W. (2013). Menu labeling regulations and calories purchased at chain restaurants. *American Journal of Preventive Medicine*, 44(6), 595–604. https://doi.org/10.1016/j.amepre.2013.01.031

Multisolving Institute. (2022, August 22). *Multisolving: One action, many benefits*. https://www.multisolving.org

Patton, M. Q. (2010). *Developmental evaluation: Applying complexity concepts to enhance innovation and use*. The Guilford Press.

Pelman v. McDonald's Corp., 237 F. Supp. 2d 512 (2003). https://law.justia.com/cases/federal/district-courts/FSupp2/237/512/2462869

Public Health Law Center. (2010). *Master settlement agreement*. https://www.publichealthlawcenter.org/topics/commercial-tobacco-control/master-settlement-agreement

Sawin, E. (2018, July 16). The magic of "multisolving." *Stanford Social Innovation Review*. https://doi.org/10.48558/W5D4-6430

APPENDIX

ADAPTATION PLANNING FOR JUSTICE, EQUITY, DIVERSITY, AND INCLUSION

These resources are designed to support the work of state, local, territorial, and Tribal health services across the nation in embedding justice, equity, diversity, and inclusion into their climate and resilience initiatives, programs, processes, and operations. The *Playbook* is a supplement to Building Resilience Against Climate Effects (BRACE) to amplify the incorporation of justice, equity, diversity, and inclusion (JEDI).

American Public Health Association. (2022). *Climate change and health playbook: Adaptation planning for justice, equality, diversity and inclusion.* https://www.apha.org/Topics-and-Issues/Climate-Change/JEDI

Centers for Disease Control and Prevention. (n.d.). *Climate and health: CDC's Building Resilience Against Climate Effects (BRACE) framework.* U.S. Department of Health and Human Services. https://www.cdc.gov/climateandhealth/BRACE.htm
> *Note:* The Centers for Disease Control and Prevention's Building Resilience Against Climate Effects (BRACE) framework was created to aid jurisdictions in navigating the health adaptation process.

Centers for Disease Control and Prevention. (n.d.). *Healthy places: Health Impact Assessment resources.* U.S. Department of Health and Human Services. https://www.cdc.gov/healthyplaces/hiaresources.htm

Centers for Disease Control and Prevention. (2016, May 31). *Tribal public health and the law: Selected resources.* U.S. Department of Health and Human Services. https://www.cdc.gov/phlp/docs/tribalph-resource.pdf

Gilbert, K. L., Ransome, Y., Dean, L. T., DeCaille, J., & Kawachi, I. (2022). Social capital, Black social mobility, and health disparities. *Annual Review of Public Health, 43,* 173–191. https://www.annualreviews.org/doi/abs/10.1146/annurev-publhealth-052020-112623

The Kresge Foundation. (2022, April). *Climate change, health, and equity message framework.* Author. https://kresge.org/wp-content/uploads/CCHE-Messaging-Framework-2022_FINAL.pdf

Madrigano, J., Shih, R. A., Izenberg, M., Fischbach, J. R., & Preston, B. L. (2021). Science policy to advance a climate change and health research agenda in the United States. *International Journal of Environmental Research Public Health, 18*(15), 7868. https://doi.org/10.3390/ijerph18157868

The Medical Society Consortium on Climate and Health. (n.d.). *Home page.* https://medsocietiesforclimatehealth.org

New Hampshire Healthcare Workers for Climate Action. (n.d.). *Home page.* https://www.nhclimatehealth.org
> *Note:* Other states have their own organizations. New Hampshire Healthcare Workers for Climate Action (NHHWCA) created climate and health webinars, spaces for interprofessional dialogue, and a Project ECHO series to support transdisciplinary health professionals in learning about climate/health concerns in a place-based context to inform policy and practice.

Rossa-Roccor, V., Giang, A., & Kershaw, P. (2021). Framing climate change as a human health issue: Enough to tip the scale in climate policy? *Lancet Planetary Health, 5*(8), e553–e559. https://doi.org/10.1016/S2542-5196(21)00113-3

Simons, J. (2022). Restorative justice as restoration of relationships. In K. Standish, H. Devere, A. Suazo, & R. Rafferty (Eds.), *The Palgrave handbook of positive peace* (pp. 1127–1147). Palgrave Macmillan, Springer Nature Reference. https://doi.org/10.1007/978-981-15-3877-3_59-1

ENVIRONMENTAL JUSTICE RESOURCES

Agency for Toxic Substances and Disease Registry. (n.d.). *Environmental Justice Index*. U.S. Department of Health and Human Services, Centers for Disease Control and Prevention. https://www.atsdr.cdc.gov/placeandhealth/eji/index.html
Note: This data tool was released by the Centers for Disease Control and Prevention (CDC) and U.S. Department of Health and Human Services (HHS) in 2022. The index is available to policy makers and public health officials and can be used to analyze the contextual, local factors driving the cumulative impacts on health to inform policy and decision-making.

American Panorama. (n.d.). *Mapping inequality: Redlining in new deal America*. https://dsl.richmond.edu/panorama/redlining/#loc=5/39.1/-94.58&text=intro

Council on Environmental Quality. (n.d.). *Climate and economic justice screening tool*. https://screeningtool.geoplatform.gov

Davis, L, & Ramírez-Andreotta, M. (2021). Participatory research for environmental justice: A critical interpretive synthesis. *Environmental Health Perspectives, 129*(2), Article 026001. https://doi.org/10.1289/EHP6274

King, R. (2022, November 11). *CMS seeks to close gaps in health equity data collection as new measures roll out*. Fierce Healthcare. https://www.fiercehealthcare.com/payers/cms-seeks-close-gaps-health-equity-data-collection-new-measures-roll-out

The Kresge Foundation. (2022, October 18). *Climate change, health & equity message framework*. https://kresge.org/resource/climate-change-health-equity-message-framework/

Levy, C. R., Phillips, L. M., Murray, C. J., Tallon, L. A., & Caron, R. M. (2022). Addressing gaps in public health education to advance environmental justice: Time for action. *American Journal of Public Health, 112*, 69–74, https://doi.org/10.2105/AJPH.2021.306560

Paine, L., de la Rocha, P., Eyssallenne, A., Andrews, C. A., Loo, L., Jones, C. P., Collins, A. M., & Morse, M. (2021). Declaring racism as a public health crisis in the United States: Cure, poison, or both? *Frontiers in Public Health, 9*, Article 676784. https://doi.org/10.3389/fpubh.2021.676784

PolicyLink. (n.d.). *GEAR—Getting equity advocacy results*. https://gear.policylink.org/book/export/html/282

U.S. Environmental Protection Agency. (2022, April 1). *EJScreen: Environmental justice screening and mapping tool*. https://www.epa.gov/ejscreen

U.S. Environmental Protection Agency. (2022, October 21). *EnviroAtlas*. https://www.epa.gov/enviroatlas
Note: This tool has an interactive feature that allows one to view the direct and indirect ways in which the environment supports health, with links to supporting literature.

Woodward, E. N., Singh, R. S., Ndebele-Ngwenya, P., Melgar Castillo, A., Dickson, K. S., & Kirchner, J. E. (2021). A more practical guide to incorporating health equity domains in implementation determinant frameworks. *Implementation Science Communications, 2*(1), Article 61. https://doi.org/10.1186/s43058-021-00146-5

HEALTH IMPACT ASSESSMENT AND HEALTH IN ALL POLICIES RESOURCES

Centers for Disease Control and Prevention. (n.d.). *Health Impact Assessment resources*. U.S. Department of Health and Human Services. https://www.cdc.gov/healthyplaces/hiaresources.htm

Health Impact Project Toolkit for HIA. The Health Impact Project provides a practical HIA toolkit containing resources that help communities, agencies, and other organizations take action to improve public health. The toolkit offers examples of Health Impact Assessments, guides, and other research to support policymakers' efforts to consider health when making decisions cross-sectors decisions.

The Pew Charitable Trusts. (n.d.). *Health Impact Project*. https://www.pewtrusts.org/en/projects/health-impact-project/health-impact-assessment

The Pew Charitable Trusts. (2018). *HIAs and other resources to advance health-informed decisions*. https://www.pewtrusts.org/en/research-and-analysis/data-visualizations/2015/hia-map?sortBy=relevance&sortOrder=asc&page=1

The Pew Charitable Trusts. (2022, July 1). *Connecting marine protected areas can improve ocean health: By linking their MPAs, regions could build climate resilience, reverse biodiversity loss, and support communities*. https://www.pewtrusts.org/en/research-and-analysis/issue-briefs/2022/07/connecting-marine-protected-areas-can-improve-ocean-health

HEALTH IMPACT ASSESSMENT EXAMPLES AND ADDITIONAL REFERENCES

American Public Health Association. (2012, October 30). *Promoting Health Impact Assessment to achieve Health in All Policies*. https://www.apha.org/policies-and-advocacy/public-health-policy-statements/policy-database/2014/07/11/16/51/promoting-health-impact-assessment-to-achieve-health-in-all-policies

Ammann, P., Dietler, D., & Winkler, M. S. (2021). Health Impact Assessment and climate change: A scoping review. *The Journal of Climate Change and Health*, 3, Article 100045. https://doi.org/10.1016/j.joclim.2021.100045

Barnes, C., McCrabb, S., Stacey, F., Nathan, N., Yoong, S. L., Grady, A., Sutherland, R., Hodder, R., Innes-Hughes, C., Davies, M., & Wolfenden, L. (2021). Improving implementation of school-based healthy eating and physical activity policies, practices, and programs: A systematic review. *Translational Behavioral Medicine*, 11(7), 1365–1410. https://doi.org/10.1093/tbm/ibab037

Chriqui J. F., & Sansone, C. N. (2016). Food, nutrition, and obesity policy. In A. A. Eyler, J. F. Chriqui, S. Moreland-Russell, & R. C. Brownson (Eds.), *Prevention, policy, and public health* (pp. 141–162). Oxford University Press.

Collins, J., & Koplan, J. P. (2009). Health Impact Assessment: A step toward Health in All Policies. *Journal of the American Medical Association*, 302(3), 315–317. https://doi.org/10.1001/jama.2009.1050

Conservation Law Foundation. (2013, September 27). *Healthy neighborhoods equity fund Health Impact Assessment*. https://www.clf.org/publication/healthy-neighborhoods-equity-fund-health-impact-assessment

Lushniak, B. D., Alley, D. E., Ulin, B., & Graffunder, C. (2015). The National Prevention Strategy: Leveraging multiple sectors to improve population health. *American Journal of Public Health*, 105(2), 229–231. https://doi.org/10.2105/AJPH.2014.302257

National Association of County and City Health Officials. (n.d.). *Home page*. https://www.naccho.org

National Prevention Council. (2011). *National prevention strategy*. U.S. Department of Health and Human Services, Office of the Surgeon General. https://www.hhs.gov/sites/default/files/disease-prevention-wellness-report.pdf

National Prevention Council. (2014, November 5). *The national prevention strategy: Prioritizing prevention to improve the nation's health*. U.S. Department of Health and Human Services, National Institutes of Health. https://prevention.nih.gov/education-training/methods-mind-gap/national-prevention-strategy-prioritizing-prevention-improve-nations-health

State of California Department of Justice, Office of the Attorney General. (n.d.). *Health in All Policies Task Force*. https://oag.ca.gov/environment/communities/policies

Rudolph, L., Caplan, J., Ben-Moshe, K., & Dillon, L. (2013). *Health in All Policies: A guide for state and local governments*. American Public Health Association, Public Health Institute. https://www.apha.org/~/media/files/pdf/factsheets/health_inall_policies_guide_169pages.ashx

INDIGENOUS AND OTHER WORLD VIEWS: POSTCOLONIAL HEALTH POLICY DISCOURSE

Alvord, L. A., & Van Pelt, E. C. (1999). *The scalpel and the silver bear: The first Navajo woman surgeon combines Western medicine and traditional healing*. Bantam Books.

Anderson-Carpenter, K. D. (2021) Black Lives Matter principles as an africentric approach to improving Black American health. *Journal of Racial and Ethnic Health Disparities*, 8(4), 870–878. https://doi.org/10.1007/s40615-020-00845-0

Cediel-Becerra, N., Prieto-Quintero, S., Garzon, A. D. M., Villafañe-Izquierdo, M., Rúa-Bustamante, C. V., Jimenez, N., Hernández-Niño, J., & Garnier, J. (2022). Woman-sensitive one health perspective in four tribes of Indigenous people from Latin America: Arhuaco, Wayuú, Nahua, and Kamëntsá. *Frontiers in Public Health*, 10, Article 774713. https://doi.org/10.3389/fpubh.2022.774713

Dodgson, J. E., & Struthers, R. (2005). Indigenous women's voices: Marginalization and health. *Journal of Transcultural Nursing*, 16(4), 339–346. https://doi.org/10.1177/1043659605278942

Edwards, M., Stagner, T. D., & Maher, S. (2021). *The great dying: Shall furnish medicine part 1*. Pulitzer Center. https://pulitzercenter.org/stories/great-dying-shall-furnish-medicine-part-1

Fine, M. (2023). *On medicine as colonialism*. PM Press.

Gilbert, K. L., Ransome, Y., Dean, L. T., DeCaille, J., & Kawachi, I. (2022). Social capital, Black social mobility, and health disparities. *Annual Review of Public Health, 43*, 173–191. https://www.annualreviews.org/doi/abs/10.1146/annurev-publhealth-052020-112623

Kimmerer, R. W. (2013). *Braiding sweetgrass: Indigenous wisdom, scientific knowledge and the teachings of plants.* Milkweed Editions.

Kozhimannil, K. B. (2020). Indigenous maternal health—A crisis demanding attention. *JAMA Health Forum, 1*(5), e200517. https://doi.org/10.1001/jamahealthforum.2020.0517

Kukutai, T., Hutchings, J., Allen, J., Allport, T., Black, A., Boulton, A., ... Foster, M., ... Hapeta, J., ... Jackson, A. M., ... Paine, S-J., ..., Parr-Brownlie, L., ... Pitama, S., Poa, D., ... Ruru, J., ... Tipene-Leach, D., Walker, G., ... Wilson-Rooy, M. (2022). *A Tiriti-based research, science and innovation system: Te Ara Paerangi: Future Pathways Green Paper submission from Te Pūtahitanga collective of Māori scientists and researchers.* Retrieved from http://www.rauikamangai.co.nz/resources-hub

Leitch, S., Corbin, J. H., Boston-Fisher, N., Ayele, C., Delobelle, P., Gwanzura Ottemöller, F., Matenga, T. F. L., Mweemba, O., Pederson, A., & Wicker, J. (2021). Black Lives Matter in health promotion: Moving from unspoken to outspoken. *Health Promotion International, 36*(4), 1160–1169. https://doi.org/10.1093/heapro/daaa121

Marya, R. & Patel, R. (2021, April 16). *Inflamed: Deep medicine and the anatomy of injustice.* Farrar, Straus and Giroux Publishers.

Megibow, E. & Powell, A. (2021). *Centering Black voices is key to addressing the Black maternal health crisis.* Urban Institute. https://www.urban.org/urban-wire/centering-black-voices-key-addressing-black-maternal-health-crisis-0

Paine, L., de la Rocha, P., Eyssallenne, A., Andrews, C. A., Loo, L., Jones, C. P., Collins, A. M., & Morse, M. (2021). Declaring racism as a public health crisis in the United States: Cure, poison, or both? *Frontiers in Public Health, 9*, Article 676784. https://doi.org/10.3389/fpubh.2021.676784

Prescod-Weinstein, C. (2021). *The disordered cosmos: A journey into dark matter, spacetime, and dreams deferred.* Bold Type Books.

Redvers, N., Celidwen, Y., Schultz, C., Horn, O., Githaiga, C., Vera, M., Perdrisat, M., Plume, L. M., Kobei, D., Kain, M. C., Poelina, A., Rojas, J. N., & Blondin, B. (2022). The determinants of planetary health: An Indigenous consensus perspective. *Lancet Planet Health, 6*, e156–163. https://www.thelancet.com/action/showPdf?pii=S2542-5196%2821%2900354-5

Simons, J. (2022). Restorative justice as restoration of relationships. In K. Standish, H. Devere, A. Suazo, & R. Rafferty (Eds.), *The Palgrave handbook of positive peace* (pp. 1127–1147). Palgrave Macmillan, Springer Nature Reference. https://doi.org/10.1007/978-981-15-3877-3_59-1

Ward, L. (2020). *America's racial karma: An invitation to heal.* Parallax Press.

NUTRITION AND OBESITY POLICY RESEARCH AND EVALUATION

Food and Nutrition Service. (2022a, August 1). *Local school wellness policy outreach toolkit.* U.S. Department of Agriculture. https://www.fns.usda.gov/tn/local-school-wellness-policy-outreach-toolkit

Food and Nutrition Service. (2022b, August 4). *A guide to smart snacks in school.* U.S. Department of Agriculture. https://www.fns.usda.gov/tn/guide-smart-snacks-school

Nutrition and Obesity Policy Research and Evaluation Network (NOPREN) is a collaborative, equity-focused applied research network that informs policies and practices designed to improve nutrition and prevent obesity. NOPREN members include researchers and practitioners interested in how policies and programs enacted at the federal, state, Tribal, and local levels impact families' food security, access to healthy food and water, and overall nutrition and health. See https://nopren.ucsf.edu/.

PARTICIPATORY ACTION RESEARCH

Arcaya, M., Schnake-Mahl, A., Binet, A., Simpson, S., Church, M. S., Gavin, V., Coleman, B., Levine, S., Nielsen, A., Carroll, L., Ursprung, S., Wood, B., Reeves, H., Keppard, B., Sportiche, N., Partirdge, J., Figueora, J., Frakt, A., Alfonzo, M., ... Youmans, T. (2018). Community change and resident needs: Designing a participatory action research study in metropolitan Boston. *Health & Place, 52*, 221–230. https://doi.org/10.1016/j.healthplace.2018.05.014

Baum, F., MacDougall, C., & Smith, D. (2006). Participatory action research. *Journal of Epidemiology and Community Health*, *60*(10), 854–857. https://doi.org/10.1136/jech.2004.028662

Davis, L., & Ramírez-Andreotta, M. (2021). Participatory research for environmental justice: A critical interpretive synthesis. *Environmental Health Perspectives*, *129*(2), Article 026001. https://doi.org/10.1289/EHP6274

Thondoo, M., De Vries, D. H., Rojas-Rueda, D., Ramkalam, Y. D., Verlinghieri, E., Gupta, J., & Nieuwenhuijsen, M. J. (2020). Framework for participatory quantitative Health Impact Assessment in low- and middle-income countries. *International Journal of Environmental Research Public Health*, *17*(20), 7688. https://doi.org/10.3390/ijerph17207688

PHYSICAL ACTIVITY POLICY RESEARCH AND EVALUATION NETWORK (PAPREN)

PAPREN is a CDC-funded network that brings diverse partners together to create environments that maximize physical activity. The network advances the evidence base and puts research into practice through collaboration across sectors with a shared vision of achieving active communities. See https://papren.org.

PLANETARY HEALTH

Fang, C., Hench, J., & Walton, A. A. (2022). *Centering equity in climate resilience planning and action: A practitioner's guide*. Antioch University. https://communityresilience-center.org/centering-equity-in-climate-resilience-planning-and-action

The Kresge Foundation. (2022). *Climate change, health, and equity message framework*. Author. https://kresge.org/wp-content/uploads/CCHE-Messaging-Framework-2022_FINAL.pdf

Planetary Health Alliance. (n.d.). *Home page*. https://www.planetaryhealthalliance.org

Price, M., Winter, K. B., & Jackson, A. (2021). Towards resilience in the Anthropocene: Transforming conservation biology through Indigenous perspectives. *Pacific Conservation Biology*, *27*(4), 309–319. https://doi.org/10.1071/PCv27n4_FO

Redvers, N., Celidwen, Y., Schultz, C., Horn, O., Githaiga, C., Vera, M., Perdrisat, M., Plume, L. M., Kobei, D., Kain, M. C., Poelina, A., Rojas, J. N., & Blondin, B. (2022). The determinants of planetary health: An Indigenous consensus perspective. *Lancet Planet Health*, *6*, e156–163. https://www.thelancet.com/action/showPdf?pii=S2542-5196%2821%2900354-5

Steinberg, N., Mazzacurati, E., Turner, J., Gannon, C., Dickinson, R., Snyder, M., & Trasher, B. (2018). *Preparing public health officials for climate change: A decision support tool. Publication No. CCCA4-CNRA-2018–012*. California's Fourth Climate Change Assessment, California Natural Resources Agency. https://www.energy.ca.gov/sites/default/files/2019-12/PublicHealth_CCCA4-CNRA-2018-012_ada.pdf

Willett, W., Rockström, J., Loken, B., Springmann, M., Lang, T., Vermeulen, S., Garnett, T., Tilman, D., DeClerck, F., Wood, A., Jonell, M., Clark, M., Gordon, L. J., Fanzo, J., Hawkes, C., Zurayk, R., Rivera, J. A., De Vries, W., Majele Sibanda, L., … Murray, C. J. L. (2019). Food in the Anthropocene: The EAT-Lancet Commission on healthy diets from sustainable food systems. *Lancet*, *393*(10170), 447–492. https://doi.org/10.1016/S0140-6736(18)31788-4

POLICY/BILL TRACKING SEARCH TOOLS AND POLICY PROCESS

Arboine, B. (2022, May 23). *Policymaking process worksheet* [Class handout]. Southern New Hampshire University, PHE610. Retrieved February 10, 2023, from https://www.coursehero.com/file/149965143/PHE-610-Policymaking-Process-Worksheet-2docx/

Ballot/referendum map. https://ballotpedia.org/States_with_initiative_or_referendum

COVID-19 health policy snapshots. https://www.ncsl.org/research/health/health-policy-snapshots-covid-19.aspx

Find bills by subject and policy area. https://www.Congress.gov/Help/faq/Find-Bills-by-Subject

Legiscan. https://Legiscan.com/About

Lodge, M., Page, E. C., & Balla, S. J. (2015). *The Oxford handbook of classics in public policy and administration.* Oxford University Press. https://doi.org/10.1093/oxfordhb/9780199646135.001.0001

Plack, M. M., Goldman, E. F., Scott, A. R., & Brundage, S. B. (2019). *Systems thinking in the healthcare professions: A guide for educators and clinicians.* The George Washington University. https://hsrc.himmelfarb.gwu.edu/cgi/viewcontent.cgi?article=1000&context=educational_resources_teaching

Tracking the U.S. Congress. https://www.govtrack.us

SOCIETY OF PRACTITIONERS OF HEALTH IMPACT ASSESSMENT (SOPHIA)

See https://hiasociety.org.

THEORETICAL APPLICATIONS FOR PUBLIC HEALTH POLICY

Baumgartner, F. R., & Jones, B. D. (1993). *Agendas and instability in American politics.* The University of Chicago Press.

Bernier, N. F., & Clavier, C. (2011). Public health policy research: Making the case for a political science approach. *Health Promotion International, 26*(1), 109–116. https://doi.org/10.1093/heapro/daq079

Brewer, G., & deLeon, P. (1983). *The foundations of policy analysis.* Brooks/Cole.

Clarke, B., Swinburn, B., & Sacks, G. (2016). The application of theories of the policy process to obesity prevention: A systematic review and meta-synthesis. *BMC Public Health, 16*(1), Article 1084. https://doi.org/10.1186/s12889-016-3639-z

Gagnon, F., Bergeron, P., Clavier, C., Fafard, P., Martin, E., & Blouin, C. (2017). Why and how political science can contribute to public health? Proposals for collaborative research avenues. *International Journal of Health Policy and Management, 6*(9), 495–499. https://doi.org/10.15171/ijhpm.2017.38

Kingdon, J.W. (1984). *Agendas, alternatives and public policies.* Little Brown and Company.

Landers, G. M., Minyard, K. J., Lanford, D., & Heishman, H. (2020). A theory of change for aligning health care, public health, and social services in the time of COVID-19. *American Journal of Public Health, 110*(S2), S178–S180. https://doi.org/10.2105/AJPH.2020.305821

Lasswell, H. (1956). *The decision process.* University of Maryland Press.

Latham, S. R. (2016). Political theory, values and public health. *Public Health Ethics, 9*(2), 139–149. https://doi.org/10.1093/phe/phv033

Lodge, M., Page, E. C., & Balla, S. J. (2015). *The Oxford handbook of classics in public policy and administration.* Oxford University Press. https://doi.org/10.1093/oxfordhb/9780199646135.001.0001

Oliver, T. R. (2006). The politics of public health policy. *Annual Review of Public Health, 27*(1), 195–233. https://doi.org/10.1146/annurev.publhealth.25.101802.123126

Ostrom, E. (2007). Institutional rational choice: An assessment of the institutional analysis and development framework. In P. A. Sabatier (Ed.), *Theories of the policy process* (2nd ed., pp. 21–64). Westview Press.

Ostrom, E., Gardner, R., & Walker, J. (1994). *Rules, games, and common-pool resources.* University of Michigan Press.

Ostrom, V., Bish, R., & Ostrom, E. (1988). *Local government in the United States.* ICS Press.

Polski, M. & Ostrom, E. (1999). *An institutional framework for policy analysis and design.* https://ostromworkshop.indiana.edu/pdf/teaching/iad-for-policy-applications.pdf

Sabatier, P. A. (Ed.). (1999). *Theories of the policy process.* Westview Press.

Sabatier, P. A. (Ed.). (2007). *Theories of the policy process* (2nd ed.). Westview Press.

Schlager, E. (2007). A comparison of frameworks, theories, and models of policy processes. In P. A. Sabatier (Ed.), *Theories of the policy process* (2nd ed.). Westview Press.

Staeheli, L. A., & Lawson, V. A. (1995). Feminism, praxis and human geography. *Geographical Analysis, 27*(4), 321–338. https://doi.org/10.1111/j.1538-4632.1995.tb00914.x

Su, Z. (2021). Rigorous policy-making amid COVID-19 and beyond: Literature review and critical insights. *International Journal of Environmental Research and Public Health, 18*(23), 12447. https://doi.org/10.3390/ijerph182312447

Thatcher, M. (1998). The development of policy network analyses. *Journal of Theoretical Politics, 10*(4), 389–416. https://doi.org/10.1177/0951692898010004002

Webster, D. G., Aytur, S. A., Axelrod, M., Wilson, R. S., Hamm, J. A., Sayed, L., Pearson, A. L., Torres, P. H. C., Akporiaye, A., & Young, O. (2022). Learning from the past: Pandemics and the governance treadmill. *Sustainability, 14*(6), 3683. https://doi.org/10.3390/su14063683

THEORETICAL CONSIDERATIONS FOR LOW- AND MIDDLE-INCOME COUNTRIES

Affleck, R. T., Gardner, K., Aytur, S., Carlson, C., Grimm, C., & Deeb, E. (2019). Sustainable infrastructure in conflict zones: Police facilities' impact on perception of safety in Afghan communities. *Sustainability, 11*(7), 2113. https://dx.doi.org/10.3390/su11072113

Lee, K., Fustukian, S., & Buse, K. (2002). *Health policy in a globalizing world.* Cambridge University Press.

Lee, K., Lush, L., Walt, G., & Cleland, J. (1998). Family planning policies and programmes in eight low-income countries: A comparative policy analysis. *Social Science and Medicine, 47*, 949–959. https://doi.org/10.1016/s0277-9536(98)00168-3

Reich, M. R. (1995). The politics of agenda setting in international health: Child health versus adult health in developing countries. *Journal of International Development, 7*, 489–502. https://doi.org/10.1002/jid.3380070310

Schneider, H., Gilson, L., Ogden, J., Lush, L., & Walt, G. (2006). Health systems and the implementation of disease programmes: Case studies from South Africa. *Global Public Health, 1*, 49–64. https://doi.org/10.1080/17441690500361083

Shiffman, J. (2007). Generating political priority for maternal mortality reduction in 5 developing countries. *American Journal of Public Health, 97*, 796–803. https://doi.org/10.2105/AJPH.2006.095455

Walt, G., & Gilson, L. (1994). Reforming the health sector in developing countries: The central role of policy analysis. *Health Policy and Planning, 9*, 353–370. https://doi.org/10.1093/heapol/9.4.353

Walt, G., Shiffman, J., Schneider, H., Murray, S. F., Brugha, R., & Gilson, L. (2008). 'Doing' health policy analysis: Methodological and conceptual reflections and challenges. *Health Policy and Planning, 23*(5), 308–317. https://doi.org/10.1093/heapol/czn024

GLOSSARY

Adelaide Statement   A declaration sanctioned by the World Health Organization that emphasizes the importance of considering health outcomes and well-being in all policy-making processes.

Administrative Procedures Act   A U.S. federal law that outlines the procedures federal agencies must follow when creating, modifying, or removing regulations.

advocacy coalition group   Individuals, groups, or organizations with shared goals or interests in shaping policy outcomes.

Agency for Healthcare Research and Quality (AHRQ)   A division of the U.S. Department of Health and Human Services. The mission of the agency is to increase quality and safety in healthcare through research and the creation of evidence-based practices.

Alexis de Tocqueville   A diplomat, author, and philosopher who examined the different political and societal constructs of the United States compared to European countries in the 19th century.

Alien and Sedition Act of 1798   Law designed to address national security concerns and opposition of political parties. The act is often seen as an example of political overreach and the importance of the protection of free speech.

allocative efficiency   An economic state that refers to the efficient distribution of resources in an economy to produce the ideal mix of goods and services to meet the consumer's needs.

American exceptionalism   An idea that the United States is exemplary and has an unparalleled and unequaled role in the world as a result of its values, political system, and historical development.

American Legislative Exchange Council (ALEC)   An organization that creates legislative models, often favoring limited government, free markets, and states' rights, for use in state legislatures.

American Rescue Plan Act of 2021   A federal law passed in response to the COVID-19 pandemic. This law provided $1.9 trillion in economic stimulus, vaccination funding, direct payments to individuals, aid to small businesses, and support for state and local governments.

amicus brief   A legal document filed by a person or organization that is not a party to the litigation but has an interest in the case and wishes to provide information to the court.

analytical functions   Tools used in analysis of data pertaining primarily to organizational capabilities; they are described as descriptive (what happened or is happening), diagnostic (why did it happen), predictive (what will happen), and prescriptive (what might happen).

analytical study   A type of research that involves identifying patterns, trends, or relationships within data that can help answer research questions or test hypotheses.

appropriation committees   Legislative committees responsible for developing and passing legislation to allocate funds for specific government programs and agencies.

Articles of Confederation   The ruling document of the United States from 1781 to 1789. It served as the Constitution of the United States until the adoption of the current Constitution in 1789.

artificial intelligence   A computer system that can perform tasks typically necessitating human intelligence, such as visual and speech perception, executive thinking, and language translation.

AstroTurf organization   A group or campaign that appears to be a grassroots movement but is organized and funded by special interest groups, political parties, individuals, or corporations.

authoritative allocation of values   The determination of values, norms, and beliefs that are most important to a society as determined by the political system.

authorization committees   Congressional committees responsible for developing and passing legislation concerning the operations of government policies, programs, and agencies, including funding needs.

Baker v. Carr **(1962)**   A landmark U.S. Supreme Court case originating in Tennessee. The Court ruled that the federal courts can hear issues regarding redistricting by population size in congressional districts.

bicameral   A system of government in which two separate chambers divide the legislative branch. The U.S. Senate and House of Representatives are an example of a bicameral system.

The Bill of Rights   A listing of the essential rights for the citizens of a country. In the United States, the Bill of Rights includes the first 10 amendments to the U.S. Constitution.

Bipartisan Safer Communities Act of 2022   A federal law that improved funding and access for mental healthcare, increased school safety initiatives, and improved gun safety laws, such as extending background checks for gun purchasers under 21 years of age.

bipartisanship A political process where both major political parties in government collaboratively work to achieve goals or pass legislation to benefit the public interest.

block grants Federal funding provided to state or local governments for broad purposes, allowing the states greater discretion regarding spending federal funds.

budget committees Legislative committees responsible for managing the budget process, passing budget proposals, and establishing fiscal objectives and spending targets in government.

Burwell v. Hobby Lobby Stores, Inc. **(2014)** A landmark U.S. Supreme Court ruling that dealt with the insurance coverage of contraceptives as mandated in the Affordable Care Act. The Court ruled that a privately held corporation could invoke a religious conviction regarding contraceptive coverage mandates, resulting in the ability of corporations to obtain waivers to contraceptive coverage in employee health insurance plans.

Bush v. Gore **(2000)** A landmark U.S. Supreme Court ruling regarding the disputed voting counts in Florida during the presidential race of 2000. The Court ruled to stop voter recount efforts, effectively awarding George W. Bush the presidency.

capitalism An economic system where private businesses or individuals own the production and distribution of goods in the economy.

Carson v. Makin **(2022)** A U.S. Supreme Court ruling that dealt with a Maine law that allowed public funding for tuition at religious schools. The Court ruled that the law did not violate the Establishment Clause, as the law did not show preferential treatment for one religion over another.

Centers for Disease Control and Prevention (CDC) The leading organization in the United States that protects the health, safety, and security of the public. The mission of the agency is to secure public health by conducting research and providing information about health threats, and responding when these threats arise.

citizen legislators Individuals who hold political office while maintaining another career or profession.

Citizens United v. Federal Election Commission **(2010)** A landmark U.S. Supreme Court ruling addressing campaign finance regulations and donations from corporations, nonprofit organizations, and unions. The Court struck down a law that restricted campaign donations from certain groups, citing the law as a violation of the First Amendment.

Civil Rights Act of 1964 A federal law that prohibits discrimination based on race, color, religion, sex, or national origin. The law bars discriminatory voter registration requirements, segregation in public schools and accommodations, and discrimination in employment.

civil service The body of nonelected government employees who work in public administration and are employed by the government or other public sector organizations.

cloture A procedure that allows legislatures to end debate on a bill and proceed with a vote on the issue.

Commerce Clause An enumerated power in the U.S. Constitution that gives Congress broad power to control and regulate commerce with "foreign Nations, and among the several States, and with the Indian Tribes" (U.S. Const. art. 1, § 8).

The Commonwealth Fund A private foundation that is dedicated to promoting a high-performing healthcare system that achieves improved access, quality, and efficiency, particularly for vulnerable populations.

The Community Guide A collection of evidence-based research developed by the U.S. Preventive Services Task Force (USPSTF) to provide recommendations for interventions to improve population health and prevent disease.

conference committee A congressional committee formed on a temporary basis to resolve differences between the House of Representatives and the Senate when different versions of a bill exist.

Congressional Budget Office (CBO) A department within the U.S. legislative branch that provides economic and fiscal analysis to Congress.

congressional calendars Daily publications composed of separate calendars from the U.S. House of Representatives and the Senate. Publications include agendas from Congress and lists of current legislation in process.

Congressional Record The official record of proceedings and debates in the U.S. Congress. The record contains transcripts of remarks made on the floor, documents submitted for the record, information about the legislative activity, and committee schedules and reports.

congressional staff Nonelected employees who work for members of the U.S. Congress in various roles. Individuals are selected by a member of Congress to serve in that member's office or on a congressional committee.

constitutional democracy A form of government where the constitution dictates the powers and limits of the political system and those retained by the people.

constitutional law A body of law that defines the role, powers, and limitations of the different government entities as outlined in the country's constitution.

Contract With America A legislative agenda created by the Republican Party during the 1994 congressional midterm elections that outlined policy proposals and legislative priorities.

core functions of public health Tasks that are fundamental to the success of public health include assessment, policy development, and assurance.

***Cruzan v. Missouri Department of Health* (1990)** A landmark U.S. Supreme Court case that dealt with the right to die. The Court ruled that individuals have a constitutional right to refuse medical care if "clear and compelling" evidence of a person's wishes can be proved. This decision led to the creation of advance health directives.

data gaps Areas in which data need to be included or completed that can hinder decision-making, policy development, and program planning.

delegated powers Powers granted to a particular branch of the U.S. government by the Constitution, also referred to as enumerated powers. At the federal level, the 10th Amendment gives residual powers to the states.

democratic pluralism A political system where there are multiple centers of power in a democracy.

determinants of health Factors that contribute to a person's overall health, including social and economic factors, health behaviors, clinical care, physical environment, and genetics.

Dickey Amendment of 1996 A provision added to the 1996 Omnibus Consolidated Appropriations Act that prohibits the Centers for Disease Control and Prevention from expending federal funds to advocate, research, or promote gun control.

Dillon's Rule A legal principle that states that local governments in the United States only have the powers delegated explicitly by state law, with no inherent sovereignty.

***District of Columbia v. Heller* (2008)** A landmark U.S. Supreme Court ruling that overturned a Washington, D.C., handgun ban and gun storage law. The Court held that the Second Amendment protects an individual's right to have a firearm for lawful purposes.

***Dobbs v. Jackson Women's Health Organization* (2022)** A landmark U.S. Supreme Court ruling that determined the Constitution does not grant a right to an abortion, overturning the previous Court rulings in *Roe v. Wade* (1973) and *Planned Parenthood of Southeastern Pennsylvania v. Casey* (1992). The ruling gives states the power to regulate or restrict abortion care.

dominant political culture A cultural practice with shared values, beliefs, and attitudes that is dominant within a society with multiple cultures present. The dominant culture often forms the norms for the society. These norms may not be shared by all. *See also* political culture.

Due Process Clause of the 14th Amendment A provision in the 14th Amendment that restricts the federal and state governments from depriving any person of life, liberty, or property without first following specific procedures and rules.

effectiveness The degree to which something achieves its intended outcomes or objections; the success of an intervention.

Electoral College The people who formally elect the president and vice president of the United States. Each state has the number of electors equal to the number of its senators and representatives.

Electronic Code of Federal Regulations A digital version of the *Code of Federal Regulations* (CFR), which is the official codification of the rules and regulations published by agencies of the federal government.

environmental determinants of health Factors in the natural and built environment that can influence individual or population health, including air and water quality, housing, climate change, the built environment, and occupational exposures to carcinogens.

equity   The quality of being fair and just in the distribution of resources and opportunities for all people.

Evidence-Based Practice for Public Health (EBPH)   An approach to public health decision-making that emphasizes using the soundest available evidence from research and experts while integrating community preferences to guide policies and programs.

executive order   A directive issued by the president of the United States that directs federal government operations, directs federal agencies and departments, or carries out executive duties. Such orders do not require congressional approval.

Executive Order 12898   An order by the president that aimed to address the disproportionately high exposure of minority and low-income populations to environmental hazards and pollution.

executive strategies   The plans, actions, and decisions made by high-level executives in an organization to achieve its goals and objectives, often focusing on long-term success.

executive summary   A brief version of a longer document or report, presented at the beginning of a document, providing an overview of key points and findings.

exposome   The cumulative environmental exposures that an individual is exposed to throughout their lifetime, which includes a range of environmental factors, such as air and water pollution, chemicals, radiation, food, stress, and social aspects.

externality   An indirect cost or benefit to an uninvolved third party that arises as an effect of another party's (or parties') activity.

faction   A group of individuals within a larger group, often marked by dissension, who share different goals or objectives than the larger group.

feasibility   The capability of a proposed project, idea, or plan to be accomplished.

federal depository libraries   Libraries within the United States that are designated by the U.S. Government Publishing Office (GPO) to receive and provide public access to government publications in various formats, guaranteeing the American people have access to government information.

Federal Register   The official daily publication of the U.S. federal government for rules, proposed rules, notices of federal agencies and organizations, executive orders, and other presidential documents.

federalism   A form of government in which power is divided and shared between a general government and a regional government, with each having its own and shared powers.

federalization of the Bill of Rights   The process by which the protections outlined in the Bill of Rights were applied through the 14th amendment to the states; also known as the nationalization of the Bill of Rights.

filibuster   An action where a legislative member speaks for a period to delay or prevent a vote on a bill or nomination.

framing The way in which reality is perceived and communicated by individuals, groups, and societies.

freedom The philosophical concept of being free or the ability to act or think without restraint.

gerrymandering The political manipulation of the boundaries of an electoral district with the purpose of generating an unfair advantage for one political party.

Government Accountability Office (GAO) An independent government agency that provides Congress with auditing, evaluation, and investigative services.

Government Publishing Office (GPO) A government agency responsible for producing, publishing, and distributing official documents for all three branches of the government and independent agencies.

grey literature Materials produced outside traditional publishing that are not peer reviewed, which may include reports, working papers, conference proceedings, dissertations, and technical documents.

Griswold v. Connecticut **(1965)** A landmark U.S. Supreme Court ruling that overturned a Connecticut law barring married women from obtaining contraceptives. The Court ruled that the right to privacy in the Constitution protects married couples when purchasing contraceptives.

guidelines A set of recommendations or instructions, often created by organizations or experts, to help ensure that best practices are followed.

Hastert Rule An informal rule in the U.S. House of Representatives that the Republican Speaker of the House will not allow a floor vote on any bill unless it has the support of the majority of the Republican caucus.

health disparities Preventable variations in health outcomes between groups of people, with disadvantaged populations experiencing more burden.

health equity The idea that every individual should have the opportunity to achieve their best health, while recognizing that individuals need resources based on personal need.

Health Impact Assessment (HIA) A systematic process that involves using interdisciplinary tools and methods to assess the potential health impacts of a proposed policy or program.

Health in All Policies (HiAP) A strategy that integrates health considerations into policy making across all sectors and levels of government.

Healthy People 2030 A national program in the United States that sets 10-year objectives for health promotion and disease prevention.

House Committee of the Whole A legislative committee where all members of the U.S. House of Representatives are considered members of the committee. The committee is used when the House wants to consider a bill under committee rules rather than those used in regular sessions.

House Rules Committee   A committee of the U.S. House of Representatives that is responsible for the rules when introducing and processing bills on the House floor.

House Ways and Means Committee   A committee of the U.S. House of Representatives with jurisdiction over all matters related to taxation, revenue, and other financial issues, including bills related to Social Security, unemployment benefits, trade agreements, and tariffs.

ideology   A set of beliefs, principles, or values that form a person's or group's perception of social, political, or economic issues.

implied powers   Powers not explicitly stated in a government's constitution but considered necessary to carry out the function of the government.

incrementalism   A process in which changes are made gradually, rather than through major or radical transformations.

initiative   A process by which citizens can propose and implement new laws or changes to existing laws directly, without the involvement of the legislature or other government officials.

Institutional Review Board   A committee that reviews proposed research involving human subjects to ensure research is conducted in an ethical manner and in compliance with federal regulations.

Interstate Commerce Clause   An enumerated power in the U.S. Constitution that gives the federal government the power to regulate commerce among the states with broad authority to regulate many forms of activity, including noncommercial activities.

Judiciary Act of 1789   A landmark federal statute that established the federal court system and defined the authority of various courts.

The Kaiser Family Foundation   A nonprofit organization that provides research and information on national health issues for journalists, policy makers, and the healthcare community.

L.E.A.D. framework   A systems-oriented framework, developed by the Institute of Medicine, designed to address complex health issues by locating evidence, evaluating evidence, assembling the evidence, and making informed decisions.

law   A system of rules that are enforced by a society or government to regulate behavior and protect the rights of individuals or populations.

Lawrence v. Texas **(2003)**   A landmark case decided by the U.S. Supreme Court concerning the right to privacy and criminalization of sexual activity. The Court struck down a Texas law that criminalized consensual same-sex activity between adults in private.

legislative strategies   Tactics used by lawmakers, lobbyists, and advocates to influence legislation in a legislative body.

Library of Congress A research library that serves as the de facto library for the United States.

litigation strategies Methods used by attorneys and their clients to resolve legal disputes through the court system.

lobbying The act of attempting to influence decisions made by a governmental official to benefit an individual, organization, or special interest group.

Loving v. Virginia **(1967)** A landmark case decided by the U.S. Supreme Court concerning the 14th Amendment. The Court invalidated laws banning interracial marriage, as they were deemed a violation of Equal Protection and Due Process clauses.

Lyng v. Northwest Indian Cemetery Protection Association **(1988)** A landmark case decided by the U.S. Supreme Court that dealt with the rights of Native Americans to practice religion on public land deemed sacred to the Indigenous Peoples. The Court ruled that the government did not violate the rights of the Indigenous Peoples, as they did not own the rights to the land.

machine learning A field of inquiry that involves the use of algorithms and models to enable computers to mimic human learning and decision-making; often seen as a form of artificial intelligence.

Marbury v. Madison **(1803)** A landmark U.S. Supreme Court ruling that occurred when a justice of the peace in the District of Columbia sued the Secretary of State for refusing to deliver a commission payment. The Court ruled the commission was warranted and issued a *writ of mandamus* to compel payment. This decision established the principle of judicial review, which gives federal courts the power to declare acts of the legislative and executive branches unconstitutional.

McDonald v. City of Chicago **(2010)** A landmark case decided by the U.S. Supreme Court that addressed the constitutionality of gun control laws. The Court ruled that the Second Amendment is enforceable to the states and that a handgun ban within a city violated the Second Amendment's protection.

Medicaid A health insurance program, funded by the federal government and administered by state governments, that provides healthcare insurance to low-income individuals and families, people with disabilities, and some elderly individuals.

Medicare A federal health insurance program that provides health insurance coverage to individuals who are 65 years or older or individuals with certain disabilities or diseases.

melting pot The concept of cultural assimilation, in which different ethnicities and cultures merge to create a common culture within a community.

MeSH (Medical Subject Headings) A vocabulary thesaurus created by the National Library of Medicine to index and search for medical and health-related information in databases, such as PubMed.

Moore v. Harper **(Pending)**   An ongoing case to be decided by the U.S. Supreme Court dealing with the redistricting of North Carolina's congressional districts. State courts had ruled that a redistricting plan adopted by the state legislature was an extreme form of gerrymandering and therefore illegal. The state legislature argues that under the independent state legislature theory, only the legislature of each state is authorized by the U.S. Constitution to set electoral districts; therefore, state courts have no ability to invalidate legislatively determined electoral districts.

National Academy of Medicine (NAM)   Formerly known as the Institute of Medicine (IOM), NAM is a nonprofit and independent organization that provides advice and guidance on issues related to medicine, health, and health policy.

National Center for Health Statistics   A division of the Centers for Disease Control and Prevention (CDC), the unit serves as the nation's principal health statistics agency that is responsible for collecting, analyzing, and disseminating health data.

National Conference of State Legislatures (NCSL)   A nonpartisan organization in the United States that serves state legislators, providing research, technical assistance, and opportunities for lawmakers to exchange ideas.

National Federation of Independent Business v. Sebelius **(2012)**   A landmark U.S. Supreme Court case that challenged the constitutionality of the Patient Protection and Affordable Care Act (2010). The Court ruled the individual mandate to obtain health insurance was a valid exercise of Congress's power to tax and spend for the general welfare. The Court also ruled that Medicaid expansion provisions of the law were unconstitutional.

natural rights   Inherent rights that are not dependent on any particular government law.

Obergefell v. Hodges **(2015)**   A landmark U.S. Supreme Court case concerning same-sex marriage and the 14th Amendment. The Court ruled state laws banning same-sex marriages were unconstitutional, thereby legalizing same-sex marriage across the country.

office of the president   The office of the executive branch of government with the president of the United States serving as the chief executive of this branch. The office comprises the offices and agencies that support the work of the executive branch.

Omnibus Budget Reconciliation Act   A series of federal laws designed to reduce the federal budget deficit and increase revenue.

partisanship   A strong allegiance to a political party, ideology, or group, often involving a deep commitment to a particular political party and the unwillingness to support oppositional positions.

Patient-Centered Outcomes Research Institute (PCORI)   A nonprofit, independent organization with the mission to empower patients, caregivers, and healthcare workers with evidence-based information about health and healthcare choices.

Patient Protection and Affordable Care Act (PPACA)   A federal law that aims to increase access to health insurance, improve the quality of healthcare, and constrain healthcare costs in the United States.

peer-reviewed literature   Academic articles that have been assessed and approved by experts and peers prior to publication in order to ensure the articles are of high quality, are accurate, and contribute to the knowledge in the field.

Pendleton Civil Service Reform Act of 1883   A federal law that establishes a merit-based system for hiring government officials, rather than selection based on political patronage.

The Pew Charitable Trusts   A nonprofit, independent organization that uses research to address challenges and issues to advance projects that lead to change.

PHRASES (Public Health Reaching Across Sectors)   A nonprofit, independent organization that provides tools for healthcare workers to communicate and integrate disciplines to improve health outcomes.

planetary determinants of health   The environmental, ecological, and interconnected sociopolitical structures that impact the health of individuals and populations.

Planned Parenthood of Southeastern Pennsylvania v. Casey **(1992)**   A landmark U.S. Supreme Court case that upheld the constitutionality of some key provisions of *Roe v. Wade* (1973). The Court upheld *Roe v. Wade* but imposed certain restrictions so long as they did not impose an undue burden on the woman.

pocket veto   A legislative maneuver when a president does not sign a bill before the end of a legislative session. If the president does not sign the bill within the time limit, the bill is automatically not enacted.

POLARIS   A portal under the Centers for Disease Control and Prevention that provides education, policy-relevant tools, and resources for healthcare providers.

policy   A set of principles, rules, or guidelines established by an organization or government to guide decision-making and behavior. Policies can cover a wide range of topics and are often created to achieve specific goals and objectives.

policy agenda   A set of issues or problems that policy makers or government officials prioritize for attention and action.

policy issue statement   A concise description of a problem that requires action or attention from policy makers, which typically includes a brief explanation of the problem, its impact, and why it requires intervention.

policy wheel   A visual tool used to illustrate the various stages involved in the policy-making process, which typically includes agenda setting, policy formulation, adoption, implementation, evaluation, and feedback.

Political Action Committee (PAC)   An organization formed by corporations, unions, trade associations, advocacy groups, or other groups that pool money and contribute funds to political campaigns or ballot initiatives.

political capital   The level of trust, goodwill, or influence that a politician or government has with the public and other political representatives.

political culture   The shared beliefs, values, attitudes, and behaviors that shape people's political actions.

political determinants of health   The social, economic, and political factors that affect the health of populations. These determinants include policies and practices that are developed and implemented by governments and other political entities.

political question   A matter that is fundamentally political in nature and is best addressed by the branches of government, rather than the courts.

political viability   The extent that a policy or action will be successful in gaining support from key stakeholders and ultimately be implemented.

politics   Action that individuals and groups make associated with decision-making, distribution of power, resources, and values in society.

population health   The health outcomes of a group or population, including the distribution of such outcomes. Population health also refers to an interdisciplinary approach to achieving positive health outcomes within a community.

population health management   An administrative approach that focuses on improving the health outcomes of a defined group or specific population by addressing their healthcare needs and risk factors through policies and programs.

positive cobenefits   The secondary or additional benefits that are achieved in addition to the primary objective of a particular policy or action.

precautionary principle   A risk management approach that aims to prevent harm to health or the environment in situations where scientific evidence is uncertain or incomplete.

PRECEDE-PROCEED   A cost-benefit planning framework used to guide the development, implementation, and evaluation of health promotion programs.

procedural democracy   A form of democracy that emphasizes majority rule.

procedural equity   The concept of fairness when delivering justice, particularly in the context of organizations and institutions.

process evaluation   A type of evaluation used to analyze the execution of a program or policy.

production efficiency   An economic concept where an economy, company, or organization cannot produce additional goods without lower production or quality of another good.

public use data   Data available to the public for use and analysis.

PubMed   An online database and search engine that provides access to abstracts, journal articles, conference proceedings, and other publications related to life sciences and biomedical research.

qualitative methods A research method that explores complex phenomena, such as human behavior, experiences, and perceptions, often by examining non-numerical patterns.

The Rand Corporation A nonprofit, global research think-tank that uses inter-disciplinary research to address a wide range of social and economic problems.

RE-AIM A planning and evaluation framework used in healthcare to assess the implementation and effectiveness of health promotion programs. It stands for Reach, Effectiveness, Adoption, Implementation, and Maintenance.

recall The process by which citizens can remove an elected official from office before their term is over; recall is usually done through a special election or referendum.

recommendation matrix A tool used in decision-making processes to evaluate and prioritize options based on certain criteria.

redlining The practice of denying financial services, such as loans or insurance, to people based on their race, ethnicity, or neighborhood.

referendum A direct vote by the people on a proposal, law, or question; a form of direct democracy.

The Religious Freedom Restoration Act of 1993 A federal law in the United States that protects the free practice of religion for individuals and religious organizations at the federal level.

right to privacy A concept referring to the right of people to be free from unwanted or unwarranted intrusion into their lives; a fundamental human right that is recognized by many countries and human rights organizations.

Robert Wood Johnson Foundation A philanthropic organization in the United States that is dedicated to improving health, access to healthcare, health equity, and leadership and training for healthcare workers.

Roe v. Wade **(1973)** A landmark decision by the U.S. Supreme Court that established the constitutional right to obtain abortion on the grounds of a right to privacy.

Rucho v. Common Cause **(2019)** A landmark decision by the U.S. Supreme Court addressing the issue of partisan gerrymandering. The Court ruled that gerrymandering is a political issue that is outside the purview of the federal courts.

rules and regulations Formal statements that outline specific requirements, procedures, or standards that must be followed for a law to be implemented; they are typically developed by governmental agencies and have the force of law.

scope and bias Scope refers to the number of participants in a decision-making process. Controlling who participates in the decision-making process tends to bias the outcome.

Second Amendment A 1791 amendment to the U.S. Constitution that establishes the right for people to bear arms.

separation of powers   A political concept that refers to the division of government into separate branches so that political power is not concentrated.

Shelby County v. Holder **(2013)**   A landmark U.S. Supreme Court decision that addressed the constitutionality of provisions in the Voting Rights Act (1965). The Court ruled that some provisions of the act are unconstitutional, as the coverage formula was based on out-of-date data.

signing statements   Written pronouncement issued by the president of the United States when signing a bill into law. With a signing statement, the president may explain their interpretation of the law, express approval or disapproval, or signal how the law will be implemented.

social determinants of health   The social and economic factors that influence the health of individuals and populations; factors can include education, income, housing, food supply, employment, access to healthcare, and social support networks.

social network analysis   The study of social structures and the relationships among individuals or groups. It involves analyzing the connections between people or groups and identifying patterns and trends in these networks.

socio-ecological model   A conceptual model used to understand and address complex health issues. The model emphasizes the interplay between individuals and their environment, recognizing that health is shaped by a variety of factors at multiple levels.

stakeholder analysis   A process of identifying and analyzing a system as it affects various stakeholders. The goal of a stakeholder analysis is to understand the interests, needs, and concerns of different stakeholders, and to develop strategies for engaging them.

stakeholder impact matrix   A tool used in a stakeholder analysis to evaluate the potential impact of a project or decision on different stakeholders.

stakeholders   Individuals, groups, or organizations that are affected by a particular action.

standing committees   Permanent committees that are established within an organization or governing body to focus on specific areas of responsibility or oversight.

states' rights   The political power and autonomy that individual states possess within a federal system of government; the powers and privileges that are reserved exclusively for the individual states and are not delegated to the national government.

strict constructionist   An individual who believes in interpreting the U.S. Constitution according to its literal text and original intent, without interpreting or expanding its meaning to fit contemporary circumstances or changing social values.

substantive equity   The concept of fairness and justice in the outcomes of a decision or action, while focusing on ensuring the results are fair and equitable, regardless of the specific procedures or rules used to arrive at those outcomes.

success in policy making   The achievement of a goal, objective, or outcome, often requiring a combination of strategic planning, evidence-based decision-making, stakeholder engagement, and effective implementation and evaluation.

Supreme Court majority opinion   The written opinion of the majority of justices expressing reasoning and rationale behind the majority decision.

Supreme Court minority dissent   The written opinion of the minority of justices expressing reasoning and rationale for nonagreement to the majority opinion.

The Surgeon General's Call to Action to Prevent and Decrease Overweight and Obesity   A report issued by the Surgeon General of the United States that outlines the public health problem of obesity and provides overarching principles to address the epidemic.

systematic reviews   A form of research involving the thorough and systematic analysis of existing research with the goal to identify and synthesize all available evidence.

term limits   Legal limits on the sum of terms or length of time that an elected official can serve in a certain office.

tragedy of the commons   An economic situation where people or groups, acting in their own self-interest, overuse a shared resource, leading to its depletion or ruin.

unanimous consent   A procedure used to obtain agreement from all members present in a legislative body without requiring a formal vote.

unintended consequences   The outcomes that were not intended or anticipated when a decision or action was taken.

United States Code   The official collection and codification of the general and permanent federal laws of the United States.

United States v. Miller **(1939)**   A landmark U.S. Supreme Court case challenging the National Firearms Act of 1934. The Court determined that the Second Amendment does not protect the right to possess a sawed-off shotgun.

veto   The power of an executive authority to stop a proposed law or policy.

Voting Rights Act of 1965   A landmark piece of federal legislation that sought to overcome legal barriers that prevented racial minorities from voting in elections, particularly in the southern states.

winner-take-all election   An electoral system in which the nominee who receives the majority of casted votes wins the election, regardless of the percentage of the population voting in the election; often referred to as single-member plurality voting.

writ of certiorari   A court process issued by a higher court, such as the U.S. Supreme Court, to a subordinate court requesting judicial review of a subordinate court's decision.

writ of mandamus   A judicial remedy issued by a court that orders any government official, lower court, public authority, or corporation to do a specific action that they are legally obligated to do.

INDEX